T0226823

Infectious Disease

Editor

MICHAEL A. MALONE

PRIMARY CARE:
CLINICS IN OFFICE PRACTICE

www.primarycare.theclinics.com

Consulting Editor
JOEL J. HEIDELBAUGH

September 2018 • Volume 45 • Number 3

ELSEVIER

1600 John F. Kennedy Boulevard • Suite 1800 • Philadelphia, Pennsylvania, 19103-2899

http://www.theclinics.com

PRIMARY CARE: CLINICS IN OFFICE PRACTICE Volume 45, Number 3
September 2018 ISSN 0095-4543, ISBN-13: 978-0-323-64214-9

Editor: Jessica McCool
Developmental Editor: Laura Fisher

Primary Care: Clinics in Office Practice (ISSN: 0095-4543) is published quarterly by Elsevier Inc., 360 Park Avenue South, New York, NY 10010-1710. Months of issue are March, June, September, and December. Periodicals postage paid at New York, NY and additional mailing offices. Subscription prices are $237.00 per year (US individuals), $474.00 (US institutions), $100.00 (US students), $289.00 (Canadian individuals), $536.00 (Canadian institutions), $175.00 (Canadian students), $355.00 (international individuals), $536.00 (international institutions), and $175.00 (international students). Foreign air speed delivery is included in all *Clinics* subscription prices. All prices are subject to change without notice. POSTMASTER: Send address changes to *Primary Care: Clinics in Office Practice*, Elsevier Periodicals Customer Service, 11830 Westline Industrial Drive, St. Louis, MO 63146. Customer Service Health Sciences Division, Subscription Customer Service, 3251 Riverport Lane, Maryland Heights, MO 63043. **Customer Service: 1-800-654-2452 (U.S. and Canada); 314-447-8871 (outside U.S. and Canada). Fax: 314-447-8029. E-mail: journalscustomerservice-usa@elsevier.com (for print support); journalsonlinesupport-usa@elsevier.com (for online support).**

Reprints. For copies of 100 or more, of articles in this publication, please contact the Commercial Reprints Department, Elsevier Inc., 360 Park Avenue South, New York, NY 10010-1710. Tel. 212-633-3874; Fax: 212-633-3820; E-mail: reprints@elsevier.com.

Primary Care: Clinics in Office Practice is covered in *MEDLINE/PubMed (Index Medicus) and EMBASE/Excerpta Medica, Current Contents/Clinical Medicine, and ISI/BIOMED.*

Contributors

CONSULTING EDITOR

JOEL J. HEIDELBAUGH, MD, FAAFP, FACG
Clinical Professor, Departments of Family Medicine and Urology, University of Michigan Medical School, Ann Arbor, Michigan

EDITOR

MICHAEL A. MALONE, MD
Associate Professor, Department of Family Medicine, Tidelands Health MUSC Family Medicine Residency Program, Myrtle Beach, South Carolina

AUTHORS

OLUMUYIWA ADEBONA, MD, MPH
Staff Physician, Family Medicine, Penn Highlands Healthcare, Dubois, Pennsylvania

SALVADOR ALVAREZ, MD
Professor, Department of Internal Medicine, Mayo Clinic School of Medicine, Jacksonville, Florida

JEFFREY H. BAKER, MD
Assistant Professor, Department of Family and Community Medicine, Penn State College of Medicine, Penn State Hershey Medical Group, State College, Pennsylvania

DEEPA BURMAN, MD, FAASM, FAAFP
Residency Faculty, Clinical Assistant Professor, Family Medicine, University of Pittsburgh Medical Center (UPMC), Latterman Family Health Center, UPMC McKeesport Family Medicine Residency, McKeesport, Pennsylvania

JEFFREY CHO, MD, MPH
Recipient of CTropMed® Certificate from ASTMH, Family and Preventive Medicine Residency Program, Loma Linda University, Loma Linda, California

KARL T. CLEBAK, MD, FAAFP
Assistant Professor, Department of Family and Community Medicine, Penn State College of Medicine, Hershey, Pennsylvania

BEVIN DOLAN, MD
Delaware Valley Infectious Disease Associates, Wynnewood, Pennsylvania

NGOZI EZINWA, MD, MPH
Assistant Professor, Loma Linda University School of Medicine, Loma Linda, California

NORMAN BENJAMIN FREDRICK, MD
Associate Professor, Family and Community Medicine and Public Health Sciences, Director, Global Health Center, Penn State College of Medicine, Hershey, Pennsylvania

ANTHONY GERMINARIO, MD
Resident, Department of Family Medicine, Tidelands Health MUSC Family Medicine Residency Program, Murrells Inlet, South Carolina

RICHARD A. GIOVANE, MD
Resident Physician, Department of Family, Internal and Rural Medicine, The University of Alabama, Tuscaloosa, Alabama

SAMUEL N. GRIEF, MD, FCFP, FAAFP
Associate Professor, Clinical Family Medicine, Department of Family Medicine, University of Illinois at Chicago, Chicago, Illinois

KRISTEN GRINE, DO
Assistant Professor, Department of Family and Community Medicine, Penn State College of Medicine, Penn State Hershey Medical Group, State College, Pennsylvania

SARA HALVERSON, MD
Assistant Professor, Loma Linda University School of Medicine, Loma Linda, California

LEESHA HELM, MD, MPH
Penn State College of Medicine, Penn State Health, Hershey, Pennsylvania

VASUDHA JAIN, MD
Resident, Department of Family Medicine, Tidelands Health MUSC Family Medicine Residency Program, Murrells Inlet, South Carolina

PAUL DRAKE LAVENDER, MD
Assistant Professor, Department of Family, Internal and Rural Medicine, The University of Alabama, Tuscaloosa, Alabama

HOBART LEE, MD, FAAFP
Assistant Professor, Loma Linda University School of Medicine, Loma Linda, California

CONNIE LEEPER, MD, MPH
Assistant Professor, Department of Family, Internal, and Rural Medicine, The University of Alabama, Tuscaloosa, Alabama

CLAUDIA R. LIBERTIN, MD
Infectious Diseases Specialist, Mayo Clinic, Jacksonville, Florida

JASON LOHR, MD, FAAFP
Recipient of CTropMed® Certificate from ASTMH, CMO, SAC Health System, San Bernardino, California; Assistant Professor, Core Faculty, Family Medicine Residency Program, Loma Linda University, Loma Linda, California

JULIE K. LOZA, MD
PGY-3, Department of Family Medicine, The University of Illinois at Chicago, Chicago, Illinois

ANDREW LUTZKANIN III, MD
Assistant Professor, Department of Family and Community Medicine, Penn State College of Medicine, Hershey, Pennsylvania

MICHAEL MALONE, MD
Associate Professor, Department of Family Medicine, Tidelands Health MUSC Family Medicine Residency Program, Myrtle Beach, South Carolina

SCOTT T. MARBERRY, MD
Sports Medicine Fellow, Family Medicine, Mayo Clinic, Jacksonville, Florida

MARTHA SHAWN MOREHEAD, MD, MPH, FAAFP
Associate Residency Director, St. Vincent's East Family Medicine Residency at Christ Health Center, Associate Professor, Volunteer Faculty, Department of Family Medicine, The University of Alabama at Birmingham School of Medicine, Birmingham, Alabama; Assistant Professor, Clinical Faculty, Alabama College of Osteopathic Medicine, Dothan, Alabama

VAN TUONG NGOC NGUYEN, DO
Assistant Professor, Department of Family Medicine, Loma Linda University, Loma Linda, California

MICHAEL OUZTS, DO
Resident, Department of Family Medicine, Tidelands Health MUSC Family Medicine Residency Program, Murrells Inlet, South Carolina

SALLY ANN L. PANTIN, MD
Assistant Professor, Department of Family Medicine, Mayo Clinic, Jacksonville, Florida

RICHARD JOHN PRESUTTI, DO
Assistant Professor, Department of Family Medicine, Mayo Clinic School of Medicine, Jacksonville, Florida

GEORGE G.A. PUJALTE, MD, FACSM
Assistant Professor, Family Medicine and Sports Medicine, Mayo Clinic, Jacksonville, Florida

JUAN QIU, MD, PhD
Professor, Department of Family and Community Medicine, Penn State College of Medicine, Penn State Hershey Medical Group, State College, Pennsylvania

CATHERINE SCARBROUGH, MD, MSc, FAAFP
Associate Residency Director, The University of Alabama Family Medicine Residency, Associate Professor, Department of Family, Internal, and Rural Medicine, College of Community Health Sciences, The University of Alabama, Tuscaloosa, Alabama

JARRETT SELL, MD, AAHIVS
Associate Professor, Department of Family and Community Medicine, Penn State Health Hershey Medical Center, Hershey, Pennsylvania

LAUREN SIMON, MD, MPH
Professor, Department of Family Medicine, Loma Linda University, Loma Linda, California

BRINTHA VASAGAR, MD, MPH
Assistant Professor, Department of Family Medicine, Medical University of South Carolina, Charleston, South Carolina

THOMAS A. WALLER, MD
Assistant Professor, Department of Family Medicine, Mayo Clinic, Jacksonville, Florida

HEBER J. WATSON, DO
Resident, Department of Family Medicine, Tidelands Health MUSC Family Medicine Residency Program, Murrells Inlet, South Carolina

JASON R. WOLOSKI, MD
Family Medicine Residency Program, Faculty, Staff Physician, Geisinger Health System, Clinical Assistant Professor of Family Medicine, Geisinger Commonwealth School of Medicine, Wilkes-Barre, Pennsylvania

ASHLEY L. YENIOR, MD
Department of Family Medicine, Mayo Clinic, Jacksonville, Florida

Contents

PRIMARY CARE: CLINICS IN OFFICE PRACTICE

FORTHCOMING ISSUES

December 2018
Women's Health
Diane M. Harper and Emily M. Godfrey, *Editors*

March 2019
Prevention and Screening
Joanna L. Drowos, *Editor*

June 2019
Urology
Gretchen Irwin and Laura Mayans, *Editors*

RECENT ISSUES

June 2018
Rheumatology
Seetha U. Monrad and Daniel F. Battafarano, *Editors*

March 2018
Cardiovascular Disease
Mark B. Stephens, *Editor*

December 2017
Gastroenterology
Rick Kellerman and Laura Mayans, *Editors*

SERIES OF RELATED INTEREST

Clinics in Geriatric Medicine (http://www.geriatric.theclinics.com)
Infectious Disease Clinics (http://www.id.theclinics.com)
Medical Clinics (http://www.medical.theclinics.com)
Physician Assistant Clinics (http://www.physicianassistant.theclinics.com)

Foreword
"Tick, Tick, Tick..."

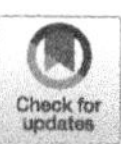

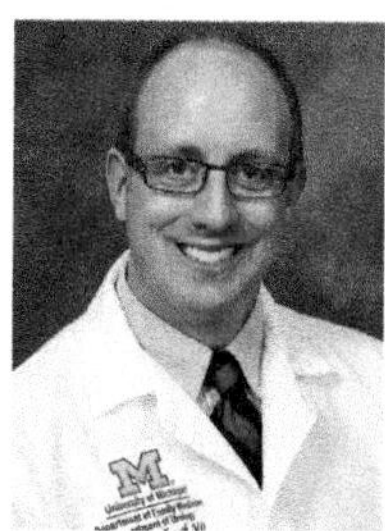

Joel J. Heidelbaugh, MD, FAAFP, FACG
Consulting Editor

The evolution of the diagnosis and treatment of infectious diseases has always been a fascination for me. The premise of a complicated puzzle to solve, compounded by a spectrum of mild to grave illnesses and uncertainty of time course or treatment success, solidifies the specialty of infectious diseases as one of constant challenge and innovation. I recently had an infectious diseases colleague describe his typical day as "finding the smoking gun and hoping to quickly extinguish it, while the pathogenic culprit always seems to either be at least one step ahead of me, or completely elusive. It's a race for time... tick, tick, tick...."

In the late 1980s, I worked in a medical laboratory in upstate New York as my summer job performing various laboratory serologic testing and preparing for my career in medicine. Not far from Connecticut where Lyme disease was first isolated, our laboratory saw hundreds of blood samples of patients to be tested, and unfortunately, many positives. A vaccine was soon developed and released, and then it faded away. The fears of tick-borne illnesses have persisted, with climbing incidence yet persistent challenges in early diagnosis. Couple this challenge with mosquito-borne and other vector-borne illnesses around the globe, and our constant quest for early diagnosis, effective treatment, and prevention.

In the late 1990s when I was a family medicine resident, I remember seeing my first case of Methicillin-resistant *Staphylococcus aureus* (MRSA). Prior to then, it was always something that we were "just colonized with," so we didn't need to worry. Now, I provide my residents with an opportunity to perform an incision and drainage of a likely MRSA abscess nearly every other week. Antibiotic resistance is often blamed on health care providers for nonjudicious use of antibiotics, while the bacteria seem to remain agile enough to morph and evade treatment.

In the present day, I see a lot of patients just prior to travel to foreign countries who request immunizations (and antibiotics to travel with "just in case"). A common pet peeve of mine is when patients continually receive antibiotics for suspected urinary tract infections without appropriate urinalysis or urine culture. During this past winter

Prim Care Clin Office Pract 45 (2018) xiii–xiv
https://doi.org/10.1016/j.pop.2018.07.002
0095-4543/18/© 2018 Published by Elsevier Inc.

when we had a record number of influenza cases, I saw increasing requests for antivirals to treat anything and everything that we didn't feel was of a bacterial cause, ranging from the common cold to suspected viral gastrointestinal illness.

I would like thank Dr Michael Malone and his authors for creating an invaluable issue of articles on infectious diseases for the *Primary Care: Clinics in Office Practice.* In addition to detailed articles on current evidence-based therapies for these topics, readers will also find reviews that highlight the great challenge of antibiotic resistance. Some rather unique topics are also presented, including aquatic skin infections and common infections during pregnancy. We hope that you will find this to be a practical collection to guide everyday practice.

Joel J. Heidelbaugh, MD, FAAFP, FACG
Departments of Family Medicine and Urology
University of Michigan Medical School
Ann Arbor, MI 48103, USA

Ypsilanti Health Center
200 Arnet, Suite 200
Ypsilanti, MI 48198, USA

E-mail address:
jheidel@umich.edu

Preface

Infectious Disease Topics for Primary Care

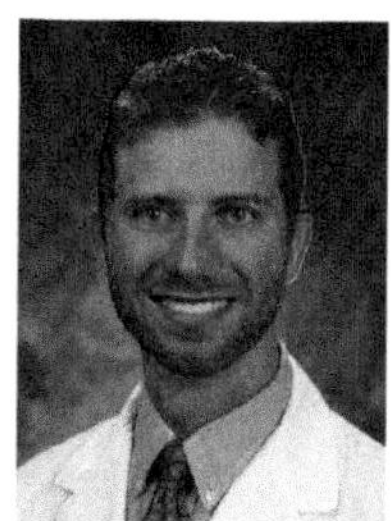

Michael A. Malone, MD
Editor

Infectious disease is an area of medicine that is commonly encountered by primary care providers. Furthermore, improving patient care and clinical outcomes in the primary care setting through prevention of disease and the timely and appropriate diagnosis and management of infections is paramount. Therefore, it is with great pleasure that I present the 2018 issue of *Primary Care: Clinics in Office Practice* devoted to the topic of Infectious Diseases. The fourteen infectious disease topics addressed in this issue were selected to cover important topics in the field of infectious disease. Each topic is structured to be evidence based and practical. The articles are written in a way that highlights key points and summarizes essential information on each topic for quick reference at the point of care. The information in this issue can be quickly utilized and applied in today's busy primary care setting. Although set up for easy reference, each article also provides a thorough overview of each topic.

This issue includes commonly seen infectious conditions, such as mite and bed bug infections, gastrointestinal infections, skin infections, CNS infections, tick-borne illnesses, infections in pregnancy, urinary tract infections, and pneumonia. It, however, also includes current and emerging issues in infectious disease, such as mosquito-borne diseases, pertussis, antibiotic resistance, and international travel.

I believe you will enjoy reading this issue of *Primary Care: Clinics in Office Practice* and will find it useful for improving your knowledge and approach to infectious disease.

Prim Care Clin Office Pract 45 (2018) xv–xvi
https://doi.org/10.1016/j.pop.2018.07.001
0095-4543/18/© 2018 Published by Elsevier Inc.

Ultimately, I hope this issue helps primary care providers improve the prevention, recognition, diagnosis, and treatment of infectious disease conditions for their patients.

Michael A. Malone, MD
Tidelands Health/
MUSC Family Medicine Residency Program
Murrells Inlet, SC 29576, USA

4320 Holmestown Road
Myrtle Beach, SC 29588, USA

E-mail address:
mimalone@tidelandshealth.org

Tick-Borne Illnesses in the United States

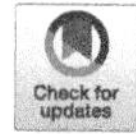

George G.A. Pujalte, MD[a,b,*], Scott T. Marberry, MD[a], Claudia R. Libertin, MD[c]

KEYWORDS

• Tick • Lyme • Babesiosis • Tularemia • Rick-borne • Ehrlichiosis • Anaplasmosis

KEY POINTS

- During febrile episodes in tick-borne relapsing fever, cerebrospinal fluid, bone marrow, or blood may have detectable spirochetes.
- Saddleback fever is the pathognomonic feature of Colorado tick fever, occurring in about 50% of patients.
- Most *Babesia* sp infections are subclinical, self-limiting, and spontaneously resolve.
- Because *Francisella tularensis* is highly infectious, it is dangerous to isolate it from sputum, lymph nodes, or skin lesions, and providers should promptly alert their laboratory of the suspicion.
- The enzyme-linked immunosorbent assay (ELISA) test is about 72% specific for Lyme and 89% sensitive; the Lyme western blot test is used to confirm a positive ELISA test.

INTRODUCTION

Close interaction with nature often leads to tick-borne infections. These cases are seen most frequently in primary care clinics when patients present symptoms. Considerable morbidity can result from untreated infections. Fortunately, they are often easily treatable when diagnosed early.

TICK-BORNE RELAPSING FEVER

History and Physical Examination

Fever is intermittent and typically greater than 40°C. Delirium may or may not be present. Signs and symptoms begin a week after tick bite. Nausea, vomiting, arthralgias, fever, chills, night sweats, and generalized malaise are usually apparent, thus, a "flulike" illness. Meningeal signs and splenomegaly may also be apparent. Splenic rupture,

The authors have nothing to disclose.

[a] Family Medicine, Mayo Clinic, 4500 San Pablo Road S, Jacksonville, FL 32224, USA; [b] Sports Medicine, Mayo Clinic, 4500 San Pablo Road S, Jacksonville, FL 32224, USA; [c] Division of Infectious Diseases, Department of Internal Medicine, Mayo Clinic, 4500 San Pablo Road S, Jacksonville, FL 32224, USA

* Corresponding author. Family Medicine, Mayo Clinic, 4500 San Pablo Road S, Jacksonville, FL 32224.

E-mail address: pujalte.george@mayo.edu

Prim Care Clin Office Pract 45 (2018) 379–391
https://doi.org/10.1016/j.pop.2018.05.011

myocarditis, pneumonitis, cranial nerve palsy, coma, iridocyclitis, hemoptysis, and epistaxis may also occur.[1,2]

Pathogen

The spirochete *Borrelia hermsii* is one causative agent for tick-borne relapsing fever. The chief vectors are ticks of the *Ornithodoros* genus. Hares, rabbits, squirrels, chipmunks, mice, and rats may serve as reservoirs. Mountainous areas west of the Mississippi River see most cases. The disease is sporadic and may appear in familial clusters.[3] Other *Borrelia* species, such as *Borrelia mayonii*, which may be found in Wisconsin and Minnesota, may cause more spirochetemia, leading to more pronounced symptoms.[4]

Diagnosis

During febrile episodes, cerebrospinal fluid, bone marrow, or blood may have detectable spirochetes. Thrombocytopenia, with or without leukocytosis, may also be noted.[1]

Management

Doxycycline is the treatment of choice, with erythromycin as a viable alternative.[5,6] If given during the late febrile stage, a Jarisch-Herxheimer reaction, characterized by seizures, rigors, sweating, fever, headache, and generalized malaise, may occur. Giving acetaminophen 2 hours before and after antibiotics may lessen the reaction's severity. Nonsteroidal anti-inflammatory drugs or steroids do not ameliorate the reaction's cardiopulmonary disturbances.

COLORADO TICK FEVER

History and Physical Examination

Colorado tick fever, also known as mountain tick fever, is caused by the Colorado tick fever virus. It is most commonly transmitted to humans by the bite of an infected adult wood tick. More than 90% of cases in the United States are from Colorado, Utah, and Montana. It is most prevalent during the summer months and is limited to mountainous elevations below 3000 m. Diagnosis can be challenging. Typically, within 1 week (usually 3–6 days) after the tick bite, the patient begins exhibiting flulike symptoms. Sore throat occurs in a third of patients. Other manifestations include chills, headache, musculoskeletal pain, and malaise. Saddleback fever is a pathognomonic feature; however, this occurs in only about 50% of patients. This biphasic fever lasts for about 3 days, followed by defervescence for 1 to 3 days, and concludes with a reappearance of the fever for another few days. A petechial, spotted rash can occur in up to a 10th of patients. The illness ranges from mild to life-threatening.

Pathogen

The wood tick, *Dermacentor andersoni*, transmits the RNA orbivirus that causes Colorado tick fever. The Rocky Mountain region sees the most cases annually, and incidence is probably higher than most reported numbers because initial presentation is generally benign.[7] Severe complications may occur in immunocompromised or asplenic patients.

Diagnosis

Thrombocytopenia and leukopenia may be present.[1] Immunofluorescence reveals the presence of the virus in blood smears. Polymerase chain reaction (PCR) is needed to confirm the diagnosis.

Management

No specific treatment exists for Colorado tick fever. Supportive treatment is indicated. As in most tick-borne illnesses, other infections need to be excluded. However, other tick-borne illnesses may have already been empirically treated with doxycycline before Colorado tick fever has been diagnosed.[1]

BABESIOSIS

History and Physical Examination

One to 4 weeks after inoculation, flulike symptoms develop as in other tick-borne illnesses. Patients may experience headaches, myalgia, sweating, and fever. In asplenic patients, babesiosis may present with renal failure, jaundice, hemoglobinuria, hemolytic anemia, and high fever, resembling falciparum malaria. In young, healthy adults or children, most *Babesia* sp infections are subclinical, self-limiting, and spontaneously resolve.[1,2]

Pathogen

Protozoans *Babesia microti* and *Babesia divergens* cause babesiosis. Babesiosis is the only tick-borne disease caused by protozoans in the United States. Various species of the *Ixodes* tick serve as the vector, but primarily *Ixodes scapularis*, the deer or black-legged tick. The northeastern United States experiences most cases.[1,2,8–11] Common hosts to these ticks include the white-tailed deer and American black bear with the reservoir being the white-footed mouse.[12]

Diagnosis

History and physical examination aid the diagnosis the most. Exposure history, including being outdoors in summer or autumn along Long Island, Nantucket, and Martha's Vineyard, should raise suspicions for diagnosis. Fever is evident. Hemolytic anemia may be present. Maltese crosses, a characteristic tetrad of merozoites in a Wright-Giemsa–stained thin blood smear, are diagnostic. PCR and serologic tests are also available.[1]

Management

Babesiosis in humans generally resolves spontaneously. Because most infected patients are asymptomatic, patients may not be aware of prior infection until serologic testing is done. Those who test positive by immunofluorescence for antibodies for *Babesia* species must be interrogated cautiously to avoid unnecessary treatment. Positive serology for *Babesia* sp immunoglobulin G (IgG) reflects exposure to the protozoan in the past. Provided the patient is asymptomatic, has a low serologic titer, and a negative smear for babesia, no treatment is indicated. If the *Babesia* PCR is positive in an asymptomatic patient, the PCR should be repeated in 3 months and treatment given only if the second test is positive. Low-level babesiosis only diagnosed by PCR probably does not require treatment initially. Symptomatic patients with a positive blood smear or PCR should be treated with atovaquone and azithromycin provided that presentation is mild and without a high level of parasitemia or significant hemolysis. Patients should be treated with quinine and clindamycin if they present with rising parasitemia, profound hemolysis, or persistent high fevers, or show more than 10% parasitemia on a smear. Children may be treated with the same medications at reduced doses. Severely ill patients with high parasitemia may benefit from exchange transfusions.[1,2,13]

TULAREMIA

History and Physical Examination

The symptoms of *Francisella tularensis* infections in humans depend on the route of bacterium entry.[14] Various syndromes describe the clinical manifestations of tularemia based on mode of infection: (1) typhoidal (ingestion of contaminated water), (2) pulmonary (inhalation of aerosolized bacteria), (3) oropharyngeal/gastrointestinal (ingestion of infected meat), (4) oculoglandular (conjunctiva exposure), and the most common, (5) ulceroglandular (direct skin inoculation).[3] Myalgias, fatigue, malaise, headache, chills, and fever rapidly ensue 3 to 6 days after inoculation. About a third of patients present with coughing. Pericarditis, acute respiratory distress syndrome, pneumonia, pleural effusions, sore throat, and skin ulcers may be noted as well.[15] Vomiting and nausea may also occur. Except in typhoidal or glandular tularemia, the infection site, which could be the roof of the mouth, eye, arm, or finger, may present with an inflamed papule within 24 to 48 hours of inoculation. An ulcer crater with colorless exudates results after the papule ulcerates and becomes pustular. Draining suppuration may be noted in regions of lymphadenopathy. Posterior auricular or cervical nodes are commonly affected in children. The femoral and inguinal nodes are more likely to be affected in adults.[1]

Pathogen

As mentioned earlier, the bacterium that causes tularemia, or rabbit fever, is called *F tularensis*. In the western United States, the tick vector is *D andersoni*, whereas in southeastern and south-central states, the tick vectors are *Dermacentor variabilis* and *Amblyomma americanum*. Contamination, inhalation, inoculation, and ingestion are the main ways of transmitting the bacteria. Infected rabbits (or other small mammals) that are skinned by hunters may have lesions from which the bacteria pass through microlesions on the hunters' skin, especially if the hands are not gloved, which is the main route of transmission in winter. Biting horse flies (Utah, Nevada, California), ticks (throughout North America), and mosquitoes (Finland, Sweden, and Russia) are the vectors of transmission in summer. Tick bites only account for about 10% of tularemia cases in the United States. Infections may also ensue from consuming contaminated water or undercooked infected meat, where the bacteria can survive for up to 3 years even when frozen.[1,2,14–16]

Diagnosis

A primary pustular lesion on an extremity, the characteristic symptoms outlined earlier, and exposure to ticks, wild rodents, or rabbits should lead to a suspicion of tularemia, particularly if in the context of correct geographic setting by history or location. Pulmonary tularemia is more likely to present with an abnormal chest radiographic finding, such as a triad of pleural effusions, hilar adenopathy, and oval opacities.[16–18] Because the organism is highly infectious, it is dangerous to isolate the organism from sputum, lymph nodes, or skin lesions, although this would be diagnostic. Providers should promptly collect appropriate specimens and alert their laboratory of the suspicion. Culture media or infected tissues should be handled with extreme caution. Growth of *F tularensis* in culture is the definitive means of confirming the diagnosis of tularemia. The diagnosis may be detected by an immunofluorescence assay test, by a single elevated serum antibody titer, by isolation of the organism from a clinical specimen, or from demonstration of an antibody titer increasing 4-fold in paired sera.[19] White blood cell count may be normal or increased. Because of the highly infectious nature of the organism, *F tularensis* is a Category A bioterrorism agent.

Management

Confirmatory laboratory test results need not be returned before treatment begins. Streptomycin and gentamicin are both bactericidal against *F tularensis* and are therefore the drugs of choice.[14,16] The dose of gentamicin needs to be reduced if renal disease is present. Fluoroquinolones, such as levofloxacin and ciprofloxacin, have been used to treat this infection.[14] Although they may not prevent node suppuration or relapses, tetracyclines or chloramphenicol may also be used.[20]

EHRLICHIOSIS AND ANAPLASMOSIS

History and Physical Examination

The clinical presentation of both human monocytotropic ehrlichiosis (HME) and human granulocytotropic anaplasmosis (HGA) is fairly similar. Fever (97% in HME and 94%–100% in HGA), myalgia, headache (81% in HME and 61%–85% in HGA), malaise, cough, and chills comprise the flulike syndrome that marks both infections.[21] HME causes a rash in up to 60% of children and less than 30% of adults. If present, the rash may appear as a petechial, macular, or maculopapular lesion on the upper extremities and trunk. Rarely (in <5% of cases), the palms and soles may have the rash. HGA rarely causes a rash and is most endemic in the Northeast and Midwest regions of the United States, usually in June and July. Differentiating clinically between ehrlichiosis and anaplasmosis is difficult in that leukopenia, thrombocytopenia, and abnormal liver function tests can occur with both infections. Geographic acquisition of the infection aids in the diagnosis as well as whether a morulae (seen on a peripheral smear) is within a monocyte (HME) or a neutrophil (HGA).

Pathogen

Anaplasma phagocytophilum (formerly classified and named *Ehrlichia equi* or *Ehrlichia phagocytophila*) is a small, gram-negative bacterium that primarily infects granulocytes and causes HGA. They are distinct epidemiologically but are clinically indistinguishable.[22] Human anaplasmosis is predominantly seen in the Northeast and Midwest regions of the United States during the months of May, June, and July. It is during this time of year that the primary vector, the ixodid tick (American deer tick), is most active and when human contact with its reservoir host is at its peak. Coinfection with Lyme disease and babesiosis is common because of a shared vector: *I scapularis*.[1,2,23–25]

HME is seen mostly in the southeastern to south-central United States. Although it can be seen year-round, most cases occur between the months of April and September, peaking in July. Its primary vectors are the American dog tick (*D variabilis*) and the lone star tick (*A americanum*).[1,2,23]

Diagnosis

Increased serum transaminases, thrombocytopenia, and leukopenia are seen in patients with either ehrlichiosis or anaplasmosis. A patient presenting with acute-onset fever and these symptoms coupled with a recent history of tick bite in an endemic area should trigger empiric treatment with doxycycline until HME or HGA has been ruled out. Specific serologies may initially be negative, and a convalescent phase serologic titer may need to be repeated in 2 to 4 weeks.[21,22,26] Seroconversion during convalescence is the principal method of diagnosing human ehrlichiosis and anaplasmosis. The diagnosis necessitates documentation of a single serum antibody titer greater than or equal to 1:128 or a 4-fold increase or decrease in antibody titer with a minimum peak of 1:64.[1,2,21] Identification of morulae within the cytoplasm of monocytes, macrophages, and neutrophils via microscopic examination of a blood smear may help in the diagnosis but requires a trained eye.

Management

Confirmation from laboratory tests should not be awaited before treatment of ehrlichiosis and anaplasmosis begins. The treatment of choice is doxycycline.[26] Tetracycline is a good alternative. Antibiotics should be given for 5 to 7 days until there is evidence of clinical improvement and after the fever subsides. It should then be continued for at least 3 more days.[26] Severe cases may require longer treatment courses.

LYME DISEASE

History and Physical Examination

Lyme disease typically presents in 3 stages. Seven to 10 days after the tick bite and concurrent inoculation of *Borrelia* sp, stage 1 (early localized Lyme disease) occurs, in which 75% of patients may develop the typical rash, called erythema migrans (EM), at the site of the tick bite. This rash consists of a red, expanding, annular papule or macule with central clearing up to 50 cm in diameter. Typically, the patient has no flulike illness; however, when present, regional lymphadenopathy, coughing, headaches, arthralgias, fatigue, and low-grade fever occur.[1,2,8,27] In the geographic distribution of the lone star tick (*A americanum*) or southeast United States, an EM -style rash with fewer systemic symptoms occurs from an unknown pathogen called southern tick-associated rash illness (STARI). The lesion is typically smaller than EM or less than 10 cm in diameter. STARI may account for the clinical diagnoses of Lyme disease in nonendemic regions of the United States because its rash mimics EM.

A few weeks after the initial infection, stage 2 (early disseminated Lyme disease) may occur. Later stages of Lyme disease (stage 2 and late/chronic Lyme disease) only occur if the infection is left untreated at stage 1. Disseminated or stage 2 Lyme disease manifests with characteristic annular lesions mainly truncal in location and anatomically. These multiple EM rashes are smaller and less red than the primary EM lesion. Disseminated Lyme disease typically does have associated constitutional symptoms, such as malaise, fever, or myalgias. Part of stage 2 Lyme disease may include Lyme carditis with primary, secondary, or tertiary (complete) heart block presenting as syncope. Complete heart block may resolve within several days of treatment with antimicrobials, and a temporary pacer may be avoided. Early Lyme neuroborreliosis occurs during the second stage of Lyme disease. There may be meningeal involvement and cranial and/or peripheral neuritis. The most classic neurologic presentation in secondary Lyme disease is Bell palsy (either unilateral or bilateral).[1,2,8,27]

Tertiary Lyme disease most typically presents as Lyme arthritis in large joints, primarily the knee. Rarely, there can be neurologic manifestations.[28] Lyme meningoencephalitis can occur by occlusive vasculitis with cerebral infarcts as the pathologic abnormality. Late Lyme disease may present as a recurrent monoarthritis or oligoarthritis afflicting 50% to 60% of untreated patients. It may remit only to recur after several weeks to months in untreated individuals.[29]

Pathogen

Lyme disease is the most common vector-borne infectious disease in the United States.[27] It is caused by the spirochete *Borrelia burgdorferi*. *I scapularis*, or the black-legged tick, is the main vector in the United States. The female tick often attaches itself to the white-tailed deer during winter, and so it is also known as the deer tick. Small to medium-sized mammals, such as the white-footed mouse and animals as large as the common raccoon, serve as principal reservoirs for *B burgdorferi*.[30] Tick nymphs or larvae become infected when they feed on such mammals. The nymphs usually infect humans, although adult ticks may also. The risk of transmission of *B burgdorferi* only becomes substantial if the infected nymph remains attached for 36 hours or longer. Adult ticks must remain attached for greater than 48 hours.[31–34] Fleas, flies, or mosquitoes cannot transmit Lyme disease. Lyme disease cannot be transmitted by blood products.[35] Geographic studies demonstrate a steady, gradual expansion of Lyme disease incidence over time emanating from 2 foci, the northeastern seaboard and the Michigan-Wisconsin region. Gradual expansion may be occurring due to favorable changing geographic conditions for tick survival or the dispersal of ticks via birds and deer.[36,37]

Diagnosis

In endemic areas, patients presenting with typical EM require no laboratory confirmation because only about 30% will have positive Lyme serologies during this early phase.[38] The enzyme-linked immunosorbent assay (ELISA) test is about 72% specific and 89% sensitive. The Lyme western blot test is used to confirm a positive ELISA test. The Lyme western blot IgG is almost 100% positive (ie, more than 5 bands positive out a total of 10 IgG bands) if the test is done in patients with an active infection longer than 1 month, as with late Lyme disease.[38] In patients who have been ill for more than 4 weeks, a positive western blot IgM test alone (negative IgG test) is most likely a false positive; therefore, the Centers for Disease Control and Prevention (CDC) recommends that only an IgG western blot be done. The CDC proposes the use of a 2-tiered testing decision tree for Lyme disease. The first required test is the enzyme immunoassay or immunofluorescence assay. If this test yields negative results, consider an alternative diagnosis. In cases where the patient has had symptoms for less than or equal to 30 days, the provider may treat the patient and follow up with a convalescent serum. If the first test yields positive or equivocal results, then, if the patient has had symptoms for less than or equal to 30 days, an IgM western blot can be performed, or, if the patient has had symptoms for greater than 30 days, an IgG western blot can be performed. IgM should not be used if the patient has been ill for more than 30 days. Lyme DNA PCR assays allow the specific diagnosis of this infection using sterile fluids such as the synovial fluid and cerebrospinal fluid for diagnosing Lyme arthritis and neuroborreliosis, respectively.[20] The PCR for *Borrelia* sp is typically used in endemic regions where prior IgG seropositivity may exist due to past infections. PCR positivity in, say, an arthrocentesis of the knee of a seropositive Lyme patient living in the northeastern United States provides further evidence of an ongoing infection. It takes weeks for the cultures from most body fluids and tissues to turn positive for *B burgdorferi*; therefore, they are not commonly used diagnostic tests.

Management

If the tick was attached for less than 36 hours, the risk of infection with *B burgdorferi* is minimal to nonexistent, and there is no need for routine antibiotic prophylaxis.[28,35] In a typical practice setting, the likelihood of infection is less than 3.5%. According to a cost-effectiveness analysis, one 200-mg dose of doxycycline is cost-effective only if the likelihood of infection is greater than this.[38–40] Antibiotic treatments are curative in most cases if symptoms develop. Doxycycline is the recommended antibiotic if the patient is older than 12 years. For 12 years old and younger, amoxicillin is the recommended antibiotic. For patients who cannot take tetracyclines or are allergic to penicillin, cefuroxime is a viable alternative. For uncomplicated cases of Lyme disease, treatment usually ranges from 14 to 21 days. Lyme meningitis and other manifestations of early neurologic Lyme disease include ceftriaxone parenterally. Although antibiotic treatment may not hasten the resolution of Bell palsy from Lyme disease, antibiotics should be given to prevent further sequelae. Patients with atrioventricular heart block and/or myopericarditis associated with early Lyme disease may be treated with either oral or parenteral antibiotic therapy for 14 days.[28] Lyme arthritis can usually be treated successfully with antimicrobial agents given by mouth. It is important to remember that *B microti* or *A phagocytophilum* or both may occur in patients with early Lyme disease in endemic areas. A key point in management is that clinical findings are sufficient for the diagnosis of EM but not for the diagnosis of extracutaneous manifestations of Lyme disease, HGA, or babesiosis.[28] Furthermore, there is no well-accepted definition of post-Lyme disease syndrome.

ROCKY MOUNTAIN SPOTTED FEVER

Pathogen

Rocky Mountain spotted fever (RMSF) is the most common rickettsial disease in the United States and is caused by *Rickettsia rickettsia*.[23] About 2000 cases of RMSF are reported in the United States every year.[41] All states except Alaska, Hawaii, and Maine have reported cases, and the disease is limited to the Western Hemisphere. Infections may occur year-round in the southern United States, although the disease is more common in the coastal Atlantic states from April to September.[20] The most common vector in the southern and eastern United States is the dog tick, *D variabilis*. In the western United States, the wood tick, *D andersoni*, is the principal vector. Person-to-person transmission does not occur, but it can be transmitted from pets via ticks. Children 5 to 9 years of age are the most commonly afflicted by RMSF.[42]

Presentation

Between 50% and 70% of patients with tick-borne disease recall getting bitten by a tick.[20,42] RMSF symptoms usually begin 5 to 7 days after inoculation. Vomiting, nausea, frontal headaches, fever, leg muscle pain, back pain, and generalized malaise are common symptoms. Abdominal pain, pleuritic chest pain, sore throat, and nonproductive cough are other symptoms. An exanthema appearing within the first few days of symptoms associated with chills, fever, and sudden headache comprise the classic presenting symptoms. The forearms, ankles, wrists, palms, and soles carry the initial lesions, which spread centripetally. Pressure applied onto the lesions, which are macular and pink, causes them to fade. The rash becomes petechial as it extends onto the neck, trunk, buttocks, and axilla. Large areas of ulceration and ecchymosis may result as the lesions coalesce. Neurologic compromise may occur along with circulatory and respiratory failure.[43] Poor outcomes and complications usually occur in patients with glucose-6-phosphate dehydrogenase deficiency.[44] RMSF outcomes are based on the day that therapy starts. Mortality is 33% if started on day 6 and 27% to 50% if started on day 7 to 9, which highlights the importance of initiating antimicrobial therapy before serologic confirmation of the disease is available.[45]

Diagnosis

History of possible outdoor exposure to ticks, geographic distribution of the disease, and physical examination are all that is needed to diagnose RMSF. RMSF should be considered in patients presenting with headaches and fever who are acutely ill with high fevers and rash in endemic areas during peak months for tick exposure. Immunofluorescent staining for *Rickettsia* after skin biopsy of rash, if present, is highly specific, although sensitivity may only be slightly more than 60%. Hyponatremia and thrombocytopenia may be noted, but laboratory testing is of limited usefulness.[44] Within the convalescence period, latex agglutination titers and increase of specific ELISA may be useful.[1]

Management

Immediate treatment is imperative when hyponatremia, thrombocytopenia, and rash are noted. A minimum of 7 days of treatment with doxycycline or tetracycline is required.[26] There is limited evidence that RMSF responds to fluoroquinolones, although there are reports that they may also be effective.[46] Early treatment is crucial to affect optimal response to antibiotics as noted above. Laboratory confirmation need not be obtained before treatment is instituted.[47]

TICK-BORNE ILLNESS PREVENTION STRATEGIES

Avoiding high-risk habitats during periods of peak tick activity is the first line of defense against tick bites.[48–50] Using bed nets when sleeping on the ground or camping, using tick repellents containing permethrin for clothing and *N*,*N*-diethyl-*m*-toluamide concentrations of 30% to 50% for the skin, wearing long pants, tucking pant legs into socks, and avoiding tick-infested areas, especially during the summer months, are some measures that may prevent tick exposure. The effectiveness of a product called Citriodiol that is derived from lemon-scented eucalyptus oil has been demonstrated.[43] Other potential tick repellents have also been identified, such as Alaska yellow cedar oil, lavender oil, and geranium oil.[51,52]

Between 24 and 48 hours of attachment to the host are required before infection occurs, and so diseases can be prevented by the early removal of ticks.[20,48] Removal of the tick can be done by applying vertical traction to its body as it is grasped gently. The best results may be achieved through forceps that are angled, medium-tipped, and blunt. Instead of tweezers, there are commercially available devices that may also be used. Passing a needle through the tick, using injected or topical lidocaine, covering the tick in petroleum jelly, nail polish, alcohol, or gasoline, or applying a hot match to the tick body are not recommended tick-removal methods. Granuloma formation and/or infection may result if parts of the proboscis remain in the skin because of improper technique.[53]

Ninety-five percent of host-seeking *I scapularis* nymphs can be killed by a single, well-timed application of deltamethrin at the forest-lawn interface of residential properties.[54] Human babesiosis, HGA, and Lyme borreliosis could theoretically be prevented by such an approach, but residents in areas highly endemic for these illnesses decline to use acaricides on their properties because of fears regarding environmental damage and toxicity to humans and animals.[48] A method for monitoring tick populations in communities is called dragging or flogging, whereby a $3' \times 3'$ white cloth is fixed to a dowel and dragged through grass and brush. The cloth should then be inspected and the ticks found clinging to the cloth identified and counted to provide a gauge of tick infestation within wilderness communities.[55]

Tests had proved the effectiveness of a recombinant vaccine in humans against the Lyme borreliosis spirochete (*B burgdorferi*) outer surface protein A (OspA), which was later approved by the US Food and Drug Administration. By 2002, it was withdrawn from the market because of low public demand, uncertainty regarding disease risk, class action lawsuits, difficult vaccination schedule, potential need for boosters, high cost, concerns of anti–vaccine groups regarding safety, and suggestions that the vaccine antigen, OspA, was arthritogenic because it served as an autoantigen.[56,57]

For centuries, vegetation management has been a method for controlling ticks. To reduce tick populations, controlled burns, brush removal, and mowing may be used, although effects may be short lived.[48] Placing a border between naturally tick-infested forested habitats and adjacent lawns on residential properties may be a more long-lasting landscape management strategy.[58,59] Because it has repellent properties, Alaska yellow cedar sawdust may be an appropriate material for such borders.[58] *I scapularis* is found in forest habitats associated with leaf litter and is the principal vector of *B burgdorferi* in the eastern United States. The population of host-seeking ticks is reduced by removal of leaf litter from the forest floor and exposes these ticks to desiccation.[60] However, the transport of exotic vectors by migratory neotropical birds causes the introduction of emerging tick species and tick-borne pathogens, particularly in southern states such as Texas, where previously uncharacterized species of *Rickettsia* and *Amblyomma* were identified between the spring seasons of 2013 and 2014, and this is likely to continue.[61]

CONCURRENT INFECTIONS

Although beyond the scope of this article, 1 bite from 1 tick may transmit different infectious pathogens that may result in concurrent infections, resulting in a clinical picture that may be mixed or more complicated.[62] Babesiosis, Lyme disease, and ehrlichiosis can all be transmitted by *I scapularis* concurrently. Lyme disease may occur concurrently with babesiosis in 23% of patients diagnosed with the former.[63] Babesiosis and/or Lyme disease may occur concurrently in 10% to 30% of patients with ehrlichiosis. More severe symptoms seem to result from such combined infections.[20,62]

REFERENCES

1. Bratton RL, Corey GR. Tick-borne disease. Am Fam Physician 2005;71:2323–30.
2. Gayle A, Ringdahl E. Tick-borne diseases. Am Fam Physician 2001;64:461–6.
3. Steve AC. Lyme borreliosis. In: Kasper DL, Harrison TR, editors. Harrison's manual of medicine. 16th edition. New York: McGraw-Hill; 2005. p. 995–9.
4. Pritt BS, Respicio-Kingry LB, Sloan LM, et al. Borrelia mayonii sp. nov., a member of the Borrelia burgdorferi sensu lato complex, detected in patients and ticks in the upper midwestern United States. Int J Syst Evol Microbiol 2016;66(11):4878–80.
5. Gilbert DN, Moellering RC, Eliopoulos GM, et al. Antimicrobial therapy. the Sanford guide to antimicrobial therapy. 34th edition. Hyde Park (VT): Blackwell Publishing; 2004. p. 39.
6. Byrd RP Jr, Vasquez J, Roy TM. Respiratory manifestations of tick-borne diseases in the southeastern United States. South Med J 1997;90:1–4.
7. Emmons RW. An overview of Colorado tick fever. Prog Clin Biol Res 1985;178:47–52.
8. Goddard J. Tick-borne diseases. In: Georgiev VS, editor. Infectious diseases and arthropods. 2nd edition. Totowa (NJ): Humana Press; 2008. p. 81–129.
9. Centers for Disease Control and Prevention. Tick-borne relapsing fever. Available at: http://www.cdc.gov/relapsing-fever/clinicians/#treatment. Accessed March 25, 2018.
10. Kazzi MG. Colorado tick fever. In: Kulkarni R, editor. Medscape. Available at: http://emedicine.medscape.com/article/786688-medication. Accessed March 25, 2018.
11. Centers for Disease Control and Prevention. Parasites: babesiosis. Available at: http://www.cdc.gov/parasites/babesiosis/health_professionals/index.html#tx. Accessed March 25, 2018.

12. Zolnik CP, Makkay AM, Falco RC, et al. American black bears as hosts of black-legged ticks (acari: ixodidae) in the northeastern United States. J Med Entomol 2015;52(5):1103–10.
13. Drugs for parasitic infections. Med Lett Drugs Ther 2010. Available at: http://secure.medicalletter.org/system/files/private/parasitic.pdfsecure.medicalletter.org/system/files/private/parasitic.pdf. Accessed March 25, 2018.
14. Ellis J, Oyston PC, Green M, et al. Tularemia. Clin Microbiol Rev 2002;15:631–46.
15. Evans ME, Gregory DW, Schaffner W, et al. Tularemia: a 30-year experience with 88 cases. Medicine 1985;64:251–69.
16. Miller RP, Bates JH. Pleuropulmonary tularemia: a review of 29 patients. Am Rev Respir Dis 1969;99:31–41.
17. Rubin SA. Radiographic spectrum of pleuropulmonary tularemia. Am J Roentgenol 1978;131:277–81.
18. Dennis DT, Inglesby TV, Henderson DA, et al. Tularemia as a biological weapon: medical and public health management. JAMA 2001;285:2763–73.
19. Centers for Disease Control and Prevention. Tickborne diseases of the United States: a reference manual for health care providers. 4th edition. Fort Collins (CO): CDC; 2017.
20. Beers MH, Berkow R. The Merck manual of diagnosis and therapy. 17th edition. Whitehouse Station (NJ): Merck Research Laboratories; 1999.
21. Dumler JS, Walker DH. Ehrlichia chaffeensis (human monocytotropic ehrlichiosis), Anaplasma phagocytophilum (human granulocytotropic anaplasmosis), and other Anaplasmataceae. In: Mandell GL, Bennett JE, Dolin R, editors. Mandell, Douglas, and Bennett's principles and practice of infectious diseases. 7th edition. Philadelphia: Elsevier Churchill Livingstone; 2010. p. 2531–8.
22. Belman AL. Tick-borne diseases. Semin Pediatr Neurol 1999;6:249–66.
23. Diaz JH. Ticks, including tick paralysis. In: Mandell GL, Bennett JE, Dolin R, editors. Mandell, Douglas, and Bennett's principles and practice of infectious diseases. 7th edition. Philadelphia: Elsevier Churchill Livingstone; 2010. p. 3649–62.
24. Centers for Disease Control and Prevention. Abstract: Consensus statement: tularemia as a biological weapon: medical and public health management. Available at: http://www.bt.cdc.gov/agent/tularemia/tularemia-biologicalweapon- abstract.asp#4. Accessed March 25, 2018.
25. Cunha BA. Ehrlichiosis. In: Bronze M, editor. Medscape. Available at: http://emedicine.medscape.com/article/235839-medication. Accessed March 25, 2018.
26. Centers for Disease Control and Prevention. Human ehrlichiosis in the United States. Available at: http://gov/ncidod/dvrd/ehrlichia/index.htm. Accessed March 25, 2018.
27. Shapiro ED. Tick-borne diseases. Adv Pediatr Infect Dis 1997;13:187–218.
28. Wormser GP, Dattwyler RJ, Shapiro ED, et al. The clinical assessment, treatment, and prevention of Lyme disease, human granulocytic anaplasmosis, and babesiosis: clinical practice guidelines by the Infectious Diseases Society of America. Clin Infect Dis 2006;43:1089–134.
29. Steere AC, Schoen RT, Taylor E. The clinical evolution of Lyme arthritis. Ann Intern Med 1987;107(5):725–31.
30. Barbour AG, Bunikis J, Fish D, et al. Association between body size and reservoir competence of mammals bearing Borrelia burgdorferi at an endemic site in the northeastern United States. Parasit Vectors 2015;30(8):299.
31. Piesman J, Mather TN, Sinsky RJ, et al. Duration of tick attachment and Borrelia burgdorferi transmission. J Clin Microbiol 1987;25:557–8.

32. Piesman J, Maupin GO, Campos EG, et al. Duration of adult female Ixodes dammini attachment and transmission of Borrelia burgdorferi, with description of a needle aspiration isolation method. J Infect Dis 1991;163:895–7.
33. Piesman J. Dynamics of Borrelia burgdorferi transmission by nymphal Ixodes dammini ticks. J Infect Dis 1993;167:1082–5.
34. Falco RC, Fish D, Piesman J. Duration of tick bites in a Lyme disease endemic area. Am J Epidemiol 1996;143:187–92.
35. Centers for Disease Control and Prevention. Lyme disease. Available at: http://www.cdc.gov/lyme/. Accessed March 25, 2018.
36. Kugeler KJ, Farley GM, Forrester JD, et al. Geographic distribution and expansion of human Lyme disease, United States. Emerg Infect Dis 2015;21(8):1455–7.
37. Kingry LC, Anacker M, Pritt B, et al. Surveillance for and discovery of Borrelia species in US patients suspected of tickborne illness. Clin Infect Dis 2017. https://doi.org/10.1093/cid/cix1107.
38. Bacon RM, Biggerstaff BJ, Schriefer ME, et al. Serodiagnosis of Lyme disease by kinetic enzyme-linked immunosorbent assay using recombinant VlsE1 or peptide antigens of Borrelia burgdorferi compared with 2-tiered testing using whole-cell lysates. J Infect Dis 2003;187(8):1187–99.
39. Magid D, Schwartz B, Craft J, et al. Prevention of Lyme disease after tick bites: a cost-effectiveness analysis. N Engl J Med 1992;327:534–41.
40. Treatment of Lyme disease. Med Lett Drugs Ther 2000;42:37–9.
41. Centers for Disease Control and Prevention. Provisional cases of selected notifiable diseases, week ending December 29, 2007. MMWR Morb Mortal Wkly Rep 2008;56:1360–71.
42. Walker DH. Tick-transmitted infectious diseases in the United States. Annu Rev Public Health 1998;19:237–69.
43. Kwitkowski VE, Demko SG. Infectious disease emergencies in primary care. Lippincotts Prim Care Pract 1999;3:108–25.
44. Centers for Disease Control and Prevention. Rocky Mountain spotted fever (RMSF). Available at: http://www.cdc.gov/rmsf/symptoms/index.html. Accessed March 25, 2018.
45. Traeger MS, Regan JJ, Humpherys D, et al. Rocky Mountain spotted fever characterization and comparison to similar illnesses in a highly endemic area—Arizona, 2002–2011. Clin Infect Dis 2015;60(11):1650–8.
46. Thorner AR, Walker DH, Petri WA Jr. Rocky mountain spotted fever. Clin Infect Dis 1998;27:1353–9.
47. Gardulf A, Wohlfart I, Gustafson R. A prospective cross-over field trial shows protection of lemon eucalyptus extract against tick bites. J Med Entomol 2004;41:1064–7.
48. Piesman J, Eisen L. Prevention of tick-borne diseases. Annu Rev Entomol 2008;53:323–43.
49. Raoult D, Fournier PE, Eremeeva M, et al. Naming of Rickettsiae and rickettsial diseases. Ann N Y Acad Sci 2005;1063:1–12.
50. Mandl CW. Steps of the tick-borne encephalitis virus replication cycle that affect neuropathogenesis. Virus Res 2005;111:161–74.
51. Dietrich G, Dolan MC, Peralta-Cruz J, et al. Repellent activity of fractioned compounds from Chamaecyparis nootkatensis essential oil against nymphal Ixodes scapularis (acari: ixodidae). J Med Entomol 2006;43:957–61.
52. Jaenson TG, Garboui S, Palsson K. Repellency of oils of lemon eucalyptus geranium, and lavender and the mosquito repellent MyggA natural to Ixodes ricinus (acari: ixodidae) in the laboratory and field. J Med Entomol 2006;43:731–6.
53. Gammons M, Salam G. Tick removal. Am Fam Physician 2002;66:643–5.

54. Schulze TL, Jordan RA, Hung RW, et al. Efficacy of granular deltamethrin against Ixodes scapularis and Amblyomma americanum (acari: ixodidae) nymphs. J Med Entomol 2001;38:344–6.
55. Cohen EB, Auckland LD, Marra PP, et al. Avian Migrants Facilitate Invasions of Neotropical Ticks and Tick-Borne Pathogens into the United States. Applied and Environmental Microbiology 2015;81(24):8366–78.
56. Steere AC, Sikand VK, Meurice F, et al. Vaccination against Lyme disease with recombinant Borrelia burgdorferi outer-surface lipoprotein A with adjuvant. N Engl J Med 1998;339:209–15.
57. Poland GA. Vaccines against Lyme disease: what happened and what lessons can we learn? Clin Infect Dis 2011;52(Suppl 3):s253–8.
58. Maupin GO, Fish D, Zultowsky J, et al. Landscape ecology of Lyme disease in a residential area of Westchester County, New York, USA. Am J Epidemiol 1991; 133:1105–13.
59. Piesman J. Response of nymphal Ixodes scapularis, the primary tick vector of Lyme disease spirochetes in North America, to barriers derived from wood products or related home and garden items. J Vector Ecol 2006;31:412–7.
60. Schulze TL, Jordan RA, Hung RW. Suppression of subadult Ixodes scapularis (acari: ixodidae) following removal of leaf litter. J Med Entomol 1995;32:730–3.
61. Cohen EB, Aukland LD, Marra PP, et al. Avian migrants facilitate invasions of neotropical ticks and tick-borne pathogens into the United States. Appl Environ Microbiol 2015;81(24):8366–78.
62. Walker DH, Barbour AG, Oliver JH, et al. Emerging bacterial zoonotic and vector-borne diseases: ecological and epidemiological factors. JAMA 1996;275:463–9.
63. Meldrum SC, Birkhead GS, White DJ, et al. Human babesiosis in New York State: an epidemiological description of 136 cases. Clin Infect Dis 1992;15:1019–23.

Mosquito-Borne Diseases

Hobart Lee, MD*, Sara Halverson, MD, Ngozi Ezinwa, MD, MPH

KEYWORDS

- Mosquitoes • Chikungunya • Dengue • Japanese encephalitis • Malaria • West Nile • Yellow fever • Zika

KEY POINTS

- Mosquito-borne diseases have become more common in the United States as globalization and urbanization have allowed previously geographically isolated diseases to spread globally.
- Patient history should include local residence, global travel, and relevant exposures, including local outbreaks.
- Diagnostic testing can vary based on symptom duration and testing availability, and should be coordinated with local public health departments or the Centers for Disease Control and Prevention.
- Treatment for most mosquito-borne diseases is supportive, and the emphasis is on reducing risk and local spread.
- Some mosquito-borne diseases require mandatory reporting in the United States.

INTRODUCTION AND BACKGROUND

The purpose of this article was to review the epidemiology, presentation, and treatment of several common and emerging mosquito-borne diseases, specifically chikungunya, dengue, Japanese encephalitis, malaria, West Nile, yellow fever, and Zika. Although the clinical presentation overlaps for several of these diseases, it is important to make an accurate diagnosis for treatment, prognosis, and prevention. Globalization, urbanization, and changes to climate and agriculture have allowed geographically isolated mosquito-borne diseases to spread globally (**Fig. 1**).[1] Patient history should include local residence, global travel, and relevant exposures, including local outbreaks.

Mosquitoes are flying, blood-sucking insects that are a common vector, taking in virulent microorganisms and passing them along to subsequent bite targets. The morbidity and mortality from mosquito-borne diseases are very high: more than 2.5 billion people are at risk to contract dengue, and more than 400,000 people die from malaria annually.[1]

Disclosure: The authors have nothing to disclose.
Department of Family Medicine, Loma Linda University School of Medicine, 1200 California Street, Suite 240, Redlands, CA 92374, USA
* Corresponding author.
E-mail address: holee@llu.edu

Prim Care Clin Office Pract 45 (2018) 393–407
https://doi.org/10.1016/j.pop.2018.05.001
primarycare.theclinics.com

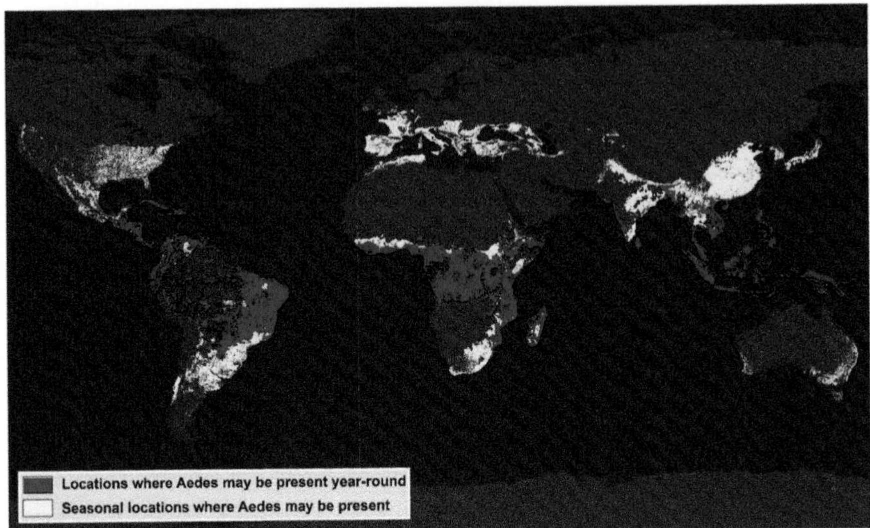

Fig. 1. Global map of the locations suitable for seasonal presence (*yellow*) and year-around presence (*red*) of hematophagous *Aedes* mosquitoes. (*From* Attaway DF, Waters NM, Geraghty EM, et al. Zika virus: endemic and epidemic ranges of *Aedes* mosquito transmission. J Infect Public Health 2017;10(1):122; with permission. CC BY-NC-ND license (http://creativecommons.org/licenses/by-nc-nd/4.0/).)

Because treatment of many mosquito-borne diseases is mainly supportive, the emphasis is on reducing risk and infection. Individuals should be encouraged to use insect repellant and mosquito netting, and to wear long-sleeved shirts and pants when local outbreaks occur or when traveling to endemic areas. Detailed, country-specific information on prevention and prophylaxis can be found on the Centers for Disease Control and Prevention (CDC) Web site. Many mosquito-borne diseases require mandatory reporting in the United States. including in 2018 chikungunya, dengue, malaria, West Nile virus, yellow fever, and Zika.[2]

Chikungunya

Epidemiology

Chikungunya affects people in more than 60 countries.[3] It is rarely fatal, but 87% to 95% of individuals suffer debilitating arthralgia, which can persist for years. Because of this chronic arthralgia, Chikungunya is called "to be contorted" in Tanzanian Kimakonde language, where the disease was first described in 1952.[4]

Chikungunya is a Togaviridae alphavirus and has a largely sylvatic life cycle, periodically causing urban human outbreaks in Africa and Asia. Its primary vectors are *Aedes aegypti* (**Fig. 2**) and *Aedes albopictus*, a more temperate-climate mosquito species, increasingly its global spread.[5] In 2004, an initial outbreak in Kenya spread to millions of people in India, with subsequent local transmission in Southeast Asia, France, and Italy.[6] The first outbreak in the Americas started on St. Martin Island in October 2013 and spread to Florida.[7] It is estimated more than 40 million people have been infected in the Americas, resulting in 23.8 million disability-adjusted life-years lost, costing more than $185 billion.[8]

Signs and symptoms

The primary clinical findings are acute-onset fever and severe arthralgia, usually within 24 to 48 hours of a mosquito bite. Headache, myalgia, conjunctivitis, nausea/vomiting,

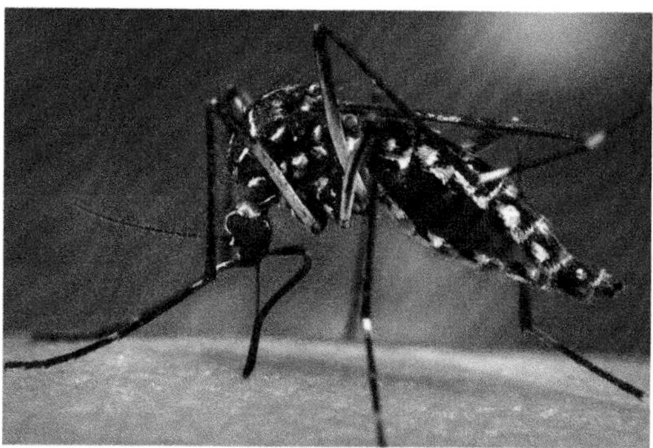

Fig. 2. *Aedes aegypti* mosquito. (*From* CDC Public Health Image Library/James Gathany.)

and maculopapular rash also may occur[8] Rare complications include uveitis, retinitis, myocarditis, hepatitis, nephritis, bullous skin lesions, hemorrhage, meningoencephalitis, myelitis, Guillain-Barré syndrome (GBS), and cranial nerve palsies. The acute viremia lasts a median of 6 days.

Children, the elderly, and patients with chronic medical conditions are at higher risk for severe disease and complications. Infection during pregnancy is not teratogenic, but acute intrapartum viremia is associated with vertical transmission in 44% of cases.[9]

Diagnosis

Reverse transcription-polymerase chain reaction (RT-PCR) is recommended days 1 to 8. After day 3, enzyme-linked immunosorbent assay (ELISA) tests can also detect immunoglobulin (Ig)M, IgG, and neutralizing antibodies. Routine complete blood counts and complete metabolic panels can show lymphopenia, thrombocytopenia, and elevated creatinine and hepatic transaminases. Thrombocytopenia less than 100×10^9/L may be used to distinguish it from severe dengue, but it is not diagnostic.

The differential diagnosis includes other mosquito-borne disease, including dengue, other alphavirus infections, and rheumatologic conditions. A potential workup algorithm to help distinguish among chikungunya, dengue, and Zika is listed in **Fig. 3**.

Treatment

The treatment of chikungunya is supportive (**Box 1**).

Prevention and control

There is no vaccine to prevent chikungunya. The focus is on reducing mosquito exposure and spread of disease (**Box 2**).[10]

Dengue

Epidemiology

Dengue is spread by the *A aegypti* and *A albopictus* mosquitoes in 100 tropical and subtropical countries in Asia, the Pacific, the Americas, Africa, and the Caribbean and is the most common and rapidly spreading mosquito-borne viral illness.[11] The endemic areas include 40% of the world population and 40% to 90% of exposed individuals will contract dengue (50–100 million infections per year), resulting in 500,000 hospitalizations (90% of hospitalizations are for children younger than 5) and 22,000 deaths.[12,13]

The dengue virus has 4 serotypes, and an infected individual has lifetime immunity only to that specific serotype.[4] Between 2006 and 2008, 244 cases of dengue were

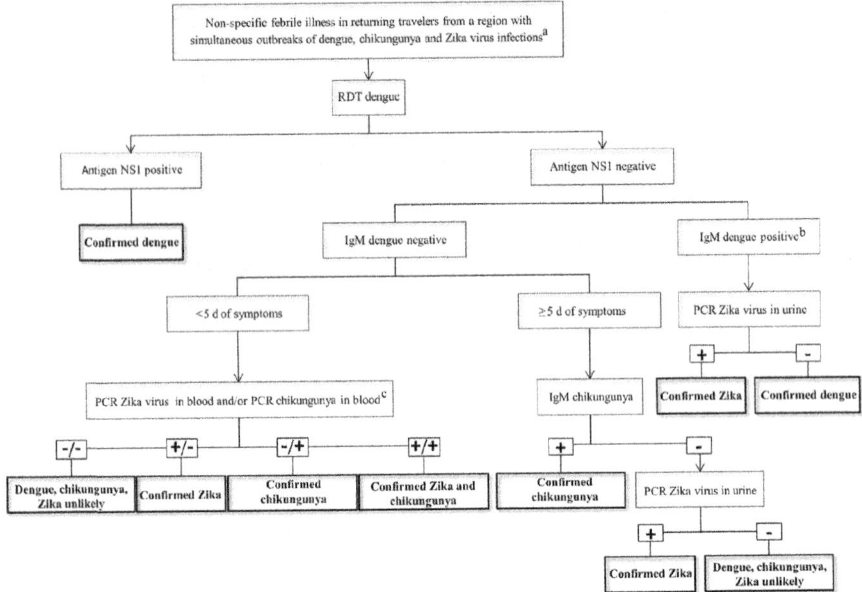

Fig. 3. Diagnostic algorithm for travelers with nonspecific febrile illness returning from regions experiencing simultaneous outbreaks of dengue, chikungunya, and Zika virus infections. RDT, rapid diagnostic test. [a] First, exclude malaria with rapid diagnostic test. [b] Cross-reactivity between Flaviviruses. [c] Sequential testing is an alternative in the absence of concerning clinical signs. (*From* Moulin E, Selby K, Cherpillod P, et al. Simultaneous outbreaks of dengue, chikungunya, and Zika virus infections: diagnosis challenge in a returning traveller with nonspecific febrile illness. New Microbes New Infect 2016;11:7; with permission. CC BY-NC-ND license (http://creativecommons.org/licenses/by-nc-nd/4.0/).)

confirmed in the United States by the CDC and all but 1 case was considered travel related.[14]

Signs and symptoms

The incubation period is 3 to 14 days after the mosquito bite and primary infections can be asymptomatic.[14] Dengue has 3 World Health Organization (WHO) classifications: without warning signs, with warning signs, and severe. Dengue without warning signs includes high fever and possible maculopapular rash (**Fig. 4**), gastrointestinal (GI) symptoms, respiratory symptoms, and bone pain.

Box 1
Supportive care for selected mosquito-borne diseases

- Rest
- Oral hydration to prevent dehydration
- Acetaminophen
- Nonsteroidal anti-inflammatory drugs (NSAIDs)
  - Note: NSAIDs and aspirin should be avoided until dengue has been ruled out
- No interferon, ribavirin, intravenous immunoglobin, or antiviral medications (limited human data, inconsistent results, and potentially harmful effects)

Box 2
How to reduce mosquito exposure and disease spread

- Use mosquito netting sprayed with mosquito repellent
- Use air conditioning or window/door screens
- Use mosquito repellents on exposed skin
- Wear long-sleeved shirts and long pants; consider permethrin-treated clothing
- Empty standing water from outdoor containers
- Support local vector control programs

Dengue with warning signs includes those in the previous sentence with severe abdominal pain, hypothermia, signs of hemorrhage, altered mentation, early signs of shock, including hemoconcentration, ascites, or pleural effusion.[13] Patients with severe dengue present in shock, respiratory distress, and with severe bleeding and organ failure.[15] A summary of nonspecific constitutional symptoms can be found in **Fig. 5**.

Diagnosis

RT-PCR is recommended within 5 days of symptom onset. After 6 days, ELISA for IgM can be done with required confirmation testing due to other flavivirus cross-reactivity.[16] IgG-to-IgM ratios can be used to differentiate between primary and secondary infections.[13]

The differential diagnosis of dengue includes other mosquito-borne diseases, leptospirosis, enterovirus, influenza, rubella, or measles.[16]

Treatment

The treatment of dengue is supportive care (see **Box 1**). Aspirin and nonsteroidal anti-inflammatory drugs should be avoided until dengue hemorrhagic complications have been ruled out. Aggressive fever reduction and pain control are recommended to reduce seizure risk.[16] Infants and children with warning signs or higher risk of severe dengue should be admitted for intravenous fluid therapy and close monitoring for shock.[17]

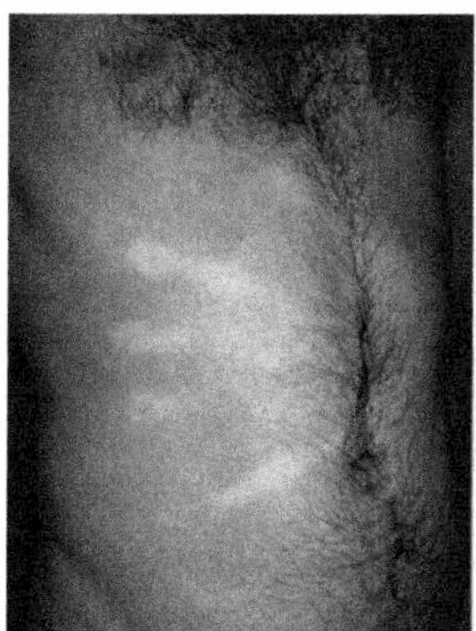
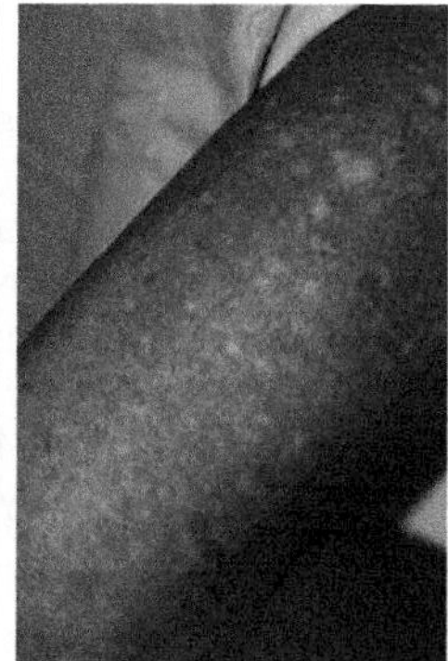
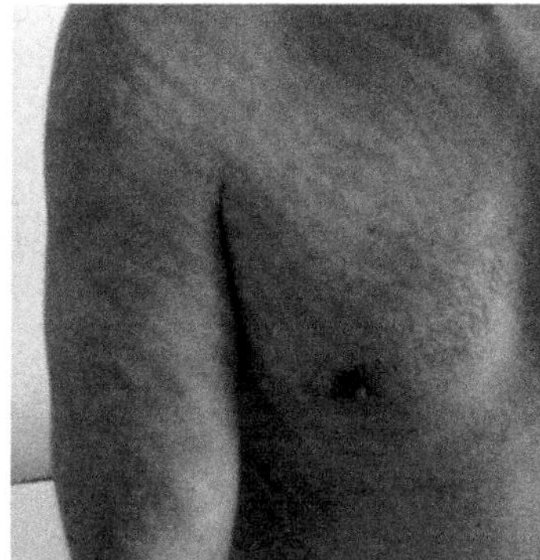

Fig. 4. Arboviral rashes. Left: maculopapular dengue rash; middle: confluent dengue rash ("white islands"); right: chikungunya rash. (*From* Neumayr A, Hatz C, Blum J. Not to be missed! Differential diagnoses of common dermatological problems in returning travellers. Travel Med Infect Dis 2013;11(6):341; with permission.)

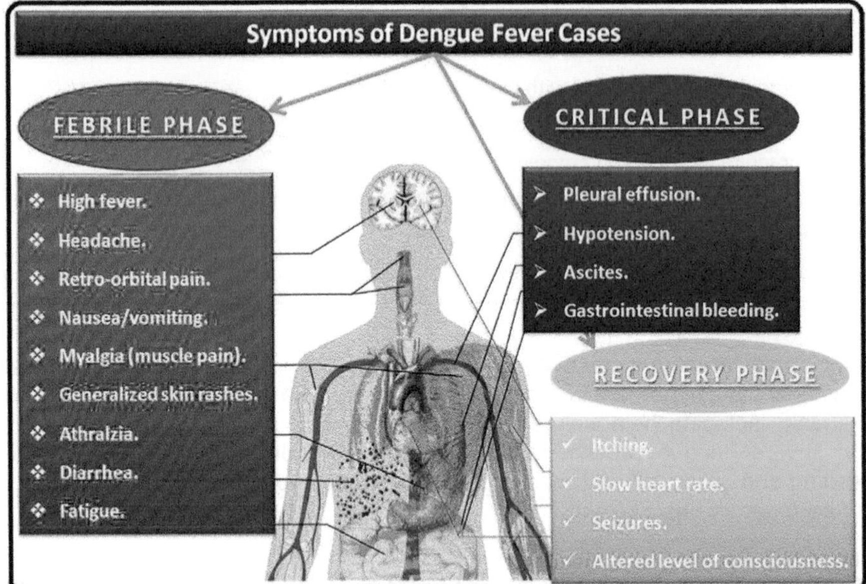

Fig. 5. Dengue nonspecific constitutional symptoms. (*From* Rao MR, Padhy RN, Das MK. Prevalence of dengue viral and malaria parasitic co-infections in an epidemic district, Angul of Odisha, India: an eco-epidemiological and cross-sectional study for the prospective aspects of public health. J Infect Public Health 2016;9(4):423; with permission. CC BY-NC-ND license (http://creativecommons.org/licenses/by-nc-nd/4.0/).)

Prevention and control

Dengvaxia is a live-attenuated vaccine indicated only for previously infected dengue patients 9 years and older living in dengue-endemic areas.[18,19] Individuals should be counseled to reduce risk of mosquito exposure and disease transmission (see **Box 2**).

Japanese Encephalitis

Epidemiology

Japanese encephalitis was first documented in Japan in 1871. It primarily affects children, with more than 68,000 cases occurring with 13,600 to 20,400 deaths annually. Fifty percent of the incidence is in China, with 75% of cases being in children younger than 15 years.[20]

Three billion people live in 24 countries in which the Japanese encephalitis virus (JEV) is endemic. The *Culex tritaeniorhynchus* mosquito is the predominant vector, and most human outbreaks follow outbreaks in farm animals or agricultural rice and flood irrigation.[21] Humans are considered dead-end hosts, as an infected individual's viremia levels are generally not high enough to transmit the infection. Risk factors include spring and fall in temperate climates, and the rainy season in the tropics.

Signs and symptoms

The average incubation period for JEV infection is 5 to 15 days (**Box 3**). JEV infection results in a rapid-onset high fever, headache, and GI symptoms. One in 250 cases develop severe disease with symptoms such as a meningitis, disorientation, seizures, spastic paralysis, parkinsonism syndrome, and coma. Twenty percent to 30% of severe cases result in death and a further 30% to 50% suffer permanent morbidity.[22]

Box 3
Incubation periods in days for selected mosquito-borne diseases

Chikungunya	3–7
Dengue	3–14
Japanese encephalitis	5–15
Malaria	9–40
West Nile	2–14
Yellow fever	3–6
Zika	3–14

Diagnosis

ELISA testing can detect JEV antibodies in serum or cerebrospinal fluid (CSF) within 3 to 8 days of symptom onset. Direct viral detection is not recommended, as the viremia is mild. IgM titers may not be detectable after 10 days but IgG antibody titers may persist for 30 to 90 days.

The differential diagnosis of JEV should include other mosquito-borne diseases and other encephalitis-causing infections (including Eastern equine encephalitis, St. Louis encephalitis, and Western equine encephalitis).[3]

Treatment

The treatment of JEV is supportive (see **Box 1**).

Prevention and control

The WHO recommends the live-attenuated virus vaccination for endemic areas.[23] In the United States, vaccination is recommended for high-risk travelers, including prolonged travel to endemic areas or during transmission season, or rural agricultural exposure. The vaccine has not been tested in pregnant women.[24] Patients should be counseled to prevent mosquito bites (see **Box 2**) and minimize risk associated with animal husbandry and irrigation flooded agriculture.

Malaria

Epidemiology

Malaria is caused by *Plasmodium* parasites (mostly commonly *Plasmodium falciparum* and *Plasmodium vivax*) transmitted by female *Anopheles* mosquitoes most commonly occurring in Africa. Malaria also can be found in Latin America, the Caribbean, Asia, Eastern Europe, and the South Pacific. In 2016, 216 million infections were reported in 91 countries. Children younger than 5 make up 70% of the 445,000 malaria deaths annually.[25] In the United States and its territories in 2013, more than 1700 cases of travel-associated malaria were diagnosed.[26]

Signs and symptoms

Symptoms (fever, headache, chills) can begin anywhere from 1 week to several months after exposure.[27] *P falciparum* can progress to severe anemia, respiratory distress from acidosis, cerebral malaria in children, or affect multiple organs in adults.[28]

Diagnosis

Smear microscopy (**Figs. 6** and **7**) is the gold standard and can help determine species, life cycle, and quantification of parasites; but should be used only if results are immediately available. Rapid diagnostic tests give a binary negative or positive result within 15 minutes and are an accurate alternative when microscopy is unavailable.[27] Follow-up PCR or microscopy confirmation testing with speciation is recommended.[26]

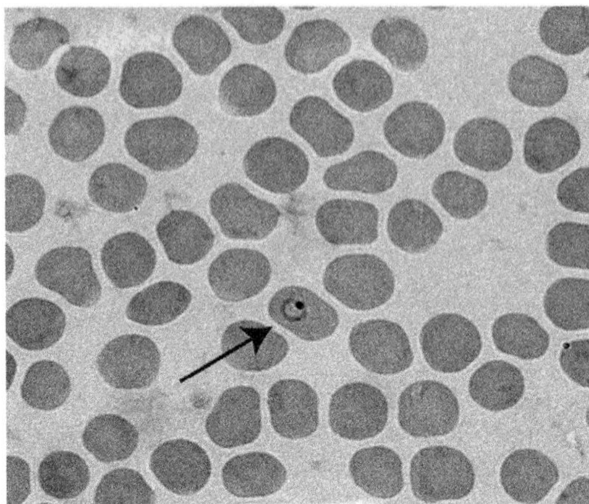

Fig. 6. *Plasmodium falciparum*–infected erythrocytes, scanty ring forms, on initial thick and thin blood films, May Grunwald Giemsa–stained peripheral blood film, ×100 objective. *Arrow* pointing to a scanty ring formation of a Plasmodium falciparum infected erythrocyte. (*From* Smith A, Denholm J, Shortt J, et al. *Plasmodium* species co-infection as a cause of treatment failure. Travel Med Infect Dis 2011;9(6):307; with permission.)

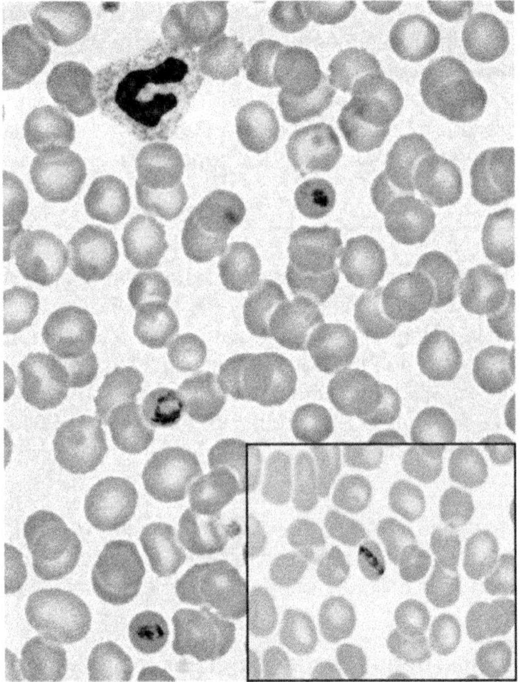

Fig. 7. *Plasmodium malariae* trophozoites and characteristic band form. Inset, detected on thick and thin blood films on second presentation, May Grunwald Giemsa–stained peripheral blood film, ×100 objective. (*From* Smith A, Denholm J, Shortt J, et al. *Plasmodium* species co-infection as a cause of treatment failure. Travel Med Infect Dis 2011;9(6):307; with permission.)

Treatment

WHO recommends artemisinin-based combination therapy for *P falciparum*, which is available in multiple formulations. Treatment regimens vary based on chloroquine resistance. Specific treatment regimens can be found at the CDC Web site.[28] Artemisinin drug resistance is a growing concern in malaria-endemic areas.[25]

Prevention and control

There is no vaccine against malaria. The prevention of malaria is primarily through mosquito bite control (see **Box 2**). Insecticide-treated mosquito nets are the most frequently used preventive tool.[29] Prophylactic antimalarial drugs are recommended for travelers, pregnant women, infants, and children younger than 5 in high-risk areas. Partial immunity to malaria can occur after years of exposure.[25]

West Nile

Epidemiology

West Nile virus (WNV) is single-stranded RNA Flavivirus discovered in Uganda in 1937, with the first case in the United States described in 1999.[30] WNV is normally transmitted from infected or dead birds, with humans being a dead-end host. WNV is now the leading cause of acquired arborviral disease in the United States.[31]

Risk factors

Risk factors include exposure to dead or infected birds, poor sanitation or standing water, and urban environments. The highest seasonal risk appears to be in the late summer or early fall.[31] Elderly patients are at high risk for developing neuroinvasive disease and long-term complications.[32] Although uncommon, human transmission has been reported through bodily fluid (blood, breast milk, conjunctival fluid), in utero, and organ transplantation.[33–36]

History

The average incubation period is approximately 10 days and most WNV-infected patients are asymptomatic.[37] Common symptoms include sudden onset of headache, generalized weakness, fever, and severe muscle or joint pain.[38] A trunk and extremity (sparing palms and soles) maculopapular, nonpruritic rash often occurs after fever resolution.[31] Approximately 40% of WNV-infected patients complain of painful eyes and chorioretinal target lesions and retinal hemorrhages are common.[38,39] Approximately 0.5% of WNV-infected patients develop neuroinvasive disease,[38] including meningitis, encephalitis, or acute flaccid paralysis.[33]

Diagnosis

Initial testing includes serum or CSF for WNV-specific IgM immunoassays. In highly suspected individuals with negative results, repeat testing should be considered. Positive WNV-specific IgM cross-reacts with other Flaviviruses, so confirmatory plaque-reduction neutralization tests (PRNTs) are recommended. CSF, serum, or urine viral RT-PCR tests are highly specific, but not sensitive, as patients have low viremia levels.[40]

Treatment

The treatment of WNV infections is supportive (see **Box 1**) and most patients with WNV infections experience a full recovery. In WNV neuroinvasive disease, recovery is highly variable, with most patients still experiencing some symptoms 6 to 12 months after initial infection. The mortality rate in WNV neuroinvasive disease is approximately 10%.[31]

Yellow Fever

Epidemiology

Yellow fever is an arbovirus transmitted by *Aedes* and *Haemagogus* mosquitoes.[41] It is endemic in 47 countries in Africa and South and Central America. Only 27,467 cases of yellow fever in Africa and 3988 cases in South America were officially diagonised 1985 to 2009, a significant underreporting according to the WHO.[42] African outbreaks, often having rural and urban components, are more widespread.[43] Travel to West Africa poses a 10 times greater risk of yellow fever than travel to South America.[44] Mortality rates, however, are higher in South America (40%–60%) compared with Africa (20%), likely from genetic factors and local immunity patterns.[42,44]

Signs and symptoms

After 3 to 6 days of incubation, patients can be asymptomatic or can have 3 to 4 days of myalgia, fever, headache, nausea, vomiting, and poor appetite. A small percentage then enter a second toxic phase with high fever, abdominal pain with jaundice and bleeding, and a 20% to 50% mortality rate within 7 to 10 days.[43,44]

Diagnosis

Yellow fever is difficult to confirm with testing. Early on, RT-PCR can detect the virus and later ELISA can detect IgM and IgG antibodies. PRNT confirmation (sensitivity 91%–100%, specificity 73%–95%) testing is usually needed.[45]

The differential diagnosis includes dengue, malaria, leptospirosis, poisoning, and other viral hepatitis.[43,44]

Treatment

The treatment for yellow fever is supportive (see **Box 1**).[43]

Prevention and control

In urban areas, mosquito control is important to decrease risk of epidemics (see **Box 2**).[43] The yellow fever vaccine is a live-attenuated vaccine that is recommended for everyone 9 months and older living in or traveling to endemic areas. The WHO currently recommends 1 vaccine dose and the CDC Advisory Committee on Immunization Practices adds a booster dose for patients pregnant during initial dose, those who have had hematopoietic stem transplantation, and patients infected with the human immunodeficiency virus.[46]

Zika Virus

Epidemiology

Zika virus is a Flavivirus first discovered in Uganda in 1952. Recent outbreaks include Micronesia in 2007 and Brazil in 2015.[47] There have been approximately 6000 cases of symptomatic Zika virus reported in the United States from 2015 to 2017.[48]

Risk factors

A Zika-infected mosquito bite is the most common method of transmission. In the United States, traveling to an endemic area represents the highest risk. Other transmission mechanisms include maternal-fetal, sexual transmission, blood transfusions, organ transplantation, and laboratory exposure.[49] Zika virus is commonly isolated from bodily fluids (sweat, saliva, and tears) and close-contact nonsexual transmission has been reported.[50]

Clinical symptoms

Most Zika-infected individuals are asymptomatic. After an incubation period of 3 to 12 days, 20% experience mild and self-limited symptoms, including low-grade fever, pruritic maculopapular rash (including palms and soles), joint pain, and non-purulent conjunctivitis (**Fig. 8**).[51,52] GBS appears to be a rare complication (0.02%) and typically appears approximately 1 week after Zika virus symptoms.[53] Newborns with congenital Zika virus infection have been noted to have severe microcephaly with partially collapsed skull, subcortical calcifications, macular scarring, focal pigmentary retinal mottling, congenital contractures, and hypertonia. The risk of any birth defect from maternal-fetal transmission appears to be approximately 10% to 15%.[54]

Diagnosis

Diagnosis is confirmed through RT-PCR or IgM serology with PRNT confirmation from CSF, serum, or other body fluid. Specific testing algorithms depend on test availability at commercial laboratories or local public health laboratories. Testing of asymptomatic, nonpregnant women is not recommended. All pregnant, symptomatic women and asymptomatic, pregnant women with on-going Zika virus exposure also should be tested. Pregnant women who have fetal findings consistent with congenital Zika virus infection should be tested.[55] Newborns born to a Zika virus–infected mother or newborns with clinical symptoms or prenatal ultrasound concerning for Zika should be tested.[56] The WHO has developed a mobile app that includes a specific section for health care workers (**Fig. 9**).

Management

The treatment of Zika virus infections is supportive (see **Box 1**). Newborns with congenital Zika virus infection will require frequent visits for management of

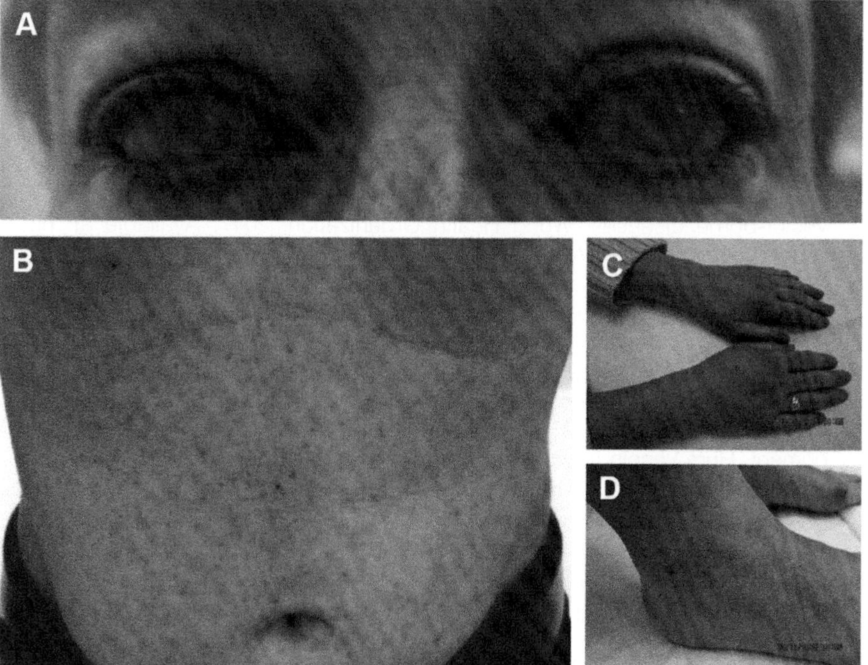

Fig. 8. Clinical features of Zika virus disease: (*A*) conjunctivitis, (*B*) maculopapular rash, (*C, D*) peripheral edema. (*From* Ginier M, Neumayr A, Günther S, et al. Zika without symptoms in returning travellers: what are the implications? Travel Med Infect Dis 2016;14(1):17; with permission.)

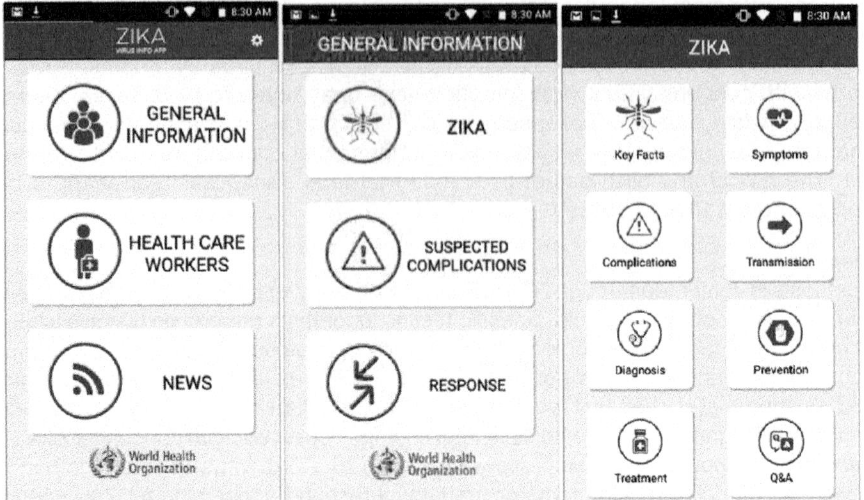

Fig. 9. WHO Zika app. (*From* Chiodini J. ZIKA App - A great resource from the World Health Organization (WHO). Travel Med Infect Dis 2016;14(5):539; with permission.)

complications, including cerebral palsy, visual and hearing loss, feeding difficulties, spasticity, and seizures. The morbidity and mortality of newborns with congenital Zika virus is not known.

Prevention

The focus of prevention is on reducing mosquito bites and transmission (see **Box 2**). To avoid sexual transmission of Zika, it is recommended that infected men wait 6 months before engaging in unprotected intercourse and infected women wait at least 8 weeks before unprotected intercourse.[57]

REFERENCES

1. Vector-borne diseases. World Health Organization; 2017. Available at: http://www.who.int/mediacentre/factsheets/fs387/en/. Accessed February 28, 2018.
2. 2018 National notifiable conditions. National notifiable diseases surveillance system. Centers for Disease Control and Prevention. Available at: http://wwwn.cdc.gov/nndss/conditions/notifiable/2018/. Accessed February 28, 2018.
3. Chikungunya. World Health Organization; 2017. Available at: http://www.who.int/mediacentre/factsheets/fs327/en/. Accessed February 28, 2018.
4. Schwameis M, Buchtele N, Wadowski PP, et al. Chikungunya vaccines in development. Hum Vaccin Immunother 2016;12(3):716–31.
5. Petersen LR, Powers AM. Chikungunya: epidemiology. F1000Res 2016;5 [pii: F1000] Faculty Rev-82.
6. Weaver SC, Lecuit M. Chikungunya virus and the global spread of a mosquito-borne disease. N Engl J Med 2015;372(13):1231–9.
7. Leparc-Goffart I, Nougairede A, Cassadou S, et al. Chikungunya in the Americas. Lancet 2014;383:514.
8. Bloch D. The cost and burden of Chikungunya in the Americas. New Haven (Connecticut): Yale University EliScholar; 2016. Available at: http://elischolar.library.yale.edu/cgi/viewcontent.cgi?article=1021&context=ysphtdl. Accessed February 28, 2018.

9. Lee VJ, Chow A, Zheng X, et al. Simple clinical and laboratory predictors of Chikungunya versus Dengue infections in adults. PLoS Negl Trop Dis 2012;6(9):e1786.
10. Thiberville SD, Moyen N, Dupuis-Maguiraga L, et al. Chikungunya fever: epidemiology, clinical syndrome, pathogenesis and therapy. Antiviral Res 2013;99(3):345–70.
11. Guzman MG, Harris E. Dengue. Lancet 2015;385(9966):453–65.
12. Epidemiology. Dengue. Atlanta (GA): Centers for Disease Control and Prevention; 2014. Available at: http://www.cdc.gov/dengue/epidemiology/. Accessed February 28, 2018.
13. Comprehensive guidelines for prevention and control of Dengue and Dengue Haemorrhagic fever. New Delhi (India): World Health Organization; 2011. Available at: http://apps.searo.who.int/pds_docs/B4751.pdf. Accessed February 28, 2018.
14. Centers for Disease Control and Prevention. Travel-associated Dengue surveillance – United States, 2006-2008. MMWR Morb Mortal Wkly Rep 2010;59(23):715–9.
15. Dengue: guidelines for diagnosis, treatment, prevention and control. Geneva (Switzerland): World Health Organization; 2009. Available at: http://www.who.int/tdr/publications/documents/dengue-diagnosis.pdf?ua=1. Accessed February 28, 2018.
16. Dengue and dengue hemorrhagic fever: information for health care practitioners. Centers for Disease Control and Prevention. Available at: http://www.cdc.gov/dengue/resources/HealthCarePract.pdf. Accessed February 28, 2018.
17. Verhagen LM, de Groot R. Dengue in children. J Infect 2014;69(S1):S77–86.
18. Khetarpal N, Khanna I. Dengue fever: causes, complications, and vaccine strategies. J Immunol Res 2016;2016:6803098.
19. Sanofi updates information on dengue vaccine. Press release. Sanofi Pasteur. Available at: http://mediaroom.sanofi.com/sanofi-updates-information-on-dengue-vaccine/. Accessed February 28, 2018.
20. Campbell G, Hills S, Fischer M, et al. Estimated global incidence of Japanese encephalitis: a systematic review. Bull World Health Organ 2011;89(10):766–74.
21. Yun SI, Lee YM. Japanese encephalitis: the virus and vaccines. Hum Vaccin Immunother 2013;10(2):263–79.
22. Fischer M, Hills S, Staples E, et al. Japanese encephalitis prevention and control: advances, challenges, and new initiatives. In: Scheld WM, Hammer SM, Hughes JM, editors. Emerging Infections 8. 1st edition. Washington, DC: ASM Press; 2008. p. 93–124.
23. Japanese encephalitis. World Health Organization; 2015. Available at: http://www.who.int/mediacentre/factsheets/fs386/en/. Accessed February 28, 2018.
24. Diagnostic testing. Japanese encephalitis. Atlanta (GA): Centers for Disease Control and Prevention; 2015. Available at: http://www.cdc.gov/japaneseencephalitis/healthcareproviders/healthcareproviders-diagnostic.html. Accessed February 28, 2018.
25. World Health Organization. World malaria report 2016. Geneva (Switzerland): World Health Organization; 2016. Available at: http://apps.who.int/iris/bitstream/10665/252038/1/9789241511711-eng.pdf. Accessed February 28, 2018.
26. Arguin PM, Tan KR. Malaria. Infectious diseases related to travel. Atlanta (GA): Centers for Disease Control and Prevention; 2017. Available at: http://wwwnc.cdc.gov/travel/yellowbook/2018/infectious-diseases-related-to-travel/malaria. Accessed February 28, 2018.
27. Abba K, Deeks JJ, Olliaro PL, et al. Rapid diagnostic tests for diagnosing uncomplicated *P. falciparum* malaria in endemic countries. Cochrane Database Syst Rev 2011;(7):CD008122.

28. Guidelines for treatment of Malaria in the United States. Atlanta (GA): Centers for Disease Control and Prevention; 2013. Available at: https://www.cdc.gov/malaria/resources/pdf/treatmenttable.pdf. Accessed February 28, 2018.
29. Gunda R, Chimbari MJ. Cost-effectiveness analysis of malaria interventions using disability adjusted life years: a systematic review. Cost Eff Resour Alloc 2017;15(1):10.
30. Kilpatrick AM. Globalization, land use, and the invasion of West Nile virus. Science 2011;334(6054):323–7.
31. Petersen LR, Brault AC, Nasci RS. West Nile virus: review of the literature. JAMA 2013;310(3):308–15.
32. Lindsey NP, Staples JE, Lehman JA, et al. Surveillance for human West Nile virus disease – United States, 1999-2008. MMWR Surveill Summ 2010;59(2):1–17.
33. Lindsey NP, Lehman JA, Staples JE, et al. West Nile virus and other nationally notifiable arboviral diseases - United States, 2014. MMWR Morb Mortal Wkly Rep 2015;64(34):929–34.
34. Centers of Disease Control and Prevention (CDC). Possible West Nile virus transmission to an infant through breast-feeding–Michigan, 2002. MMWR Morb Mortal Wkly Rep 2002;51(39):877–8.
35. Fonseca K, Prince GD, Bratvold J, et al. West Nile virus infection and conjunctival exposure. Emerg Infect Dis 2005;11(10):1648–9.
36. Paisley JE, Hinckley AF, O'Leary DR, et al. West Nile virus among pregnant women in a northern Colorado community, 2003-2004. Pediatrics 2006;117(3):814–20.
37. Pealer LN, Mafin AA, Petersen LR, et al. Transmission of West Nile virus through blood transfusion in the United States in 2002. N Engl J Med 2003;349(13):1236–45.
38. Zou S, Foster GA, Dodd RY, et al. West Nile fever characteristics among viremic persons identified through blood donor screening. J Infect Dis 2010;202(9):1354–61.
39. Chan CK, Limstrom SA, Tarasewicz DG, et al. Ocular features of West Nile virus infection in North America: a study of 14 eyes. Ophthalmology 2006;1132(9):1539–46.
40. WNV antibody testing. Atlanta (GA): Centers for Disease Control and Prevention; 2015. Available at: http://www.cdc.gov/westnile/healthcareproviders/healthCareProviders-Diagnostic.html. Accessed February 28, 2018.
41. Garske T, Van Kerkhove MD, Yactayo S, et al. Yellow fever in Africa: estimating the burden of disease and impact of mass vaccination from outbreak and serological data. PLoS Med 2014;11(5):e1001638.
42. Monath TP, Vasconcelos PFC. Yellow fever. J Clin Virol 2015;64:160–73.
43. Yellow fever. World Health Organization; 2016. Available at: http://www.who.int/mediacentre/factsheets/fs100/en/. Accessed February 28, 2018.
44. Gershman MD, Staples JE. Yellow fever. Infectious diseases related to travel. Atlanta (GA): Centers for Disease Control and Prevention; 2017. Available at: https://wwwnc.cdc.gov/travel/yellowbook/2018/infectious-diseases-related-to-travel/yellow-fever. Accessed February 28, 2018.
45. Simões M, Camacho LA, Yamamura AM, et al. Evaluation of accuracy and reliability of the plaque reduction neutralization test (micro-PRNT) in detection of yellow fever virus antibodies. Biologicals 2012;40(6):399–404.
46. Staples JE, Bocchini JA Jr, Rubin L, et al. Yellow fever vaccine booster doses: recommendations of the Advisory Committee on Immunization Practices, 2015. MMWR Morb Mortal Wkly Rep 2015;64(23):647–50.
47. Gatherer D, Kohl A. Zika virus: a previously slow pandemic spreads rapidly through the Americas. J Gen Virol 2016;97(2):269–73.

48. Zika cases in the United States. Atlanta (GA): Centers for disease control and prevention; 2017. http://www.cdc.gov/zika/reporting/case-counts.html. Accessed February 28, 2018.
49. Musso D, Gubler DJ. Zika virus. Clin Microbiol Rev 2016;29(3):487–524.
50. Brent C, Dunn A, Savage H, et al. Preliminary findings from an investigation of Zika virus infection in a patient with no known risk factors — Utah, 2016. MMWR Morb Mortal Wkly Rep 2016;65:981–2.
51. Plourde AR, Bloch EM. A literature review of Zika virus. Emerg Infect Dis 2016; 22(7):1185–92.
52. Petersen LR, Jamieson DJ, Power AM, et al. Zika virus. N Engl J Med 2016;374: 1552–63.
53. Cao-Lormeau VM, Blake A, Mons S, et al. Guillain-Barre syndrome outbreak caused by Zika virus infection in French Polynesia. Lancet 2016;387:1531–9.
54. Reynolds MR, Jones AM, Petersen EE, et al. Vital signs: update on Zika virus–associated birth defects and evaluation of all U.S. infants with congenital Zika virus exposure — U.S. Zika Pregnancy Registry, 2016. MMWR Morb Mortal Wkly Rep 2017;66:366–73.
55. Testing guidance. Zika virus. Atlanta (GA): Centers for Disease Control and Prevention; 2018. Available at: http://www.cdc.gov/zika/hc-providers/testing-guidance.html. Accessed February 28, 2018.
56. Adebanjo T, Godfred-Cato S, Viens L, et al. Update: interim guidance for the diagnosis, evaluation, and management of infants with possible congenital Zika virus infection — United States, 2017. MMWR Morb Mortal Wkly Rep 2017;66: 1089–99.
57. Petersen EE, Meaney-Delman D, Neblett-Fanfair R, et al. Update: interim guidance for preconception counseling and prevention of sexual transmission of Zika virus for persons with possible Zika virus exposure — United States, 2016. MMWR Morb Mortal Wkly Rep 2016;65:1077–81.

Mite and Bed Bug Infections

Jason R. Woloski, MD[a,*], Deepa Burman, MD[b],
Olumuyiwa Adebona, MD, MPH[c]

KEYWORDS

• Mite • Bed bug • Scabies • Chiggers • House dust mites • Grain itch

KEY POINTS

- Common mite infections encountered in the primary care office include scabies, chiggers, grain itch, and allergic responses from house dust mites.
- Scabies is one of the 50 most prevalent diseases worldwide, with the mite burrowing under skin, especially interdigital web spaces, causing intensely pruritic, urticated papules.
- House dust mites are a well-known trigger for chronic allergic disease, especially respiratory allergic disease.
- Bed bugs live in dark crevices, such as mattresses, feed at night, and cause a maculopapular immune/allergic skin response in humans.
- Treatment of bed bug bites is largely symptomatic (antihistamines, topical steroids) with the focus being on eradication of the infestation, often requiring skilled exterminators.

INTRODUCTION

Patients with suspected bites or skin rashes regularly present to their primary care physician. For this reason, proper identification of the trigger for the skin reaction is essential to guide treatment and eradication. Mite infections and bed bugs are 2 such groups of organisms commonly encountered. Common mite reactions include scabies, chiggers, grain itch, and allergic responses from dust mites. Bed bugs are also becoming increasingly common with increased global travel, causing an immune mediated allergic skin response in humans.

SCABIES

Scabies is one of the 50 most prevalent diseases worldwide, and as recently as 2010 was estimated to affect more than 100 million people globally.[1,2] It has been

Disclosure Statement: The authors have nothing to disclose.
[a] Family Medicine Residency Program, Geisinger Health System, Geisinger Commonwealth School of Medicine, 1000 East Mountain Drive, Wilkes-Barre, PA 18711, USA; [b] Family Medicine, University of Pittsburgh Medical Center (UPMC) McKeesport, Latterman Family Health Center, UPMC McKeesport Family Medicine Residency, 2347 Fifth Avenue, McKeesport, PA 15132, USA; [c] Family Medicine, Penn Highlands Healthcare, 100 Hospital Avenue, Dubois, PA 15801, USA
* Corresponding author.
E-mail address: jwoloski@geisinger.edu

Prim Care Clin Office Pract 45 (2018) 409–421
https://doi.org/10.1016/j.pop.2018.05.002

recognized as a disease in humans as far back as 3000 years ago and was reported in ancient India, China, and the Middle East.[3] This condition is characterized by pruritus, which can be debilitating in some cases. Unlike in developing countries where the greatest burden of disease rests with the pediatric population, scabies in North America is more evenly distributed across all age groups, including the elderly, with outbreaks often occurring in nursing homes.[3–5]

Scabies is caused by the mite *Sarcoptes scabiei* and occurs as a result of the invasion of the skin by the parasite (**Fig. 1**). The female mite burrows into the epidermis of the skin, where she lays her eggs, with full-grown adult mites subsequently emerging within 2 weeks.[3,6] These adult mites mate and may reinfect the host or another host. The mites are transferred from person to person by prolonged contact, usually after about 20 minutes,[6–8] although fomites, particularly clothing items and beddings, have also been implicated.[3]

Presentation

There is often a 4- to 6-week period between initial contact with the organism and onset of symptoms.[9] Patients typically present with intensely itchy, urticated papules, nodules, and vesicles, which are due to a hypersensitivity reaction to the mites, their saliva, and other products, as well as the direct effect of the mite invasion.[10,11] The lesions are typically located in the interdigital web spaces, around the male genitalia, and the groin, but they may also be found elsewhere on the body.[6,12] The number of mites colonizing a human host is usually between 10 to 20 in classic scabies because the healthy host immune system is able to limit mite numbers.[2,3]

Crusted scabies (also known as Norwegian scabies) is a rare variant of scabies, thought to be associated with an immunosuppressed state and has been reported in patients with HIV as well as those undergoing organ transplantation[2,6,11,13–15] (**Fig. 2**) The colonizing mites may be as many as hundreds and even millions in this case.[3,13] It is highly contagious on account of the large number of mites present in affected individuals, although itching may be a less prominent complaint in up to 50% of cases.[6,11]

The itching in scabies also leads to defects in the integrity of the skin, and as a result, may also be associated with secondary bacterial infections,[4,11] *Staphylococcus*

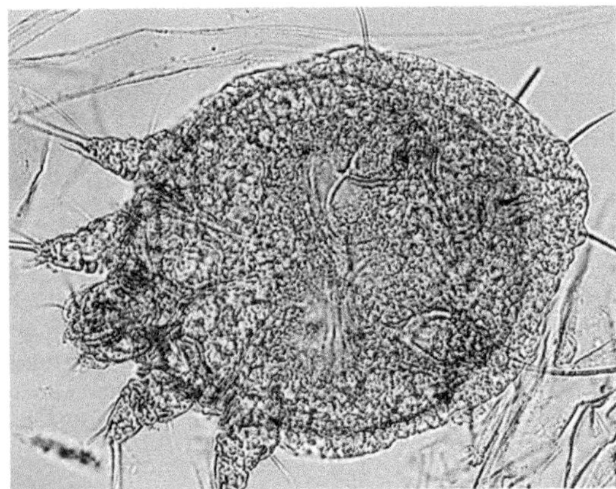

Fig. 1. A *S scabiei* mite obtained from a skin scraping (mineral oil, original magnification ×100). (*From* Jaramillo-Ayerbe F, Berrío-Muñoz J. Ivermectin for crusted Norwegian scabies induced by use of topical steroids. Arch Dermatol 1998;134(2):144; with permission.)

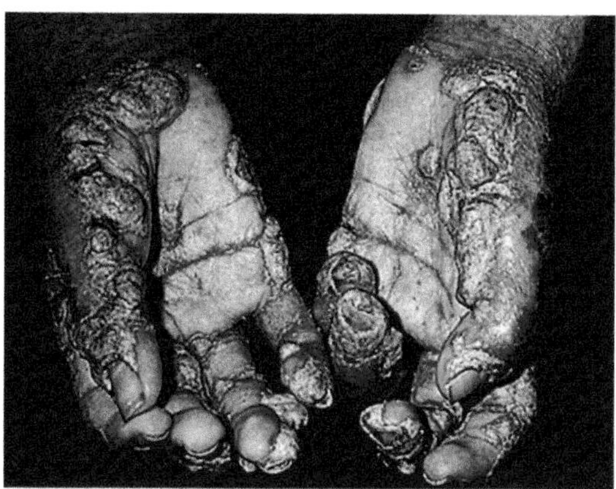

Fig. 2. Crusted Norwegian scabies: prominent hyperkeratotic and fissured plaques and nodules on patient's palms. (*From* Jaramillo-Ayerbe F, Berrío-Muñoz J. Ivermectin for crusted Norwegian scabies induced by use of topical steroids. Arch Dermatol 1998;134(2):144; with permission.)

aureus and *Streptococcus pyogenes* being common culprits. Possible secondary infections include erysipelas and cellulitis. Sequelae of Streptococcal infections, including glomerulonephritis and rheumatic fever, have also been known to occur following the secondary infections.[2,3,7,9]

Diagnosis

The clinical presentation of a history of pruritic rash, typically worse at night, coupled with characteristic lesions present in typical locations is often enough to make the diagnosis.[6,9,16,17] There may be similar symptoms in family members as well. Identification of the characteristic mite burrow on the skin is pathognomic, but these are not easily seen.[6,8,17] Other diagnostic methods include skin scraping and visualization of the mite with microscopy, burrow ink testing, and direct visualization of the skin under magnification.[6,12,17]

Management

Topical permethrin 5% is the first-line treatment of scabies[18] and is applied to the skin (neck to toes) for about 8 to 14 hours, usually overnight, and then washed off.[6,7,12] A repeat of therapy 7 days afterward increases the likelihood of cure because this agent does not kill mite eggs. Other alternatives include topical benzyl benzoate, lindane, malathion, precipitated sulfur, and oral ivermectin.[3,6,9,12] Secondary bacterial infections may also be treated with topical or oral antibiotics, depending on severity.[6] There is, however, a risk of reinfestation without treatment of close contacts and proper care of all clothing. All household members should, therefore, be treated to prevent recurrence of the symptoms.[3,6]

CHIGGERS

Chiggers belong to the Trombiculidae family and are also known as harvest mites.[19,20] The condition "chiggers" specifically describes the larval stage of the organism, which is the only stage in the mite's lifecycle that is responsible for the presenting symptoms.[19]

The adult female lays its eggs in the soil; these eggs hatch within 6 to 12 days. Afterward, the larval form is ready and waits on grass blades for a suitable host to pass. They then attach to the skin and begin migrating toward an appropriate site on the skin for feeding.[19,20] This migration is, however, hindered by constrictions and bands in clothing. Hence, the bites tend to be found in clusters around areas where these constrictions usually are, for example, around the ankles or the waistline.[19–21] In the Northern parts of the United States, transmission may be limited to the spring/summer seasons, but in the South, may be continuous all year round.[22]

Patients typically present with itching, and on physical examination, papules and/or pustules may be found in clusters at areas of tight-fitting sections of clothing as mentioned[20]. These symptoms occur as a result of host response to digestive enzymes introduced by the larvae when feeding.[19,20]

The lesions tend to be self-limiting in most cases, with itching resolving for the most part within 72 hours.[19] In rare cases, the infected individual may develop a hypersensitivity reaction to the organism, characterized by swelling and urticaria with a prolonged duration of symptoms.[19] The summer penile syndrome has been noted in boys who develop a local hypersensitivity reaction to the organism, characterized by penile swelling and pruritus, as well as some dysuria.[23]

Prevention is the mainstay of treatment and can be accomplished by the application of DEET (*N*,*N*-diethyl-meta-toluamide or *N*,*N*-diethyl-3-methylbenzamide) to the skin and clothing.[19,20] Topical permethrin is an alternative that can also be applied to clothing to prevent latching of the larval mites. For patients with lesions, symptomatic relief can be obtained with common topical antipruritics (for example, calamine lotion, menthol) as well as systemic antihistamines.[21] In some cases, steroids may also be required for more severe cases.[19]

GRAIN ITCH

Grain itch is typically seen in agricultural workers who handle straw.[22] Most cases are caused by *Pyemotes ventricosus*, a mite typically found on wheat and other grain-producing plants.[20] Although insects are its usual hosts, the mite readily attach to nearby humans as well.[22,24] Lesions are characterized by intensely pruritic, erythematous wheals with vesicles that may progress to pustules.[24] Patients may also complain of fever, headache, or vomiting.[20,24] Sustained infestation on human hosts is unusual. Topical permethrin can also be used to eliminate the mites from the skin.[20]

MITES AND ALLERGIES

House Dust Mites

House dust mite (HDM) is a major perennial source of allergy. It is a significant cause of allergic rhinitis and allergic asthma. Dust mites (*Dermatophagoides pteronyssinus* and *Dermatophagoides farinae*) are globally ubiquitous arthropods that belong to class Arachnida. They are commonly present in human dwellings and especially abundant in bedding, sofas, carpets, or any woven material. Dust mites do not bite, and aside from causing allergic disease, they are not known to pose other harm to humans. Many mite allergens have been purified, sequenced, and cloned. All species present in the home environment and capable of inducing immunoglobulin E (IgE) mediated sensitization are called domestic mites.[25]

Dust mites absorb humidity[26] from the atmosphere (so higher concentrations are found in damp homes) usually with the aid of fungal degradation. Therefore, in areas that have prolonged cold winters, indoor environments are so dry that they are usually free of dust mites. The prevalence of HDM allergy is linked to exposure to the mite itself primarily by close proximity to dust mite debris during time spent in bed, on the floor, or on upholstered furniture.

Allergenic effects in HDM allergy are thought to be orchestrated through 2 main routes: through the $CD4^+$ TH2 cells that induce and drive the IgE-dependent allergic response and through the innate immune system.[27] The fecal particles contain allergenic dust mite-derived proteins, endotoxin, enzymes, and dust mite and bacterial DNA, all of which can be immunostimulatory.[28] These particles are large and heavy and become transiently airborne after vigorous disturbance, but then settle rapidly, so no allergen is detectable in the air within 15 minutes. As a result, air filtration plays a small role in controlling exposure to dust mite.

Asthma Control and House Dust Mites

HDM allergy is strongly implicated in the pathogenesis of respiratory allergic disease,[29,30] particularly allergic asthma and allergic rhinitis due to sensitization[31,32] to HDM, predominantly the species *D pteronyssinus* and *D farina*.[33–36] The sensitization to HDM in children less than 5 years of age is a significant risk factor for asthma later in childhood.[37,38]

The best outcomes for patients might be achieved by focusing directly on the HDM and its allergens. Identifying HDM allergy as the underlying cause of respiratory allergic disease is an important step in managing clinical control of symptoms as well as potentially preventing disease progression.

Allergen-specific strategies may have a role in altering the progression of respiratory allergic disease and enabling the long-term prevention of asthma in children with HDM allergy.

Treatment for Respiratory Allergic Disease by House Dust Mite Allergy

The 3 therapeutic options that are currently available for respiratory allergic disease caused by HDM allergy are (1) allergen avoidance, (2) pharmacologic intervention, and (3) allergen immunotherapy (AIT). Allergen avoidance and AIT can be implemented only after the identification of the specific underlying allergy.[33]

Allergen avoidance

Successful controlled trials have used combinations of physical measures, including pillow covers, mattress covers, washing bedding in hot water, and carpet removal, rather than chemical treatments. In one study by Murray and colleagues,[39] mite-impermeable encasings reduced acute care attendance, but not steroid use. Compared with adults, the main impact of avoidance may be more in babies with a familial genetic predisposition to asthma because childhood intervention is effective in controlling asthma in atopic children.[40]

Effective avoidance measures include physical barriers, humidity control, and reducing areas that can harbor dust mite colonies. Some other ways to reduce exposure to dust mite allergens include heat treatment, acaricides, and allergen-denaturing agents. **Table 1** shows different measures to avoid allergen exposure.

Because of extensive education needed to acquire successful results from the treatment, many clinicians are not convinced that avoidance should be a primary part of the treatment. Certainly, all mite-allergic patients should be advised that if their wheezing does not improve sufficiently, they should take steps to decrease exposure in the home.

Pharmacotherapy

Pharmacotherapy for rhinitis includes oral or intranasal second-generation antihistamines and nasal corticosteroids, along with other add-on options including oral leukotriene antagonists and antihistamine eye drops. Asthma treatment is a stepwise progression through inhaled corticosteroids, long-acting β2-agonists, leukotriene modifiers, theophylline, and anti-IgE.

Table 1
Measures for house dust mite allergen avoidance

Physical method	Allergen impermeable cover for mattress, pillows, and box springs Weekly washing of bedding with hot/warm water and detergent Replace carpet with polished flooring and area rugs Vacuum weekly with HEPA (high-efficiency particulate air) filtration system
Minimize fabric and upholstery reservoirs	Washable window covers Minimize soft toys No upholstered furniture
Regulation of humidity	Maintain relative humidity <50% Use of dehumidifier in the basement
Heat treatment	Dry heat or steam treatment of carpets
Insecticides and allergen denaturing agents	Benzyl benzoate and tannic acid, but prolonged eradication is not possible

Although strong evidence supports pharmacologic treatment of rhinitis and asthma in general, direct evidence of pharmacologic impact on HDM allergy-related conditions is heterogeneous and weaker.

Allergen immunotherapy

AIT can modify the natural history of respiratory allergic disease. It is safe and effective with lasting effect even after the end of treatment.[41] Developments in immunotherapy are continuing to build on the successful demonstration of the safety and efficacy of both subcutaneous immunotherapy (SCIT) and sublingual immunotherapy (SLIT) in both reducing symptom burden and use of pharmacotherapeutic medication. Both of them require treatment over several years.

SCIT must be given under medical supervision. SLIT has a superior safety profile with lesser risk of anaphylaxis, the advantage of home self-administration, and less time commitment.[42] Recent double-blind placebo-controlled studies on SLIT tablets have shown them to be beneficial for treatment of patients with allergic rhinitis and/or mild to moderate HDM-induced allergic asthma.[43,44]

Accurate diagnosis of the species of dust mite and preferably the allergen group is one of the major limiting factors in the provision of adequate treatment of HDM-related respiratory disease.

BED BUG INFECTIONS

Epidemiology

A rather rapid resurgence of bed bugs has been documented since the mid-1990s.[45,46] A previous renaissance was documented around the time of World War II, infecting upwards of 30% of American homes.[47] Some commonly cited reasons for this most recent reappearance include increased pesticide resistance, increased travel, and insecticide overuse.[46,48] Bed bugs are known to be resilient and adaptable, with reports indicating that bed bugs may have been around dating back to the Ice Age and much of recorded history.[48,49]

Bed bugs belong to the family "Cimicidae," which are exclusively "blood feeding" obligate parasites.[45,46] Hence, humans serve as very suitable hosts for bed bug bites. There are also several documented species of bed bugs, but those most commonly feeding on human hosts include "*Cimex lectularius*" (common bed bug) and "*Cimex hemipterus*" (tropical bed bug).[45,46]

One analogy for the appearance of a bed bug is that of an "apple seed," due to its wingless, flat, oval, darker brown appearance of about 0.5 cm in length.[45,48] Bed bugs are known to have 5 juvenile stages.[50] In a lifespan, a single adult female can produce upwards of several hundred eggs.[46,50] Bed bugs are rather enduring, surviving more than a few months without a blood meal once in the adult stage, thus complicating eradication attempts.[48,50,51]

Precipitating Factors

The word "bed bug" can often produce a visual image of uncleanliness. However, given the ease of domestic and international travel, insects can be found in hotels, luggage, and other tourist destinations. Nevertheless, low-income housing units still remain a popular site for bed beg infestations.[45]

Bed bugs prefer dark locations and feed during the evening, with carbon dioxide and warmth of human hosts serving as an enticing stimulant for the bugs.[46,48,50] For this reason, after feeding bed bugs return to popular locations, including bed frames and the gaps of furniture and walls, as well as other dark crevices such as picture frames and suitcases.[46,49,52] Bed bugs, therefore, frequent highly populated tourist sites, such as hotels, cruise ships, and trains.[51,53]

Although bed bugs are found across all demographics, one study performed in the emergency room setting identified patients presenting with bed bugs to be more likely men, older, and with higher triage emergency severity index scores.[54]

Diagnostic Evaluation

Bed bugs, because of their blood feeding nature, freely predispose humans to bites. Bed bugs feed on humans but fortunately do not live on humans.[50] As a result of the bite, a skin reaction occurs. The saliva introduced by the bed bug during feeding on human hosts results in a skin immune/allergic response to the proteins contained within the saliva.[45,47] During the actual bite/feed, occurring nocturnally, anesthetic and anticoagulant compounds are also released, thus allowing the feeding to go undetected by the human host for several minutes.[46,49] Feeding by bed bugs only takes place for up to 10 minutes every 3 to 5 days.[49]

Because the reaction may be a delayed hypersensitivity type reaction, a skin response may not be seen until the morning after a bite or even a few days later.[45] Several individuals exposed to bed bug bites may not produce a skin reaction from a bite. Although a true incidence of these cases varies due to poor availability of data, it is estimated to be around 20%.[45,49] However, subsequent exposures nearly always produce a skin reaction, which also tends to be more immediate.[45,46]

The appearance of the rash/bite reaction on human skin is the key to the diagnosis of bed bug infections. The rash may also change because of the timing of the bite, ranging from an early small faint red macular appearance to pruritic wheals, papules, or vesicles.[45,46] The "wheal" is often greater than 1 cm and may actually last a few days before subsiding.[45] Similarly, with more extensive exposure, the rash may take on a bullous appearance, similar to erythema multiforme, and even in rare circumstances result in an anaphylaxis reaction.[45,48] There have even been reports of extensive exposure leading to iron deficiency anemia.[48]

The location of the skin rash resulting from bed bugs is typically the exposed areas of the body during sleep, such as the arms, face, neck, legs, and shoulders.[45,46,49] A clinical clue to bed bug bites can be a "linear pattern," although absence of this pattern should not cause a physician to dismiss the possibility of a bed bug bite

(**Figs. 3** and **4**). This linear pattern has often been described as a "breakfast, lunch, and dinner" pattern, where a set of 3 bites occurs in a row.[46,48] In the hands of a skilled provider, dermoscopy may also prove valuable to identifying bed bug bites through identification of maculopapules with a central hemorrhagic punctum.[55]

Differential Diagnosis

Rashes in the primary care setting can be quite challenging because of similar rash appearance and symptoms, including pruritus. Typical differential diagnosis should include other insect bites (mosquitoes, spiders, fleas, lice, ticks, scabies mites), allergic reactions (antibiotics, foods), and varicella infection.[45] The location in unclothed areas, pruritic maculopapular appearance, and accumulation in clusters or lines helps distinguish bed bug bites.[46] In addition, if the rash has been present for several weeks and has not spread (for example, to the trunk), that can also be helpful in the diagnoses. Briefly, some key characteristics of other insect bites include a target rash from tick bites, a predisposition for the feet/ankles from flea bites, and scabies in the interdigital regions.[48]

Disease Transmission

Fortunately, there is no proven evidence that human pathogens can be transmitted by bed bug bites, although it has been suggested that the possibility exists.[45–48,56,57] This hypothesis stems from the fact that ticks, mosquitoes, and other blood-feeding arthropods have this capability.[58] For this reason, research is continuing, particularly relating to arboviruses and bed bugs.[58] Although no proven transmission exists, the bed bugs themselves have been known to be infected with human pathogens and capable of carrying more than 40 microorganisms.[49,56]

Treatment

Based on the notion that bed bugs are not vectors for human disease, most of the treatment is focused on symptomatic care, followed by attention to the eradication of the bed bug infestation. Commonly used therapies include antihistamines and topical corticosteroids, with systemic corticosteroids being reserved for more blistering infections.[45,48] However, even without treatment, as long as no subsequent exposures occur, the skin reaction will likely resolve in one to 2 weeks.[46–48]

Bed bug bites triggering asthmatic reactions are also documented.[45] Therefore, primary care physicians should perform a comprehensive physical examination, so that

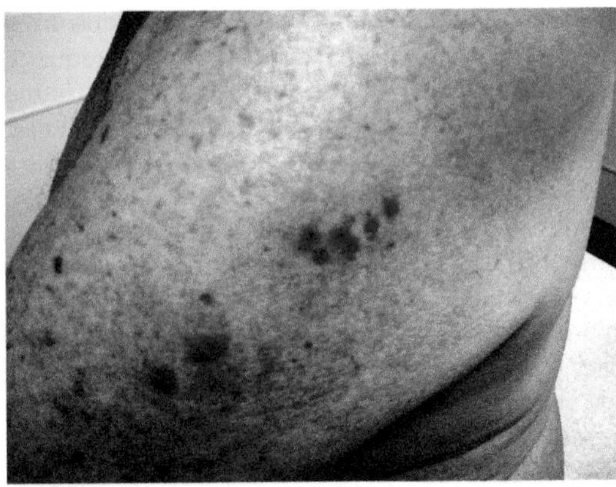

Fig. 3. Bed bug bites. (Copyright © Thomas Jefferson University.)

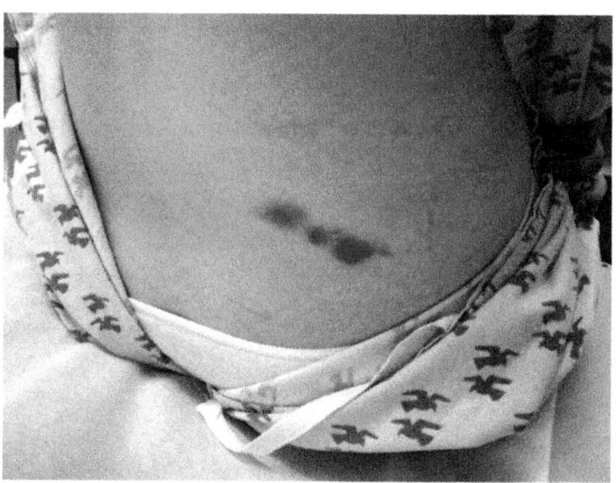

Fig. 4. Bed bug bites. (Copyright © Thomas Jefferson University.)

possible more subtle findings, for example, mild wheezing, are not missed. Similarly, the pruritic nature of bed bug bites can often lead to secondary skin infections from host scratching, such as impetigo and cellulitis, as well as scarring.[46,48]

Primary care physician also have the unique skill of attention to the biopsychosocial model of care. Not surprisingly, the diagnosis of bed bugs can often lead to emotional distress by patients, so attention to a patient's psychological well-being is also paramount. It has been suggested that individuals exposed to bed bugs may be prone to insomnia, nightmares, fear, panic, and even posttraumatic stress disorder.[59] Discussion of the widespread nature of bed bugs, and focusing the discussion on "how do we solve this," can help patients cope with the diagnosis. With increased knowledge regarding transmission, it is hoped that the stigma associated with bed bug diagnoses will be curtailed.

Infestation Identification and Eradication

Identifying the specific location of the infestation can often be the most challenging task during eradication. Not surprisingly, infestation along mattress beading is a popular site for bed bugs.[45,47] Adult bed bugs can often be seen with the naked eye.[47] However, if visual inspection does not reveal any insects, looking for "dark spotting," that is, evidence of bed bug fecal deposition, can be helpful.[45] Similarly, bedding should be examined for any reddish blood stains or a sweet smell from emitted oils by the bed bugs.[21,48] Using white-colored linens and a magnifying glass can help.[46,47] Quickly shining a light before dawn, when they are actively looking for a feed, can also assist with visualization of live bed bugs searching for food.[46,48] Clinicians should also take a careful history to identify possible sources of infection, such as recent travel, new furniture, recent visitors.[48]

Bed bugs can easily migrate, through crawling or passively on inanimate objects, to other locations, even via ventilation ducts and electric wiring.[46,50,51] Therefore, by the time a central infestation is located, secondary locations may have begun to take hold. Fortunately, no travel by bed bugs directly on humans has been discovered.[46]

Because of increasing insecticide resistance, trained pest control professionals are often needed when an infestation is suspected.[45] A multistage treatment method should focus not only on pesticide delivery, but also on removal of clutter and old furniture, sealing of crevices, vacuuming, plastic mattress and pillow covers, and even novel bed bug trapping devices.[46,48] Canine detection of bed bugs is another commonly used method by exterminators.[46]

Because of their ability to survive at a wide temperature range, if items are nonwashable, it has been suggested that they undergo heat treatment of at least 120°F for at least 2 hours or cold treatment of at least 23°F or lower for 5 days.[46]

Following the multifaceted eradication approach, follow-up inspections should also be completed within a few weeks in case all the eggs were not removed and subsequently hatched.[49]

Health Care Setting Bed Bug Infections

Health care settings, by nature of the many visitors and patients seen on a daily basis, are also vulnerable to bed bug infestations. There is also likely underreporting by health care institutions.[50] For this reason, training hospital personnel regarding the recognition of bed bugs and bites is important.[50] Some hospitals have developed formalized "Bedbug Procedures," which may involve inspection and collection of bugs for confirmation by microbiology and blocking a room for 72 hours following extermination.[53]

Prevention

Improving sanitation, particularly in high-traffic living quarters, along with improved pest control strategies can improve the control of bed bug populations. However, as mentioned, the difficultly lies in the increasing resistance of bed bugs to pesticides and intercontinental travel. Thus, an attempt at avoidance, for example, through cautious inspection of bedding, luggage, and furniture, particularly for frequent travelers, is an important strategy.[46] There are some data to support possible deterring of bites through application of oil of lemon eucalyptus orDEET.[46] Implementation of routine inspections in high prevalence areas, such as low-income apartments, can also be useful given the high percentage of residents often unaware of infestation.[60] Last, increasing public health education is needed because of the documented meager level of knowledge regarding bed bugs in the public and the economic impact associated with pest control.[52,61]

REFERENCES

1. Hay RJ, Johns NE, Williams HC, et al. The global burden of skin disease in 2010: an analysis of the prevalence and impact of skin conditions. J Invest Dermatol 2014;134(6):1527–34.
2. Fischer K, Walton S. Parasitic mites of medical and veterinary importance–is there a common research agenda? Int J Parasitol 2014;44(12):955–67.
3. Thomas J, Christenson JK, Walker E, et al. Scabies-An ancient itch that is still rampant today. J Clin Pharm Ther 2017;42(6):793–9.
4. Karimkhani C, Colombara DV, Drucker AM, et al. The global burden of scabies: a cross- sectional analysis from the Global Burden of Disease Study 2015. Lancet Infect Dis 2017;17(12):1247–54.
5. Scheinfeld N. Controlling scabies in institutional settings: a review of medications, treatment models, and implementation. Am J Clin Dermatol 2004;5(1):31–7.
6. Banerji A. Scabies. Paediatr Child Health 2015;20(7):395–402.
7. Hay RJ, Steer AC, Engelman D, et al. Scabies in the developing world–its prevalence, complications, and management. Clin Microbiol Infect 2012;18(4): 313–23.
8. Gunning K, Pippitt K, Kiraly B, et al. Pediculosis and scabies: treatment update. Am Fam Physician 2012;86(6):535–41.

9. Hardy M, Engelman D, Steer A. Scabies: a clinical update. Aust Fam Physician 2017;46(5):264–8.
10. Chosidow O, Fuller LC. Scratching the itch: is scabies a truly neglected disease? Lancet Infect Dis 2017;17(12):1220–1.
11. Bhat SA, Mounsey KE, Liu X, et al. Host immune responses to the itch mite, Sarcoptes scabiei, in humans. Parasit Vectors 2017;10(1):385.
12. Anderson KL, Strowd LC. Epidemiology, diagnosis, and treatment of scabies in a dermatology office. J Am Board Fam Med 2017;30(1):78–84.
13. Elosua-González M, García-Zamora E. Crusted Scabies. N Engl J Med 2017; 377(5):476.
14. Hulbert TV, Larsen RA. Hyperkeratotic (Norwegian) scabies with gram-negative bacteremia as the initial presentation of AIDS. Clin Infect Dis 1992;14(5):1164–5.
15. Tirado-Sanchez A, Bonifaz A, Montes de Oca-Sanchez G, et al. Crusted scabies in HIV/AIDS infected patients. Report of 15 cases. Rev Med Inst Mex Seguro Soc 2016;54(3):397–400 [in Spanish].
16. Schmidt-Guerre AR, Aranda-Hulin B, Maumy-Bertrand M, et al. Diagnosis and treatment of scabies by general practitioners: a survey of practices in France. Ann Dermatol Venereol 2017;145(2):89–94 [in French].
17. Thompson MJ, Engelman D, Gholam K, et al. Systematic review of the diagnosis of scabies in therapeutic trials. Clin Exp Dermatol 2017;42(5):481–7.
18. Workowski KA, Bolan GA. Sexually transmitted diseases treatment guidelines, 2015. MMWR Recomm Rep 2015;64(3):102–3.
19. Hohenberger ME, Elston DM. What's eating you? Chiggers. Cutis 2017;99:386–8.
20. Ken KM, Shockman SC, Sirichotiratana M, et al. Dermatoses associated with mites other than Sarcoptes. Semin Cutan Med Surg 2014;33(3):110–5.
21. Juckett G. Arthropod bites. Am Fam Physician 2013;88(12):841–7.
22. Goddard J. Physician's guide to arthropods of medical importance. 6th edition. Boca Raton (FL): CRC press, Taylor and Francis Group; 2013.
23. Smith GA, Sharma V, Knapp JF, et al. The summer penile syndrome: seasonal acute hypersensitivity reaction caused by chigger bites on the penis. Pediatr Emerg Care 1998;14(2):116–8.
24. Booth BH, Jones RW. Epidemiological and clinical study of grain itch. J Am Med Assoc 1952;150(16):1575–9.
25. Platts-mills T, Vervloet D, Thomas W, et al. Indoor allergens and asthma:report of the third international workshop. J Allergy Clin Immunol 1997;100(6):S2–24.
26. Simpson A, Simpson B, Custovic A, et al. Household characteristics and mite allergen levels in Manchester, UK. Clin Exp Allergy 2002;32(10):1413–9.
27. Wang J-Y. The innate immune response in house dust mite-induced allergic inflammation. Allergy Asthma Immunol Res 2013;5(2):68.
28. Ghaemmaghami AM, Robins A, Gough L, et al. Human T cell subset commitment determined by the intrinsic property of antigen: the proteolytic activity of the major mite allergen Der p 1 conditions T cells to produce more IL-4 and less IFN-γ. Eur J Immunol 2001;31(4):1211–6.
29. Blomme K, Tomassen P, Lapeere H, et al. Prevalence of allergic sensitization versus allergic rhinitis symptoms in an unselected population. Int Arch Allergy Immunol 2013;160(2):200–7.
30. Arshad SH. Does exposure to indoor allergens contribute to the development of asthma and allergy? Curr Allergy Asthma Rep 2009;10(1):49–55.
31. Shaaban R, Zureik M, Soussan D, et al. Rhinitis and onset of asthma: a longitudinal population-based study. Lancet 2008;372(9643):1049–57.

32. Masoli M, Fabian D, Holt S, et al. The global burden of asthma: executive summary of the GINA dissemination committee report. Allergy 2004;59(5):469–78.
33. Calderón MA, Linneberg A, Kleine-Tebbe J, et al. Respiratory allergy caused by house dust mites: what do we really know? J Allergy Clin Immunol 2015;136(1): 38–48.
34. Andiappan AK, Puan KJ, Lee B, et al. Allergic airway diseases in a tropical urban environment are driven by dominant mono-specific sensitization against house dust mites. Allergy 2014;69(4):501–9.
35. Biagtan M, Viswanathan R, Bush RK. Immunotherapy for house dust mite sensitivity: where are the knowledge gaps? Curr Allergy Asthma Rep 2014;14(12):482.
36. Gandhi VD, Davidson C, Asaduzzaman M, et al. House dust mite interactions with airway epithelium: role in allergic airway inflammation. Curr Allergy Asthma Rep 2013;13(3):262–70.
37. Holt PG, Rowe J, Kusel M, et al. Toward improved prediction of risk for atopy and asthma among preschoolers: a prospective cohort study. J Allergy Clin Immunol 2010;125(3):653–659 e7.
38. Lodge CJ, Lowe AJ, Gurrin LC, et al. House dust mite sensitization in toddlers predicts current wheeze at age 12 years. J Allergy Clin Immunol 2011;128(4): 782–788 e9.
39. Murray CS, Foden P, Sumner H, et al. Preventing Severe Asthma Exacerbations in Children. A Randomized Trial of Mite-Impermeable Bedcovers. Am J Respir Crit Care Med 2017;196:150–8.
40. Toelle BG, Ng KKW, Crisafulli D, et al. Eight-year outcomes of the childhood asthma prevention study. J Allergy Clin Immunol 2010;126(2):388–389 e3.
41. Pawankar R, Bunnag C, Khaltaev N, et al. Allergic rhinitis and its impact on Asthma in Asia Pacific and the ARIA Update 2008. World Allergy Organ J 2012;5(S3):S212–7.
42. Cox L, Compalati E, Kundig T, et al. New directions in immunotherapy. Curr Allergy Asthma Rep 2013;13(2):178–95.
43. Calderón MA, Kleine-Tebbe J, Linneberg A, et al. House dust mite respiratory allergy: an overview of current therapeutic strategies. J Allergy Clin Immunol Pract 2015;3(6):843–55.
44. Moingeon P. Progress in the development of specific immunotherapies for house dust mite allergies. Expert Rev Vaccines 2014;13(12):1463–73.
45. Doggett SL, Russell R. Bed bugs - what the GP needs to know. Aust Fam Physician 2009;38(11):880–4.
46. Studdiford JS, Conniff KM, Trayes KP, et al. Bedbug infestation. Am Fam Physician 2012;86(7):653–8.
47. Shmidt E, Levitt J. Dermatologic infestations. Int J Dermatol 2012;51(2):131–41.
48. McMenaman KS, Gausche-Hill M. Cimex lectularius ("Bed Bugs"): recognition, management, and eradication. Pediatr Emerg Care 2016;32(11):801–6.
49. Kolb A, Needham GR, Neyman KM, et al. Bedbugs. Dermatol Ther 2009;22(4): 347–52.
50. Munoz-Price LS, Safdar N, Beier JC, et al. Bed bugs in healthcare settings. Infect Control Hosp Epidemiol 2012;33(11):1137–42.
51. Bernardeschi C, Le Cleach L, Delaunay P, et al. Bed bug infestation [review]. BMJ 2013;346:f138.
52. Heukelbach J, Hengge UR. Bed bugs, leeches and hookworm larvae in the skin. Clin Dermatol 2009;27(3):285–90.
53. Hurst S, Humphreys M. Bedbugs: not back by popular demand. Dimens Crit Care Nurs 2011;30(2):94–6.

54. Sheele JM, Gaines S, Maurer N, et al. A survey of patients with bed bugs in the emergency department. Am J Emerg Med 2017;35:697–8.
55. Shirato T, Iwata H, Yoshimoto N, et al. Dermoscopy is useful for bed bug (Cimex lectularius) bites. J Eur Acad Dermatol Venereol 2016;30:539–40.
56. Delaunay P, Blanc V, Del Giudice P, et al. Bedbugs and infectious diseases. Clin Infect Dis 2011;52(2):200–10.
57. Ho D, Lai O, Glick S, et al. Lack of evidence that bedbugs transmit pathogens to humans. J Am Acad Dermatol 2016;74(6):1261.
58. Adelman ZN, Miller DM, Myles KM. Bed bugs and infectious disease: a case for the arboviruses. PLoS Pathog 2013;9(8):e1003462.
59. Ashcroft R, Seko Y, Chan LF, et al. The mental health impact of bed bug infestations: a scoping review. Int J Public Health 2015;60(7):827–37.
60. Wang C, Singh N, Zha C, et al. Bed bugs: prevalence in low-income communities, resident's reactions, and implementation of a low-cost inspection protocol. J Med Entomol 2016;53(3):639–46.
61. Kaylor MB, Wenning P, Eddy C. Prevalence, knowledge, and concern about bed bugs. J Environ Health 2015;78(1):20–4.

Pertussis: The Whooping Cough

Van Tuong Ngoc Nguyen, DO*, Lauren Simon, MD, MPH

KEYWORDS

- Bordetella pertussis • Whooping cough • Tdap and DTaP vaccine
- Paroxysmal cough

KEY POINTS

- Pertussis is characterized by 3 stages: catarrhal, paroxysmal, convalescent.
- Pertussis vaccine or infection does not confer lifelong immunity and thus requires booster immunizations.
- Infants are the most susceptible to infection and have the highest morbidity and mortality from pertussis.
- The prevalence of pertussis is likely higher than suspected due to its nonspecific presentation, but is still a cause of significant morbidity including missed work.

INTRODUCTION

Before the advent of the pertussis vaccine in the 1940s, there were up to 266,000 reported cases of pertussis in the United States. In the 1980s, the number of reported cases reached its nadir, dipping to just more than 1000 reported cases.[1] Unfortunately, in the past decade, the number of reported cases has risen to 20,000 to 40,000 confirmed and presumed cases a year.[1] Overall, the incidence of pertussis has decreased more than 80% with introduction of this vaccine (**Fig. 1**).[1] However, this number is likely underestimated, as these incident rates are dependent on clinician recognition and report of the disease. The long duration of the disease, possibly spanning months, can make the prevalence of pertussis difficult to track.[2]

It is spread via infectious droplets and is extremely contagious. Due to its highly infectious nature, most patients will be required to abstain from work for 5 to 7 days after starting antimicrobial treatment, resulting in significant personal and economic morbidity. On average, however, adults missed 9.8 days of work. Adolescents, on the other hand, missed 5.5 days from school. Thirty-eight percent of adolescents were still coughing 106 days after cough onset and adults 94 days after.[3]

Disclosure Statement: The authors have nothing to disclose.
Department of Family Medicine, Loma Linda University, 1200 California Street, Suite 240, Redlands, CA 92374, USA
* Corresponding author.
E-mail address: vatnguyen@llu.edu

Prim Care Clin Office Pract 45 (2018) 423–431
https://doi.org/10.1016/j.pop.2018.05.003

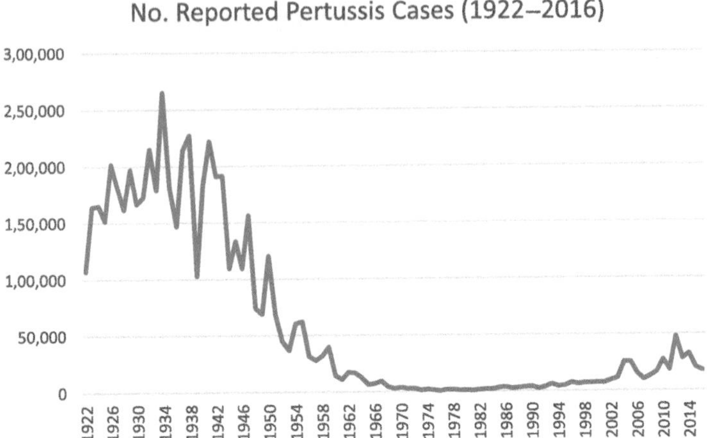

Fig. 1. Number of reported pertussis cases to CDC. (*Data from* Centers for Disease Control and Prevention. Pertussis cases by year (1922–2015). Available at: https://www.cdc.gov/pertussis/surv-reporting/cases-by-year.html. Accessed February 11, 2018.)

BACKGROUND AND PATHOPHYSIOLOGY

Pertussis, also known as whooping cough and the 100-day cough, is an infection caused by the bacterium, *Bordetella pertussis*.[1] *B pertussis* is a gram-negative bacterium that requires special media for isolation. It produces various toxins and multiple antigens that attacks respiratory cells, causing inflammation and paralysis of cilia.[1] It is these various antigens that contribute to the different stages of pertussis.[1] Recent research has detected the bacterium in alveolar macrophages. This interferes with pulmonary secretion clearance and is the basis of the clinical symptoms.[1]

It is spread via infectious droplets and is extremely contagious, infecting approximately 80% of household contacts in one identified case.[1] There is no temporal, seasonal pattern associated with pertussis, but it does have a slight increase in incidence in the summer and fall.[1]

Before the introduction of the pertussis vaccine, children were naturally susceptible to the infection. Childhood infection would confer immunity to adolescents and adults. The transmission of maternal antibodies would provide natural immunity to neonates until these antibodies waned. As the infants aged, they would become susceptible to pertussis infection. In contrast, during this postvaccination time, children are immune to pertussis after childhood vaccinations but will then develop waning vaccine immunity as they get older. Thus, adolescents and adults are susceptible to pertussis infection and can transmit it to infants.[4]

The pertussis vaccine is 95% effective initially and then reduces to 42% efficacy after 5 years.[5] Other observational studies note that the pertussis vaccine confers immunity for 4 to 20 years, but not lifelong. Local reactions to the vaccine (redness, swelling, pain at injection site) was more common in those patients receiving whole-cell DTP (diphtheria, tetanus, pertussis) vaccines. Due to the frequency of these local reactions, a more purified, acellular, vaccine was created. Acellular vaccines have fewer side effects.[6] Only the acellular vaccine is available in the United States.[1,7] The vaccine contains inactivated components of *B pertussis*. It is combined with diphtheria and tetanus toxoids and is approved for administration to infants as young as 6 weeks old.[1] In a study of 1391 persons, 195 adverse reactions were reported, ranging from

5 deaths to 145 hospitalizations; none of these were deemed attributable to the vaccine. No neonatal abnormalities were noted in 60 pregnant patients.[8]

If possible, the same brand of vaccine should be used, but there are no data that suggest mixed administration can cause decreased immunogenicity. Completing the series is the most important, but there is no need to restart the series if there is a missed dose.[1] If a patient has had pertussis, this does not confer lifelong immunity and the patient should still receive the *B pertussis* vaccine when indicated.[1,9]

CLINICAL PRESENTATION

The presentation of pertussis can vary according age and immunization status.[4,10] The clinical presentation of pertussis can vary between the immunized and nonimmunized patient.[11]

In the immunized patient, pertussis can be a milder disease, ranging from asymptomatic to paroxysmal cough for 1 to 2 weeks.[1] Immunized patients may present with only a prolonged cough that does not have the characteristic "whoop."[11] These patients may have more pharyngeal symptoms and episodes of sweating.[11,12] Although a milder disease process may occur when the patient has been immunized, these patients are often identified as the first case in transmitting the infection to more susceptible people, including the nonimmunized and infants.[1]

In the nonimmunized patient, the presentation of pertussis can be divided into 3 stages: catarrhal, paroxysmal, and convalescent stages.

The catarrhal, first stage of pertussis presents with nonspecific symptoms, such as coryza, conjunctival irritation, and a slight cough. This also may be accompanied by a low-grade fever, but it is not a prominent symptom of this illness. Unfortunately, all of these symptoms are similar to those of the common cold.

Approximately 7 to 10 days later, in the nonimmunized patient, the paroxysmal stage begins with the classic paroxysms of cough, with or without the inspiratory "whoop." These paroxysms can cause the patient to become cyanotic and is often followed by vomiting. This cycle of paroxysmal coughing and vomiting leads to exhaustion and can be particularly distressing to patients. These paroxysms are more frequent at night and is usually the symptom that leads to even the consideration of pertussis on the differential diagnosis.[1] This stage can last up to 10 weeks, with symptoms peaking 2 to 3 weeks into the stage.[1]

The convalescent stage is marked by slow and gradual resolution of these paroxysms. The paroxysms tend to resolve within 2 to 3 weeks, but can recur with subsequent infections, regardless of etiology of the upper respiratory infection. This cough is more similar to that noted in other upper respiratory infections.[1] These patients are still infectious, even in this late stage.

DIAGNOSIS

The goal of diagnosing pertussis in the clinical setting is to expedite its correct diagnosis to ensure appropriate treatment and prevent transmission. With this in mind, the Centers for Disease Control and Prevention (CDC) National Notifiable Diseases Surveillance System uses a standardized case definition for reporting of suspected cases of pertussis:

Paroxysms of coughing, or
Inspiratory "whoop," or
Post-tussive vomiting, or
Apnea, with or without cyanosis, in infants 0 to 12 months of age.

Although laboratory evaluation is typically not done unless hospitalized, in severe cases, laboratories may show an elevated white blood cell count, often greater than 20,000. This lymphocytosis may be absent in those with milder cases.[1]

In the public health setting, the goal is to correctly identify and report true cases to avoid unnecessary public health interventions. Although culturing *B pertussis* is still the gold standard, it also can be isolated from sputum and confirmed via polymerase chain reaction (PCR) or serology.[1] Culture is more specific and best done in the first 2 weeks of the cough, whereas PCR is more sensitive and best done within 4 weeks of the cough.[1] Serology is best used for confirming the diagnosis of pertussis in its later stages, up to 8 weeks after cough onset but up to 12 weeks. Cultures can take up to 2 weeks to be positive in only 30% to 50% of all cases.[1] Untreated and unvaccinated infants can remain culture-positive for more than 6 weeks.

TREATMENT

The mainstay of clinical treatment of pertussis is early treatment. Treatment with antibiotics during the first 1 to 2 weeks, before coughing paroxysms occur, is specifically with macrolide antibiotics, such as azithromycin, clarithromycin, or erythromycin. Administered early, appropriate antibiotic treatment of pertussis can reduce the duration and severity of symptoms and reduce its communicability.[4]

Before choosing a specific antibiotic for pertussis treatment, the clinician must consider the potential for adverse events, drug interactions, cost, ease of use, and tolerability of the selected antibiotic. Consideration of the risk for adverse events is particularly important with use of macrolide antibiotics because they have a black box warning for their association with QT interval prolongation.[13] Specifically, in March 2013, the US Food and Drug Administration issued a warning that azithromycin may cause electrical activity changes leading to potentially fatal cardiac arrhythmias. Azithromycin should thus be avoided in patients with known prolonged QT interval, history of torsades de pointes, bradyarrhythmias, or uncompensated heart failure. Caution should be taken with patients who have increased risk for cardiac arrhythmia, such as electrolyte imbalance and chronic antiarrhythmic medication use.[14]

It is important to use the macrolide antibiotics early in treatment of pertussis within the first 2 weeks of infection before the onset of the coughing/paroxysmal phase for them to be effective in the illness. For patients older than 1 year, treatment should occur within 3 weeks of the cough's onset. Infants younger than 1 year and pregnant patients should be treated within 6 weeks of the cough's onset.

The CDC guideline recommends azithromycin, clarithromycin, or erythromycin for 5, 7, or 14 days, respectively. Azithromycin and clarithromycin are better tolerated than erythromycin. Azithromycin is the preferred agent because clarithromycin and erythromycin are cytochrome P450 enzyme inhibitors and can have many drug interactions. If macrolide antibiotic use is contraindicated, a 14-day course of trimethoprim-sulfamethoxazole (TMP-SMX) may be substituted as an alternative in patients older than 2 months.[15] TMP-SMX is contraindicated in patients younger than 2 months due to its increased risk of kernicterus. Some trials have shown that short versus long-term antibiotics have similar clinical outcomes.[16]

For infants younger than 1 month, only the macrolide azithromycin (dose 10 mg/kg per day for 5 days) is preferred because it has not been associated with infantile hypertrophic pyloric stenosis. TMP-SMZ is contraindicated in those younger than 2 months because of risk for kernicterus.

For infants age 1 to 5 months, prescribe azithromycin 10 mg/kg in a single daily dose for 5 days or clarithromycin 15 mg/kg in 2 divided dosages daily for 7 days or erythromycin 40 to 50 mg/kg per day divided in 4 dosages for 14 days. If age 2 months or older and allergic to macrolides, alternatively use TMP-SMZ (TMP 8 mg/kg per day and SMZ 40 mg/kg per day each in 2 divided doses) for 14 days.

The dosage for infants 6 months or older and children is azithromycin 10 mg/kg in a single dose day 1 followed by 5 mg/kg per day (maximum 500 mg) on days 2 to 5, or clarithromycin 15 mg/kg per day in 2 divided doses (maximum 1 g per day) for 7 days, or erythromycin 40 to 50 mg/kg per day (maximum 2 g/d) in 4 divided doses (6 hours apart) for 14 days. For TMP-SMZ, the dosage is TMP 8 mg/kg per day with SMZ 40 mg/kg per day in 2 divided doses for 14 days.

The dosage for adults is azithromycin 500 mg single on day 1 followed by 250 mg on days 2 to 5, or clarithromycin 1 g divided twice daily for 7 days, or erythromycin 2 g/d in 4 divided doses (6 hours apart) for 14 days. Alternatively, if macrolide allergy or intolerance, can use TMP 320 mg and SMZ1600 mg per day in 2 divided doses for 14 days.

Antibiotics are the mainstay of pertussis treatment. Symptomatic treatment of the cough associated with pertussis has not been very effective in trials. Pertussis immunoglobulin reduces the number of whoops in a day by 3 on average. Diphenhydramine and beta-agonist did not change the number of coughing paroxysms in a day. Dexamethasone did not decrease hospital length of stay.[17]

PROGNOSIS

Factors that can reduce the severity of *B pertussis* infection include having some residual immunity to a prior pertussis infection or vaccination and use of macrolide antimicrobial in the early catarrhal phase of pertussis illness.[4] The immune response to 1 or more antigenic or biologically active products of pertussis induces immunity, but it is not lifelong.

Infants and those with untreated pertussis remain infectious for more than 6 weeks. The infectious period is reduced to approximately 21 days in older children and adults with history of prior immunization or infection.[18] Patients treated early in the infection, however, remain infectious for 5 days after beginning an effective antibiotic regimen.

COMPLICATIONS

The most common complication of pertussis, and cause of most of the pertussis-related deaths, is secondary bacterial pneumonia. The pertussis biotoxin attaches to cilia on the respiratory epithelial cells. The cilia become paralyzed and inflammation of the respiratory tract occurs, resulting in impaired ability to clear respiratory secretions.

Very young infants are at the highest risk for developing pertussis-related complications, such as pneumonia, hypoxemia, anorexia, vomiting and dehydration, otitis media, pneumothorax, epistasis, and rectal prolapse from the severity of coughing. Neurologic complications, such as seizures, encephalopathy, and subdural hematomas, also can occur. In addition to bacterial pneumonia, persistent cough, and encephalopathy complications, adolescents and adults also may develop pertussis-related trouble sleeping, urinary incontinence, and rib fractures.[1,4]

PREVENTION

Pertussis is transmitted via respiratory droplets when coughing and sneezing. The bacteria may even stay on surfaces as fomites in the form of respiratory secretions. Hand hygiene and avoidance of known infections is thus crucial in decreasing the transmission of pertussis. Moreover, the act of cocooning, the term used to describe immunization of all household and close contacts of infants, can significantly decrease the risk of pertussis transmission to infants. Caregivers and close contacts of infants should be immunized at least 2 weeks before contact with the infant. Also, routine vaccination beginning at age 2 months and practicing basic infection precautions, such as avoiding sick contacts and decreasing exposure to respiratory droplets from infected individuals, can also decrease the risk of pertussis transmission.

One of the essential elements to reduce risk of pertussis is through vaccination. The Advisory Committee on Immunization Practices (ACIP) recommends that children receive immunizations to reduce risk for acquiring pertussis. The recommended childhood immunization schedule for pertussis prevention is a series of 5 vaccinations of diphtheria, tetanus, and acellular pertussis (DTaP) beginning at 2, 4, and 6 months of age, followed by DTaP between 15 and 18 months of age, and again between ages 4 and 6 years (**Table 1**). A combination vaccine, such as Pediarix, which also includes hepatitis B and polio vaccine components (DTaP-HepB-IPV), may be used for the first 3 doses in children between 6 weeks and 6 years of age. Another combination vaccine, such as Pentacel, which also contains Haemophilus influenzae type B and polio vaccine components (HIB-DTaP-IPV), may be used for the first 4 doses in children between 6 weeks and 4 years of age. The fifth dose of DTaP and fourth dose of IPV can be administered as a combination vaccine, Kinrix, or as individual vaccines.[19]

The current immunization schedule for adolescents includes a preteen immunization, between 11 and 12 years of age, with adult tetanus reduced diphtheria and acellular pertussis (Tdap). Since 2005, there are 2 licensed Tdap vaccines in the United States: Adacel for those 11 to 64 and Boostrix for those aged 10 to 18 years.

Adults are advised to get the Tdap vaccine instead of 1 dose of their adult tetanus toxoid and reduced diphtheria toxoid (Td) vaccine booster if they did not receive the preteen or teen dose of Tdap.[20] Adolescents and adults and those who are exposed to infants younger than 12 months old are advised to get the Tdap vaccine at their routine health examination if Tdap has not been received previously.

Immunity to pertussis, whether induced from vaccination or from having pertussis infection, wanes over time, so it is advised that teens and adults receive a pertussis vaccination booster. It is unclear exactly how long immunity to pertussis lasts following vaccination. Klein and colleagues[5] used data from Kaiser Permanente Northern California for children with a positive pertussis PCR during their study

Table 1
Pertussis vaccination schedule

	Age	Minimum Interval	Other Notes
Dose 1	6 wk–2 mo	—	All forms of pertussis-containing vaccines may be interchanged if needed (ie, Pediarix, Pentacel).
Dose 2	4 mo	4 wk	
Dose 3	6 mo	4 wk	Severe allergic reaction to a vaccine component or following a prior dose or encephalopathy not due to another cause within 7 d of vaccination are the only contraindications to vaccine administration.
Dose 4	15–18 mo	6 mo	
Dose 5	4–6 y	—	
Dose 6	11–12 y	—	Administered in adult Tdap immunization (ie, Adacel, Boostrix).

Data from Centers for Disease Control and Prevention. Pertussis vaccination: use of acellular pertussis vaccines among infants and young children. Recommendations of the Advisory Committee on Immunization Practices (ACIP). Morb Mortal Wkly Rep 1997;46(No. RR-7):1–25.

period, who had received their fifth dose of DTaP within 47 to 84 months of age, and found that the risk of contracting pertussis increased annually by approximately 42% per year after receiving their fifth dose of DTaP. Of note, this study used data from children who received the acellular pertussis vaccine. According to the CDC, immunity induced by the acellular pertussis vaccine wanes more rapidly that the previously used whole-cell vaccines. Since the late 1990s, due to safety concerns and an improved side-effect profile, whole-cell vaccines are no longer used in the United States.

At least 25% of early infancy cases of pertussis are due to their mother having the illness. Because of the increased frequency of pertussis and its high infant morbidity, there are specific recommendations for administering the Tdap vaccine to pregnant women in their third trimester of pregnancy. Since 2012, the ACIP recommends the administration of Tdap vaccine to pregnant women between 27 and 36 weeks' gestation of *each* pregnancy, regardless of the woman's prior Tdap immunization status.[20] This strategy protects the mother from getting pertussis, passing it to the infant, and confers passive immunity to the infant. It is no longer recommended to give Tdap postpartum, which protects only the mother, unless the patient has never received Tdap. One study notes immunizing pregnant women between 27 and 36 weeks' gestation is 85% more effective at preventing pertussis in infants younger than 2 months than immunizing a woman in the hospital after giving birth.[9,18,20,21]

A pregnant woman can receive the Tdap vaccine earlier in her pregnancy as needed (eg, wound, community outbreak of pertussis). If Tdap is given earlier than 27 weeks' gestation, it should not be repeated during that pregnancy.[20] The protection from pertussis immunization or prior pertussis infection lasts approximately 5 to 10 years, after which immunity wanes and risk of pertussis infection increases. It is uncertain whether maternal transplacental antibodies contribute to infant protection against pertussis.

POSTEXPOSURE PROPHYLAXIS

The CDC supports using postexposure prophylaxis (PEP) in people at high risk for developing severe pertussis and people who will have close contact with those at high risk for pertussis, defined as those within 21 days of exposure to a person with infectious pertussis.[15] High-risk persons are defined as those who are personally at high risk for developing severe illness or will have close contact with people at high risk of severe illness. Examples of high-risk persons include infants and those with preexisting health conditions that may be worsened by pertussis, such as those with immune compromise or severe asthma. Also at high risk are women in the third trimester of pregnancy, as they transmit their own pertussis infection to their neonates. Individuals who are exposed to infants younger than 12 months, such as those who work in childcare, maternity wards, and neonatal intensive care units, are at high risk for contracting pertussis.[15] In addition to initiating prompt treatment, all cases of pertussis should be quickly reported to local and state health officials so that those exposed can be promptly offered PEP. Azithromycin remains the antibiotic of choice for chemoprophylaxis to *B pertussis*.[15]

SUMMARY

B pertussis can cause serious and potentially fatal complications, especially in very young infants. Early diagnosis and treatment of pertussis with a macrolide antibiotic, such as azithromycin, before the paroxysmal stage of disease can help mitigate complications and reduce the spread of this highly contagious disease.

REFERENCES

1. Center for Disease Control and Prevention. Epidemiology and prevention of vaccine-preventable diseases. In: Hamborsky J, Kroger A, Wolfe S, editors. 135th edition. Washington (DC): Public Health Foundation; 2015. Available at: https://www.cdc.gov/vaccines/pubs/pinkbook/index.html. Accessed November 17, 2017.
2. Kurt TL, Yeager AS, Guenette S, et al. Spread of pertussis by hospital staff. JAMA 1972;221:264–7.
3. Lee G, Lett S, Schauer S, et al. Societal costs and morbidity of pertussis in adolescents and adults. Clin Infect Dis 2004;39(11):1572–80.
4. Hewlett E, Edwards K. Pertussis – not just for kids. N Engl J Med 2005;352: 1215–22.
5. Klein K, Bartlett J, Rowhani-Rahbar A, et al. Waning protection after fifth dose of acellular pertussis vaccine in children. N Engl J Med 2012;367:1012–9.
6. Zhang L, Prietsch SO, Axelsson I, et al. Acellular vaccines for preventing whooping cough in children. Cochrane Database Syst Rev 2014;(9):CD001478.
7. Center for Disease Control and Preventioin. Updated recommendations for use of tetanus toxoid, reduced diphtheria toxoid, and acellular pertussis vaccine (Tdap) in pregnant women-Advisory Committee on Immunization Practices (ACIP), 2012. MMWR Morb Mortal Wkly Rep 2013;62:131–5.
8. Ward JL, Cherry JD, Chang SJ, et al. Efficacy of an acellular pertussis vaccine among adolescents and adults. N Engl J Med 2005;353:1555–63.
9. Centers for Disease Control and Prevention. Summary of DTaP and Tdap vaccine recommendations across the lifespan. Available at: www.cdc.gov/vaccines/vpd/pertussis/recs-summary.html. Accessed November 17, 2017.
10. American Academy of Pediatrics. Pertussis. In: Pickering L, Baker CJ, Kimberlin D, et al, editors. Red book: 2009 report of the committee on infectious diseases. 28th edition. Elk Grove Village (IL): American Academy of Pediatrics; 2009. p. 504–19.
11. Deeks S, De Serres G, Boulianne N, et al. Failure of physicians to consider the diagnosis of pertussis in children. Clin Infect Dis 1999;28:840–6.
12. von Konig CH, Halperin S, Riffelmann M, et al. Pertussis of adults and infants. Lancet Infect Dis 2002;2:744–50.
13. Ray W, Murray K, Hall K, et al. Azithromycin and the risk of cardiovascular death. N Engl J Med 2012;366:1881–90.
14. U.S. Food and Drug Administration. FDA drug safety communication: Azithromycin (Zithromax or Zmax) and the risk of potentially fatal heart rhythms. Silver Spring, MD. 2013. Available at: https://www.fda.gov/drugs/drugsafety/ucm341822.htm. Accessed February 12, 2018.
15. Center for Disease Control and Prevention. Recommended antimicrobial agents for the treatment and postexposure prophylaxis of pertussis: 2005 CDC guidelines. MMWR Morb Mortal Wkly Rep 2005;54(RR-14):1–16.
16. Altunaiji SM, Kukuruzovic R, Curtis N, et al. Antibiotics for whooping cough (pertussis). Cochrane Database Syst Rev 2007;(3):CD004404.
17. Wang K, Bettiol S, Thompson MJ, et al. Symptomatic treatment of the cough in whooping cough. Cochrane Database Syst Rev 2014;(9):CD003257.
18. Centers for Disease Control and Prevention. Prevention of pertussis, tetanus and diphtheria among pregnant and postpartum women and their infants. Recommendations of the Advisory Committee on Immunization Practices. MMWR Morb Mortal Wkly Rep 2008;57(No.RR-4):1–18.

19. Center for Disease Control and Prevention. Pertussis vaccination: use of acellular pertussis vaccines among infants and young children. Recommendations of the Advisory Committee on Immunization Practices (ACIP). MMWR Morb Mortal Wkly Rep 1997;46(No. RR-7):1–25.
20. Center for Disease Control and Prevention. Updated recommendations for use of tetanus toxoid, reduced diphtheria toxoid and acellular pertussis vaccine (Tdap) in pregnant women and persons who have or anticipate having close contact with an infant aged <12 months—Advisory Committee on Immunization Practices (ACIP), 2011. MMWR Morb Mortal Wkly Rep 2011;60:1424–6.
21. Winter K, Glaser C, Watt J, et al. Pertussis epidemic—California 2014. MMWR Morb Mortal Wkly Rep 2014;63(48):1129–32.

Skin Infections

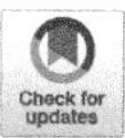

Karl T. Clebak, MD, FAAFP[a,*], Michael A. Malone, MD[b]

KEYWORD

- Bacterial, fungal, and Viral skin infections • Impetigo • Bullous impetigo • Erysipelas
- Cellulitis • Methicillin-resistant *Staphylococcus aureus* • Periorbital cellulitis
- Orbital cellulitis

KEY POINTS

- Skin and soft tissue infections can be organized by their underlying etiology: bacterial, fungal, and viral causes.
- The primary care provider will commonly see skin and soft tissue infections in the outpatient setting.
- Skin and soft tissue infections range from the uncomplicated impetigo to the potentially lethal necrotizing fasciitis.

INTRODUCTION

The primary care provider will commonly see skin and soft tissue infections in the outpatient setting. Skin and soft tissue infections range from the uncomplicated impetigo to the potentially lethal necrotizing fasciitis. This article reviews these infections based on their underlying etiology: bacterial, fungal, and viral causes.

BACTERIAL SKIN INFECTIONS

Impetigo

Impetigo (**Fig. 1**) is a common bacterial skin infection of superficial epidermis. It is caused by *Staphylococcus aureus*, group A beta-hemolytic *Streptococcus pyogenes*, or less commonly, anaerobic bacteria.[1] Although impetigo can occur at any age, it most commonly affects children aged 2 to 5 and is the most common bacterial skin infection. Impetigo is the third most common skin disease in children after dermatitis and viral warts.[2] Impetigo accounts for 50% to 60% of all bacterial skin infections.[3] Summer months in temperate regions and humid, tropical climates are predisposing

Disclosure: The authors have nothing to disclose.

[a] Department of Family and Community Medicine, Penn State College of Medicine, 121 North Nyes Road, Harrisburg, PA 17112, USA; [b] Department of Family Medicine, Tidelands Health MUSC Family Medicine Residency Program, 4320 Holmestown Road, Myrtle Beach, SC 29588, USA
* Corresponding author.
E-mail address: kclebak@pennstatehealth.psu.edu

Prim Care Clin Office Pract 45 (2018) 433–454
https://doi.org/10.1016/j.pop.2018.05.004

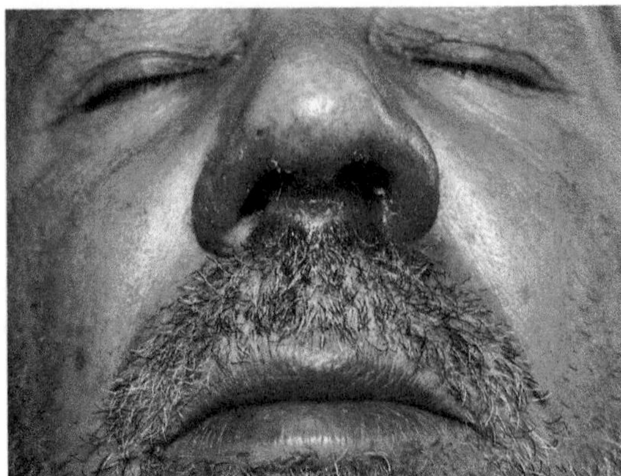

Fig. 1. Impetigo of nares. (*Courtesy of* Klaus D. Peter, Gummersbach, Germany.)

factors. Insect bites, varicella, herpes simplex virus, and other conditions that involve breaks in the skin predispose patients to the formation of secondary impetigo.[2]

Nonbullous impetigo typically begins as a single red maculopapular lesion that quickly becomes a vesicle. The vesicle may rupture and the contents dry to form the characteristic honey-colored crusts.[2]

Treatment of nonbullous impetigo consists of topical antibiotics.[4] Two antibiotic creams, mupirocin and fusidic acid, are at least as effective as oral antibiotics where the disease is not extensive.[4] Systemic antibiotics may be needed if there are numerous lesions, outbreaks affecting several people, or ecthyma (ulceration extending into dermis).[5] Options for oral treatment include beta-lactamase–resistant penicillins (cloxacillin, dicloxacillin and flucloxacillin), broad-spectrum penicillins (ampicillin, amoxicillin with clavulanic acid), cephalosporins. or macrolides.[5] Acute poststreptococcal glomerulonephritis is a serious complication that affects between 1% and 5% of patients irrespective of antibiotic treatment.[2]

Bullous impetigo is caused exclusively by toxin-producing *S aureus*, representing a localized form of staphylococcal scalded skin syndrome.[6] It most commonly affects the neonate. Initially, large, superficial, fragile bullae can develop on the trunk and extremities. Bullous impetigo may affect the anogenital area and buttocks of infants, being one of the most common causes of ulceration in these regions.[1] Antibiotic coverage for *Staphylococcus* is the mainstay of treatment. Dicloxacillin and cephalexin are recommended because susceptibility of found *S aureus* isolates.[5]

Erysipelas

Erysipelas has been defined in 3 different ways. First, the distinction between erysipelas and cellulitis is the depth of infection. Erysipelas is a more superficial infection affecting the superficial dermis, including the superficial lymphatics. This is in contrast to cellulitis, which involves the deeper reticular dermis and subcutaneous fat. Erysipelas has more clearly defined borders of inflammation. A second definition of erysipelas refers only to facial cellulitis. The third definition from European countries considers erysipelas a synonym for cellulitis affecting any skin area.[5]

Group A beta-hemolytic streptococci is believed to be the most common cause of erysipelas, in particular *S pyogenes*.[5] Traditionally, penicillin has been the treatment of choice for erysipelas. Other treatment options include a cephalosporin, such as cephalexin, dicloxacillin, orclindamycin.[5] The recommended duration of antibiotic therapy is 5 days; however, treatment should be extended if the infection has not improved.[5]

Cellulitis

Cellulitis is a bacterial infection that involves the subcutaneous tissue and may extend to the dermis of the skin. It presents as a rapidly spreading, painful indurated area of subcutaneous tissue with overlying warmth and erythema. The borders of the cellulitis lesion are not distinct in contrast to the sharp borders associated with erysipelas (**Fig. 2**). Cellulitis (**Fig. 3**) occurs after the protective integrity of the epidermis has been compromised (eg, trauma, ulcers, eczema), allowing bacterial access to the subepidermal tissues. It also may occur as a result of seeding from a distant source or generalized bacteremia.[7] Systemic symptoms, such as fevers, chills, and malaise, may give rise to a toxic appearance of the patient.

Group A beta-hemolytic *Streptococcus* and *S aureus* are the 2 most common causes of cellulitis.[7] Methicillin-resistant *S aureus* (MRSA) is becoming increasingly more common. MRSA is the most common bacteria isolated from purulent skin and soft tissue infections.[8] Animal or human bites can cause cellulitis, resulting from the skin flora of the recipient of the bite or the oral flora of the biter.[7] Pneumococcal cellulitis can occur in patients with diabetes mellitus, alcohol abuse, systemic lupus erythematosus, the nephrotic syndrome, or a hematologic cancer.[9] Cellulitis due to *Pseudomonas* is seen after nail punctures through sneakers and auricular ear piercings.[10,11]

Diagnosis is usually made clinically. Identification of specific organisms may be possible through Gram stain and culture of material aspirated from the wound. Blood cultures may be drawn if systemic signs are present.

To limit the spread of the infection, treatment should be initiated as soon as possible. Antibiotics should include empiric coverage against *S aureus* and streptococci. β-Lactam (eg, cephalexin, dicloxacillin) antibiotics are recommended first-line treatment for patients without suspicion for MRSA. In patients with suspected MRSA, Sulfamethoxazole-Trimethoprim, clindamycin, doxycycline, minocycline, or

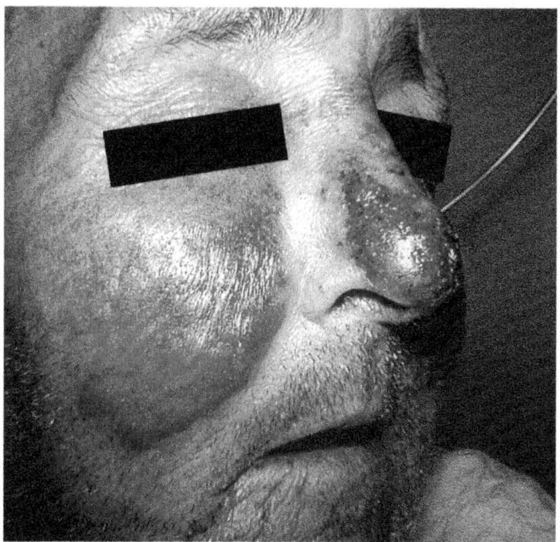

Fig. 2. Facial erysipelas. (*Courtesy of* CDC/Thomas F. Sellers, Emory University, Atlanta, Georgia.)

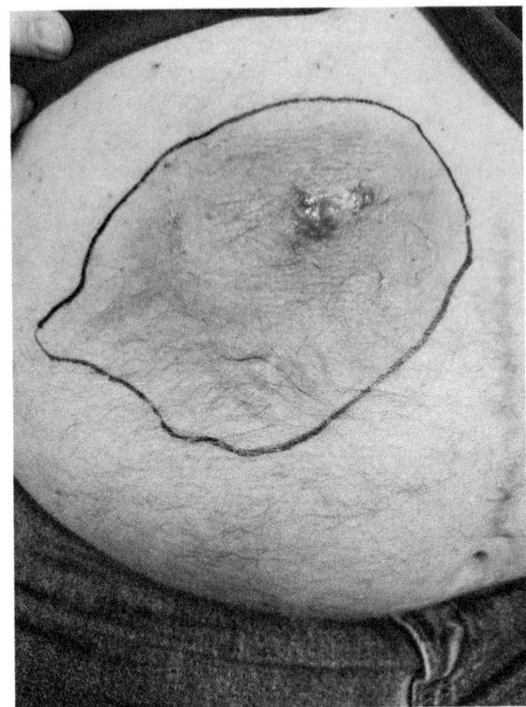

Fig. 3. Abscess with surrounding cellulitis. (*Courtesy of* Kenyetta Givans, MD, Hershey, Pennsylvania.)

third-generation or fourth-generation fluoroquinolones are recommended.[12] Patients with systemic symptoms (eg, fever, rigors, emesis), unstable vital signs (eg, hypotension, tachycardia), or no improvement with an appropriate course of oral antibiotics require admission to the hospital and administration of parenteral antibiotics. Stable patients requiring intravenous antibiotics can be safely treated outpatient.[13] Vancomycin and linezolid are intravenous drug therapies that can be used in suspected MRSA infections.[14]

Methicillin-Resistant Staphylococcus aureus

MRSA refers to the isolates that are resistant to β-lactam antibiotics, including penicillins and cephalosporins.[15] After being first identified during the 1960s in the health care setting, community-acquired MRSA has become more prevalent. Community-acquired MRSA may be responsible for up to 60% of skin and soft tissue infections (SSTIs) seen in US emergency departments.[8] Children, ethnic minorities, intravenous drug users, recent antibiotic use, men who have sex with men, residents of long-term care facilities and prisons, and patients receiving hemodialysis are all risk factors for MRSA infection.[15]

There are no reliable signs and symptoms to distinguish MRSA infections from other purulent SSTIs.[16] Necrotic skin lesions, necrotizing pneumonia, pleural empyema, necrotizing fasciitis, septic thrombophlebitis with pulmonary embolization, myositis, severe sepsis with purpura fulminans, and the Waterhouse–Friderichsen syndrome have been associated with community-associated MRSA.[15]

The recommended treatment of community-associated MRSA infection depends severity of the clinical presentation. Purulent SSTIs without associated systemic signs, such as fever, tachycardia, or hemodynamic instability, are generally managed with incision and drainage, with or without oral antibiotic therapy.[15] As compared with health care–associated MRSA isolates, community-associated MRSA isolates are usually susceptible to clindamycin, less often resistant to other non–β-lactam antibiotics.[17] Clindamycin, trimethoprim-sulfamethoxazole, and tetracyclines all may be used to treat mild to moderate community-acquired MRSA infections.[18] Clindamycin use is associated with *Clostridium difficile* infection. Caution is recommended in using trimethoprim-sulfamethoxazole in elderly and renally compromised patients due to risk of hyperkalemia. Trimethoprim-sulfamethoxazole is contraindicated in pregnant or breastfeeding women and in patients with megaloblastic anemia. Tetracyclines are not recommended in pregnant women or children younger than 8 years. Options to treat severe MRSA infections include intravenous therapy vancomycin, linezolid, daptomycin, tigecycline, telavancin, and ceftaroline.[19]

Preseptal/Orbital Cellulitis

Preseptal (periorbital) cellulitis is bacterial infection of the soft tissues that surround the eye that lay anterior to the orbital septum and may include the eyelid. Orbital cellulitis is the infection of the soft tissues, fat, and intraocular muscles posterior to the orbital septum.[20] Preseptal cellulitis most commonly affects patients younger than 5 and is almost 3 times more common than orbital cellulitis.[20] Orbital bacterial infections can present in all ages; however, are seen more often in the pediatric population and a 2:1 male predominance has been noted. Orbital cellulitis occurs more during the winter months when it is associated with sinus and upper respiratory tract infections. Most cases have a unilateral presentation.[20]

Preseptal and orbital cellulitis due to *Haemophilus influenzae* type B has declined after the advent of the *Haemophilus influenzae* type B vaccination.[21,22] Most common causes of bacterial infection include the skin flora *Staphylococcus*, *Streptococcus*, and anaerobes.[20] Community-acquired MRSA has emerged as a cause of preseptal and orbital cellulitis.[23] Rhinosinusitis is the most common predisposing factor for pediatric orbital cellulitis. However, preseptal and orbital cellulitis also can result from extension of external ocular infection, such as a hordeolum (stye) or dacryocystitis (infection of the lacrimal system), an upper respiratory tract infection, a dental abscess, a superficial break in the skin due to an infected insect bite, impetigo, acne, eczema, periocular surgery, direct penetrating injury to the orbit, or hematogenous seeding.[20]

Preseptal cellulitis typically presents with unilateral swelling, erythema, and tenderness of the upper and lower eyelids with or without fever. Orbital cellulitis presents similarly; however, the patient also may have proptosis, pain, or limitation of extraocular movement, decreased visual acuity, chemosis, or papilledema.[24] Orbital computed tomography (CT) with contrast can help distinguish between periorbital and orbital cellulitis.[25,26]

Management of simple periorbital cellulitis should cover *Staphylococcus* and *Streptococcus*.[20] In the management of periorbital cellulitis, no evidence suggests that intravenous antibiotics are superior to oral antibiotics in terms of recovery time or prevention of complications.[25] The choice of antibiotic route should be based on general appearance of the patient, ability to take oral medication, compliance, and clinical progression of the disease.[20] Appropriate antibiotics for outpatient therapy should cover beta-lactamase–producing organisms (eg, amoxicillin/clavulanate, cefuroxime axetil, cefpodoxime proxetil, and cefdinir). The typical length of therapy is 7 to 10 days or until symptom resolution.

The management of suspected orbital cellulitis includes hospital admission for close monitoring, intravenous antibiotic therapy, and surgical consultation with ophthalmology and/or otolaryngology. Empiric coverage of *Staphylococcus* and *Streptococcus* (second-generation or third-generation cephalosporins, ampicillin/sulbactam, or nafcillin may be considered). If anaerobes are suspected from a sinus or odontogenic source, clindamycin or metronidazole offer anaerobic coverage. MRSA coverage should be considered as well. Intravenous antibiotics can be switched to oral antibiotics to complete a 10-day to 14-day course once the eyelid edema and erythema have improved. If anaerobes are suspected (from a sinus or odontogenic source), clindamycin or metronidazole offer anaerobic coverage. MRSA coverage should be considered as well. The primary goals of surgical intervention if needed include draining abscesses, releasing pressure on the orbit, and obtaining cultures to guide antimicrobial therapy.[27]

Preseptal cellulitis complications may include local abscess formation. Untreated orbital cellulitis may lead to permanent vision loss, neurologic deficits, or death.[28]

Folliculitis

Folliculitis (**Fig. 4**) is defined as inflammation of hair follicles. It is characterized by superficial inflammation of hair follicles with perifollicular papules or pustules on an erythematous base.[29] It may be caused by infection, chemicals, or physical injury.

Infectious causes are more the most common, and include bacterial, fungal, and other causes. Bacterial causes are the most common infectious etiology, and *S aureus* is the most common bacterial pathogen. Other common bacteria include *Streptococcus* and *Pseudomonas aeruginosa*, seen after exposure to water or hot tubs, leading to the frequently referred to "hot tub folliculitis."[29] Bacterial folliculitis may be more common in men due to beard area and shaving. Fungal causes of folliculitis include *Malassezia*, which is reported to be most common fungal cause. *Malassezia* is more frequent in adolescents and men, associated with travel to tropical climates, often presents on chest or back, and can be associated with human immunodeficiency virus (HIV) or immunosuppression.[29] *Candida* can be seen in immunocompromised states and in heroin users.[29] *Pseudofolliculitis barbae* is characterized by a chronic, inflammatory reaction to shaving. *Pseudofolliculitis* appears when the hair shaft penetrates the wall of the hair follicle or enters the epidermis. It appears more common in darkly pigmented skin due to coarseness of the hair shaft.[29]

Diagnosis of folliculitis is usually made clinically and testing is not required unless there is a failure to respond to treatment. Testing may include: bacterial, fungal, or viral cultures; histopathologic examination; polymerase chain reaction; or cytology.[30]

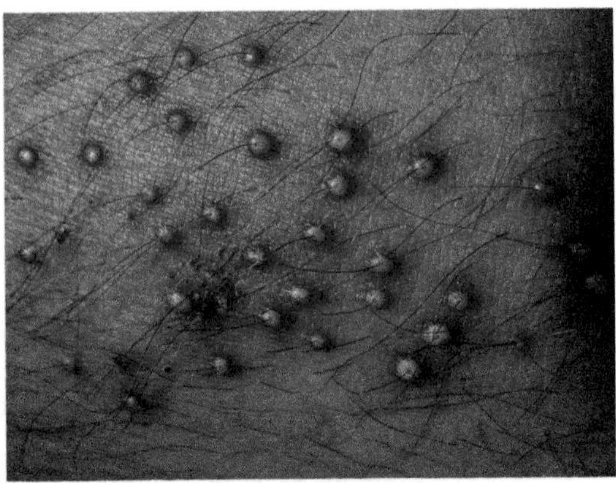

Fig. 4. Folliculitis.

Folliculitis treatment involves treating the underlying cause. Topical therapy, such as mupirocin or fusidic acid ointment, or benzoyl peroxide, is commonly considered first-line empiric treatment. If symptoms fail to respond to topical therapy, consider a 7-day course of oral antibiotics with cephalosporins, dicloxacillin, or flucloxacillin. Consider MRSA infection treatment if infection worsens. Pseudomonas folliculitis generally resolves spontaneously, however if symptoms persist, ciprofloxacin may be used. For fungal folliculitis, itraconazole can be used. *P barbae* is typically treated by not shaving the affected area for at least 4 weeks.[31]

Furuncles/Carbuncles/Other Skin Abscess

A skin abscess (see **Fig. 2**) is a collection of pus within dermis and deeper skin tissues, most often due to bacterial infection from skin flora or organisms from mucous membranes. A furuncle (also known as a boil) is an infection of the hair follicle with purulent extension into the adjacent subcutaneous tissue leading to abscess formation. A carbuncle is a collection of furuncles that converge and drain through a follicular opening.[32] Most commonly furuncles, carbuncles, and abscesses are caused by *S aureus*. MRSA was found to be the most common identifiable cause of SSTIs in patients presenting to emergency departments in 11 US cities.[33] Consider furuncles/carbuncles/other skin abscess in the differential for patients who present with a "spider bite," as prevalence of MRSA skin infections has increased.

Surgical intervention remains the mainstay of therapy for simple cutaneous abscesses; data do not support routine antibiotic use.[34] Incision and drainage is superior to ultrasound-guided needle aspiration for abscess treatment.[35] Incision and drainage should include expression of all purulent material and lysis of all loculations if possible. Guidelines recommend considering antibiotics in the case of multiple lesions, gangrene, immunocompromised patients, surrounding cellulitis, or systemic signs of infection.[32]

If MRSA is identified, recommended coverage includes trimethoprim-sulfamethoxazole, clindamycin, doxycycline, or minocycline. If methicillin-susceptible *S aureus* is identified, treatment options include 5 to 14 days of dicloxacillin or cephalexin. For severe infections failing incision and drainage with oral antibiotic therapy, intravenous antibiotic options for MRSA include cefazolin, clindamycin, linezolid, nafcillin, telavancin, or vancomycin.[32]

Necrotizing Fasciitis

Necrotizing fasciitis is a rare but serious bacterial infection involving the deeper layers of skin characterized by widespread necrosis of the skin, subcutaneous tissue, and superficial fascia spreading across the fascial planes. Fournier gangrene is a subtype of necrotizing fasciitis of the perineal and perianal regions that often involves the genital regions.[5] Early identification of suspected necrotizing fasciitis is important, as it represents a surgical emergency. The mortality in patients with group A streptococcal necrotizing fasciitis, hypotension, and organ failure is high, ranging from 30% to 70%.[5] Suspect necrotizing fasciitis if there are signs of systemic toxicity (such as fever, hypotension, leukocytosis, or acute renal failure), pain disproportionate to examination, bullae or cutaneous necrosis, tense edema, tissue crepitus, loss of sensation, or rapid progression despite antimicrobial therapy.[36] Diabetes, smoking, and alcohol abuse are common comorbidities.

Necrotizing fasciitis usually develops from an initial break in the skin related to trauma or surgery. The infection can be monomicrobial, from streptococci or less commonly community-acquired MRSA, *Aeromonas hydrophila*, or *Vibrio vulnificus*, or polymicrobial, involving a mixed aerobe-anaerobe bacterial flora.[5] There is often a predisposing condition, such as diabetes, arteriosclerotic vascular disease, venous insufficiency with edema, venous stasis or vascular insufficiency, ulcer, or injection drug use.[5] Cases of necrotizing fasciitis that arise after varicella or trivial injuries, such as minor scratches or insect bites, are usually due to *S pyogenes* or, far less commonly, community-acquired MRSA.[5] Polymicrobial infection is most commonly associated with clinical settings: perianal abscesses, penetrating abdominal trauma, surgical procedures involving the bowel, decubitus ulcers, injection sites in illicit drug users, and spread from a genital site such as Bartholin abscess, episiotomy wound, or a minor vulvovaginal infection.[5] In the polymicrobial infections, numerous different anaerobic and aerobic organisms can be cultured from the involved fascial plane, with an average of 5 pathogens from each wound. Most of the organisms originate from the bowel or genitourinary flora, including coliforms and anaerobic bacteria.[5]

Suggested blood tests for suspected necrotizing fasciitis that may aid in the diagnosis of include complete blood count with differential; coagulation studies;, comprehensive metabolic panel, including glucose, calcium, and albumin; liver function tests; lactate, C-reactive protein (CRP); creatinine kinase; or blood cultures.[36] The Laboratory Risk Indicator for Necrotizing Fasciitis (LRINEC) score may help differentiate necrotizing fasciitis from cellulitis and abscess.[37] The LRINEC score: 4 points if CRP $\geq$150 mg/L, 1 point if white blood cell count 15 to 25/mm^3, 2 points if >25/mm^3, 1 point if hemoglobin 11 to 13.5 g/dL, 2 points if <11 g/dL, 2 points if sodium <135 mmol/L (135 mEq/L), 2 points if creatinine >141 mmol/L (1.85 mg/dL), 1 point if glucose >10 mmol/L (180 mg/dL). An LRINEC score $\geq$6 corresponds to an increased risk of necrotizing fasciitis.[37] Imaging studies may support clinical suspicion; however, should not delay surgical evaluation when suspicion is high.[5] Imaging studies may include MRI or CT.

Urgent surgical exploration, debridement, and fasciotomies are critical for prognosis and survival. In most cases, repeat surgical debridement is necessary, with an average of 3 debridements per patient.[38] Empiric broad-spectrum intravenous antibiotic coverage is recommended when there is suspicion of necrotizing fasciitis.[5] Empiric antibiotic treatment should be broad. Regimens for suspected necrotizing fasciitis include vancomycin or linezolid plus piperacillin-tazobactam or plus a carbapenem, or plus ceftriaxone and metronidazole.[5] Penicillin plus clindamycin is recommended for treatment of documented group A streptococcal necrotizing fasciitis.[5] Adjunctive therapy may include hyperbaric oxygen and intravenous immunoglobulin treatment.

FUNGAL SKIN INFECTIONS

Sporotrichosis

Sporotrichosis is a skin infection due to the fungus *Sporothrix schenckii*. Sporotrichosis is also referred to as gardener's disease, as it is typically acquired via inoculation of skin with soil, plant, or other matter contaminated with the fungus as can happen while gardening. Domestic cat and dog bites also may be a cause of sporotrichosis.[39] Alcoholism and diabetes have been found to be risk factors. Immunosuppression is a risk for disseminated or systemic disease. The time from inoculation to signs of infection varies from days to months. Sporotrichosis is more common in children and young adults; however, may present at any age.[39]

Lymphocutaneous sporotrichosis is the most common presentation, first presenting as a small hard nodule at the site of injury. Secondary regional lymphadenopathy later develops.[39] The lymphangitic form of sporotrichosis is characterized by first developing an erythematous necrotic or ulcerated nodule. After a few weeks, nodules develop along the lymphatic drainage tract. Sporotrichosis may present at any age, but it is more common in children and young adults. In children, facial lesions are more common; in adults, lesions typically involve hands and arms.[39]

Diagnosis is usually made based on clinical suspicion. Suspect sporotrichosis in patients with the presence of an abscess, pustule, or ulcer with nodules in nearby lymphatics and a history of recent travel to tropical regions, history of animal bites, or activities involving contact with soil, plants, wood, or animals.[39] Diagnosis is confirmed by isolation of *S schenckii* from fungal culture.

For cutaneous and lymphocutaneous sporotrichosis, itraconazole is the drug of choice. The recommended course of antifungals is for 2 to 4 weeks after resolution of all lesions, with the duration of a typical course of treatment lasting a total of 3 to 6 months.[40] Patients who do not respond to initial treatment with itraconazole should receive a higher dosage or change therapy to terbinafine or a saturated solution of potassium iodide. Fluconazole may be used if the patient does not tolerate these treatments. Local hyperthermia can be used for treating pregnant and nursing women who cannot safely receive other antifungal treatments.[40]

Tinea Capitis

Tinea capitis is an infection of hair follicles on the scalp and the surrounding skin caused by a dermatophyte, usually *Microsporum* or *Trichophyton*.[41] Tinea capitis usually affects children 3 to 7 years old; however, cases in adults may occur.[42] There is higher incidence of tinea capitis in children of African American and Caribbean descent.[42] Risk factors for tinea capitis include crowded living conditions, large family size, and low socioeconomic status.[42]

Usual presentation includes areas of hair loss with different degrees of inflammation. The black dot form of tinea capitis involves the hair breaking off at the base, leaving a "black dot" appearance on a hairless base. In the gray type of tinea capitis, there is usually one or more circular patches with marked scaling. In the diffuse scale type, there is fine, widespread scaling similar to dandruff in seborrheic dermatitis, with minimal or no hair loss present. The favus form is characterized by scaly erythematous patches with scutula, a yellow honey cup-shaped crust pierced by a central hair. Scutula in different areas may combine to form a single mass. A cheesy or mouselike odor may be present. The inflammatory type of tinea capitis is kerion. Kerion consists of an indurated, boggy swelling with vesicles and pustules usually localized to one spot. Kerion may be accompanied by purulent discharges as well as cervical lymphadenopathy, malaise, and fever.[43] An id reaction may occasionally be seen with inflammatory tinea capitis early in treatment. The id reaction typically occurs on the face, neck, or upper chest.[44]

Diagnosis is typically made from history and physical examination. Examination with a Wood lamp is not routinely useful, as only *Microsporum* species produce fluorescence. Microscopic analysis of hair and skin scrapings may reveal fungi; however, it has low sensitivity. A negative result requires culture in fungal medium.[44]

Topical therapy alone is not recommended for the management of tinea capitis. The recommended course of griseofulvin is for 6 to 8 weeks. Terbinafine may be used for children older than 4 years.[41] Itraconazole is licensed to treat pediatric tinea capitis across Europe.[41]

Tinea Corporis/Cruris/Pedis

Tinea infections are caused by the dermatophytes *Trichophyton*, *Microsporum*, and *Epidermophyton*. Tinea corporis is the cutaneous fungal infection of the trunk, extremities, or face, commonly referred to as ringworm. Tinea corporis typically presents as a pruritic red, annular patch with central clearing and a leading edge of scale. Lesions may be single or multiple, ranging in size from 1 to 5 cm.[45]

Tinea cruris, also referred to as jock itch, most commonly affects adolescent and young adult male individuals and involves the upper thigh opposite the scrotum. A

Wood lamp examination may be helpful to distinguish tinea from the other skin infection erythrasma, because the causative organism of erythrasma (*Corynebacterium minutissimum*) exhibits a coral red fluorescence. However, results of the Wood lamp examination can be falsely negative if the patient has recently bathed.[45]

Tinea pedis (athlete's foot) is the cutaneous fungal infection of the foot. Tinea pedis typically involves the skin between the toes, but may include the sole, sides, and dorsum of the foot. The acute form may present with erythema and maceration between the toes, sometimes accompanied by painful vesicles. The more chronic form is characterized by scaling, peeling, and erythema between the toes and can spread to other areas of the foot. The "moccasin pattern" of tinea pedis refers to the erythema and hyperkeratosis involving the plantar and lateral aspects of the foot.[45]

Although tinea infections are usually diagnosed based off of history and physical examination, microscopic examination of skin scraping using a potassium hydroxide (KOH) may be helpful.[46] Fungal culture is usually not necessary. Skin biopsy may be used to rule out other dermatologic conditions.[47]

The first choice for treatment of tinea corporis, tinea cruris, and tinea pedis is topical antifungal medication.[47] Topical antifungal preparations include terbinafine and butenafine. Extensive or resistant tinea infections may be treated with courses of oral terbinafine or itraconazole.[47] If a rash worsens after treatment with a topical steroid, suspicion should be raised for a dermatophyte infection.[45]

CANDIDAL INTERTRIGO

Candidal intertrigo is the most common cutaneous candidal infection of hair-bearing skin.[48] Risk factors include obesity, repetitive skin friction, hyperhidrosis, immunodeficiency, diabetes mellitus, and frequent antibiotic use.[49–51]

Presentation

Candidal intertrigo typically presents with erythematous plaques and erosions with fine peripheral scaling and erythematous satellite lesions.[48,50] The plaques are often pruritic and occasionally painful.

Diagnosis

Candidal intertrigo is commonly diagnosed clinically, based on the characteristic appearance (noted previously), but may be confirmed with KOH examination or culture of skin scrapings.[51] Direct microscopic examination reveals oval budding yeasts with septate hyphae and pseudohyphae.[52] Biopsy reveals parakeratotic scale with underlying subcorneal pustules.[53]

Treatment

There is relatively little evidence regarding the best therapy for candidal intertrigo, but topical antifungals, including topical nystatin, clotrimazole, ketoconazole, miconazole, or econazole are considered the first-line therapy.[51,54] Topical antifungal agents are typically applied twice daily until resolution; usually 2 to 4 weeks.

After antifungal treatment, adding drying agents, such as miconazole, nystatin, undecylenic acid, and tolnaftate, Domeboro solution, carbol-fuchsin solution (Castellani's paint), and potassium permanganate solution can reduce recurrence.[55–57] Talcum powder should be avoided due to ovarian cancer risk.[58]

Systemic antifungal medication for severe or resistant cases include oral fluconazole 50 to 100 mg daily or 150 mg weekly for adults and fluconazole 6 mg/kg once, then 3 mg/kg per day or itraconazole 5 to 10 mg/kg per day divided in 2 doses for children.[51,59–63] Oral ketoconazole risks outweigh the benefit and it should be avoided.[64] Low-potency topical corticosteroids may be used in conjunction with antifungal therapy to treat pruritus and discomfort but higher potency steroids should be avoided.[48]

Candidal Diaper Dermatitis

Candidal diaper dermatitis is a common skin eruption in infant and toddlers.[65,66]

Presentation

Candidal diaper dermatitis typically occurs on skin surfaces in direct contact with a wet diaper, including the buttocks, lower abdomen, genitalia, and upper thighs.[65] It classically presents with beefy red plaques, satellite papules, and superficial pustules that leave a scale once ruptured.[67] In contrast to simple irritant diaper dermatitis, candidal infections *involve the skin folds*, whereas irritant diaper dermatitis spares the skin folds.[66]

Diagnosis

Diagnosis usually is based on clinical presentation, but may be confirmed by KOH preparation or a fungal culture of skin scrapings. Persistent infection suggests type 1 diabetes mellitus or immunodeficiency.

Treatment

In most cases, treatment involves frequent diaper changes, air exposure, gentle cleansing, use of topical barrier preparations, and topical antifungals, such as nystatin, clotrimazole, miconazole, ketoconazole, and sertaconazole with little known difference in efficacy among these antifungals.[68,69]

Pityriasis (Tinea) Versicolor

Pityriasis versicolor (PV), also known as tinea versicolor (**Fig. 5**), is a common superficial fungal infection caused by *Malassezia* species, which is part of the normal skin flora.[70,71]

Presentation

Patients with PV typically present with pigmentation skin changes involving the trunk, back, abdomen, and proximal extremities. The face, the scalp, and the genitalia are less commonly involved.[72] Occasionally, mild pruritus occurs.[73]

Diagnosis

Diagnosis is typically based on history and physical examination, but skin scraping examination with KOH, Wood lamp examination, or rarely, culture can confirm diagnosis.

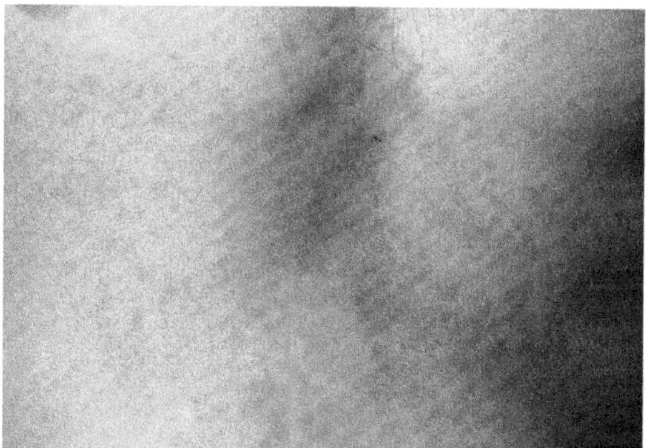

Fig. 5. Pityriasis (tinea) versicolor. (*Courtesy of* CDC/Lucille K. Georg, Atlanta, Georgia.)

Treatment

Ketoconazole possesses the strongest in vitro activity against *Malassezia*, and represents the topical treatment of choice for PV.[71] Other first-line topical treatments includes zinc pyrithione, ketoconazole, and terbinafine.[71,73,74] In cases of severe or recalcitrant PV, the drug of choice is oral itraconazole, although an effective alternative is oral fluconazole.[71]

VIRAL SKIN INFECTIONS

Herpes Simplex Virus Infections

Herpes simplex virus (HSV)-1 and HSV-2 both produce clusters of tense blisters on an erythematous base that evolve into crusted ulcerations. The lesions can be painful and last for 10 to 14 days and there can be associated fever and maliase.[75] Once HSV infection occurs, the virus lives in a latent state in nerves and can reactivate. In general, the severity of illness is less with reactivation.[76] Recurrence rates are lower for HSV-1 infection compared with HSV-2. HIV infection increases risk for contracting HSV and recurrent or extensive HSV infections.

Presentation

Orofacial herpes simplex, also known as herpes labialis or cold sores, are common during childhood and adolescence and present with clustered blisters along the lip vermillion border. Genital herpes simplex infections often involve bilateral blisters and ulcerative lesions in the anogenital region.

HSV infection of the finger, known as herpetic whitlow, can occur due to the spread of oral or genital herpes or to dentists and health care workers through infected secretions.[77] Often misdiagnosed as a bacterial skin infection, herpetic whitlow heals over 2 to 3 weeks, but can recur.[77,78] Outbreaks of HSV-1 skin infections have also occurred among wrestlers on the face, neck, and arms, and is referred to as herpes gladiatorum.

Diagnosis

Diagnosis of HSV is often based on clinical presentation. Viral culture can be obtained if uncertainty exists.[79] Although not typically utilized, various serologic assays can be used for HSV diagnosis. The Tzanck smear is not sensitive or specific and is typically not useful.[79] Scraping slides may be examined for herpes antigens via immunofluorescence microscopy.

Treatment

There is no cure for herpes, but antiviral medications can prevent or shorten outbreaks. In addition, daily suppression for herpes can reduce the likelihood of transmission to partners.

Prevention of genital herpes

There is currently no vaccine for genital herpes infection, so antiviral medication is the mainstay of prevention. The Centers for Disease Control and Prevention (CDC) guidelines recommend the following antivirals for prophylaxis:[80]

- Acyclovir 400 mg twice a day
- Famciclovir 500 mg twice daily
- Valacyclovir 500 mg twice daily

Episodic treatment

Oral acyclovir can reduce the duration of symptoms for genital herpes, but there is no evidence to support topical treatments.[81] The 2015 CDC guidelines recommend the following oral antivirals for episodic therapy[80]:

- Acyclovir: 800 mg 3 times daily for 2 days; or 800 mg twice daily for 5 days; or 400 mg 3 times daily for 5 days.
- Famciclovir: 1000 mg twice daily for a single-day duration; or 125 mg twice daily for 5 days; or 500 mg once, followed by 250 mg twice daily for 2 days.
- Valacyclovir: 500 mg twice daily for 3 days or 1000 mg once daily for 5 days.

Prevention of herpes labialis outbreaks

Long-term use of oral antivirals reduced cold sores by 0.09 episodes per person per month.[82] Effective preventive oral antiviral regimen studies include acyclovir (400 mg twice daily) and valacyclovir 500 mg daily.[83,84] The preventive effect of long-term acyclovir cream and sunscreen is uncertain.[82]

Treatment of herpes labialis

Lidocaine and prilocaine cream (25 mg of each per 1 g) reduced symptom and eruption duration in a small randomized controlled trial.[85] Topical acyclovir (5 times daily for 5 days) and penciclovir (every 2 hours for 5 days) may reduce episode duration, but does not improve pain.[86] Episodic oral antiviral medications (Acyclovir 400 mg 3 times a day or 200 mg 5 times a day, Famciclovir 500 mg 3 times a day for 7 days, and valacyclovir 1000 mg 2 times a day for 7 days) appear to reduce symptom duration and resolution time.[86]

Varicella-Zoster Virus

Varicella-zoster virus (**Fig. 6**) infection causes 2 clinically distinct forms of disease: a primary infection results in varicella, also known as chickenpox, and reactivation is known as shingles or zoster.[87] Varicella is more common in children, but shingles is more frequent in adults older than 60.[87]

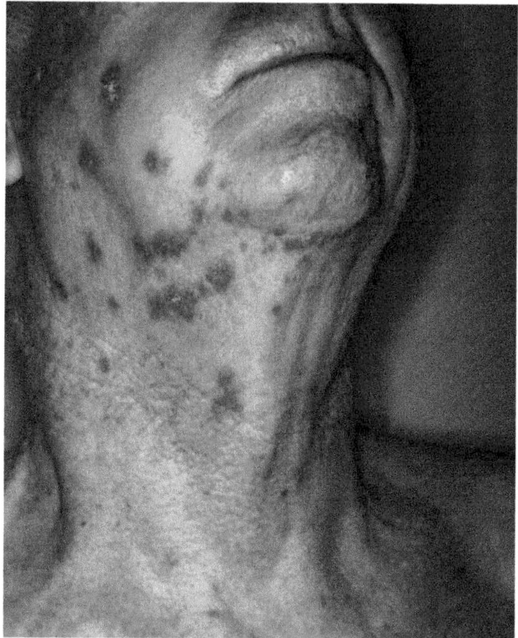

Fig. 6. Varicella-zoster virus. (*Courtesy of* the National Institute of Allergy and Infectious Diseases, Bethesda, Maryland.)

Clinical manifestations

Varicella is characterized by vesicular lesions in different stages of development on the face, trunk, and extremities.[87,88] The prodrome of fever, malaise, pharyngitis, or loss of appetite is followed closely by the vesicular pruritic rash that begins macular, rapidly become papular, and evolves into vesicles that become crusted.[88]

Zoster (shingles) is characterized by a painful, unilateral vesicular eruption on an erythematous base, which usually occurs in a restricted dermatomal distribution.[87] The rash is generally limited to one dermatome, but can occasionally affect 2 or 3 neighboring dermatomes.

Treatment

Varicella Most healthy children have self-limited infection with primary varicella. Therefore, primary treatment is supportive care, including antihistamines for the pruritic rash and nonsteroidal anti-inflammatory drugs or acetaminophen for fever. Varicella can cause severe complications, such as soft tissue infection, pneumonia, hepatitis, and encephalitis. Antiviral treatment with acyclovir, valacyclovir, or famciclovir should be initiated for high-risk groups (adolescents, adults, pregnant women, and immunocompromised hosts) to decrease morbidity and mortality.[89]

Zoster Evidence suggests that oral antiviral therapy (acyclovir, valacyclovir, and famciclovir) hastens resolution of lesions and pain, if initiated within 72 hours of symptoms[90] (**Table 1**). Antiviral therapy should be initiated in all immunocompromised patients with herpes zoster, even if they present after 72 hours, and immunocompromised patients with disseminated zoster should be hospitalized for intravenous acyclovir therapy.[91,92] Antiviral agents, used at the time of the rash, have been proposed as an intervention to prevent the development of post herpetic neuralgia (PHN), but there is little evidence to support this.[93] Patients with recurrent zoster should be treated with antiviral therapy similar in dose and duration as their initial treatment. Nonsteroidal anti-inflammatory drugs, acetaminophen, and tramadol are useful for mild to moderate pain, but more severe pain may warrant stronger opioid analgesics, such as oxycodone.[92]

Adjuvant therapies, such as gabapentin, tricyclic antidepressants (TCAs), or glucocorticoids do not have a significant role in the acute zoster treatment, although further studies are needed to see if TCAs or gabapentin can help reduce PHN risk.[94,95]

Preventing transmission Patients with zoster are not infectious before vesicles appear and after the lesions have crusted and reepithelialized. Those with active lesions should keep the rash covered and avoid contact with both pregnant and immunocompromised individuals. Vaccination can help reduce outbreaks.

Table 1
Treatment of acute herpes zoster

Medication	Dosing	Duration, d
Valacyclovir	1000 mg 3 times a day	7
Famciclovir	500 mg 3 times a day	7
Acyclovir	800 mg 5 times a day	7

Data from Dworkin RH, Johnson RW, Breur J, et al. Recommendations for the management of herpes zoster. Clin Infect Dis 2007;44 Suppl 1:S1; and Saguil A, Mercada M, Lauters R. Herpes zoster and postherpetic neuralgia: prevention and management. Am Fam Physician 2017;96(10):656–63.

Molluscum Contagiosum

Molluscum contagiosum (**Fig. 7**) is a common childhood disease cause by a poxvirus infection manifesting as flesh-colored, dome-shaped papules on the skin.[96,97] It is associated with immunodeficient states such as HIV infection and immunosuppressive agents,[98] but also occurs in healthy adolescents and adults related to sexually transmitted disease (STD), shared bathing or swimming areas,[99] or contact sports.[97] Molluscum contagiosum is spread by direct human skin-to-skin contact and thus can occur anywhere on the body, except the palms and soles. Genital lesions in sexually active individuals are classified as STDs, but most anogenital lesions in children are from autoinoculation.[100] Children with molluscum contagiosum can attend daycare or school, but lesions should be covered to reduce transmission.

Presentation and diagnosis

The diagnosis of molluscum contagiosum is usually made by the characteristic appearance of single or multiple 2-mm to 5-mm, firm, flesh-colored, dome-shaped papules on the skin with central umbilication.[101,102] Pruritus may be present or absent, and the most common areas of involvement include the trunk, axillae, antecubital and popliteal fossae, and crural folds.[101,102] Sexually transmitted molluscum contagiosum typically involves the groin, genitals, proximal thighs, and lower abdomen. When necessary, histologic examination can confirm the clinical diagnosis. Sexually active adolescents and adults with genital lesions should be evaluated for other STDs.

Treatment

Molluscum contagiosum usually resolves in immunocompetent individuals within months, but treatment may be preferred by the patient.[103] However, evidence supporting the various treatments is lacking.[103] A 2017 Cochrane review evaluated treatments including 5% imiquimod, cryospray, 10% potassium hydroxide,10% Australian lemon myrtle oil, 10% benzoyl peroxide cream, 0.05% tretinoin, 5% sodium nitrite, 5% salicylic acid, calcarea carbonica, and 10% povidone iodine plus 50% salicylic acid plaster, but concluded there is little evidence for their effectiveness, and natural resolution of molluscum contagiosum is a reasonable treatment.[103] Other treatment options with little evidence include topical cantharidin (beetle juice), curettage, and

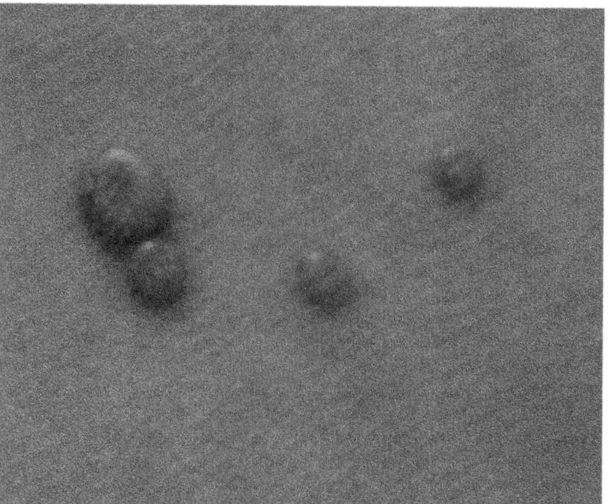

Fig. 7. Molluscum contagiosum. (*Courtesy of* CDC, Dave Bray, Walter Reed Medical Center, Bethesda, Maryland.)

topical corticosteroids.[102,104] Molluscum in the genital region is typically treated due to the potential for sexual transmission, although the use of cantharidin should be avoided in the genital area.[105]

Warts

Warts (also known as verrucae) are benign skin growths caused by the human papillomaviruses (HPV) virus.

Cutaneous warts (common, plantar, and flat warts)

Cutaneous warts occur most commonly in children and young adults and may manifest as common warts (verruca vulgaris), plantar warts (verruca plantaris), and flat (plane) warts (verruca plana). Warts may occur singly, in groups, or as coalescing warts forming plaques.[106]

Diagnosis The diagnosis of cutaneous warts is based on clinical appearance, but biopsy can be used for confirmation. The presence of thrombosed capillaries after paring hyperkeratotic debris on plantar or common warts can help with diagnosis.[107] Common warts, also called verruca vulgaris, appear as hyperkeratotic papules with a rough, irregular surface. They range from 1 mm to larger than 1 cm. They can occur on any part of the body but are seen most commonly on the knees, fingers, and dorsal surface of the hand. Filiform warts are long slender growths, usually seen on the face around the lips, eyelids, or nares. Plantar warts are typically hyperkeratotic lesions on the heels or other weight-bearing areas on the plantar aspect of the feet. Flat warts (verruca plana) are typically flesh-colored, small (1–5 mm), and smoother than other warts. They are more common in children and can present in large numbers (>100). They can occur anywhere, but common areas are the face, hands, and shins.

Treatment Treatment of cutaneous warts may not be necessary, as spontaneous remission of warts occurs in two-thirds of children within 2 years.[108] However, resolution in adults tends to be slower and may take up to several years.[108] Common reasons for treatment include pain, functional impairment, or cosmetic reasons. Topical salicylic acid and cryotherapy with liquid nitrogen are the most common treatments for common and plantar warts and have the most evidence for efficacy.[108,109] However, lack of high-quality studies of therapeutic interventions limit recommendations on treatments.[109] Other treatment options include cantharidin, trichloroacetic acid, surgery, laser therapy, imiquimod, topical or intralesional immunotherapy, and 5-fluorouracil.[108] Many treatments for common and plantar warts may be effective for flat warts, but there is little evidence specifically for flat warts. The best treatment for refractory warts is also unclear.

Condyloma acuminatum (anogenital warts)

Condyloma acuminatum refers to skin lesions attributed to HPV, the most common STD worldwide.[110] Symptoms begin approximately 2 to 3 months after initial contact.[111] Approximately 90% of anogenital warts (AGW) are related to HPV types 6 and 11.[110]

Diagnosis Diagnosis is typically made based on the clinical presentation.

Lesions can be highly variable in appearance.[111] AGWs begin as small, nondistinctive 1-mm to 2-mm flesh-colored papules on the skin, but can grow very large.[111] They can be smooth (particularly on the penile shaft), verrucous, or lobulated, and may be flat, dome-shaped, cauliflower-shaped, or pedunculated.[111] Color can be highly variable and multiple sites of the anogenital region can be involved simultaneously. Particularly with anal lesions, there may be a history of immunosuppression, anal intercourse, or other STDs. They can manifest individually but are more frequently found in large clusters.

In men, genital warts have a propensity for the penile glans and in women they are typically in the vulvovaginal and cervical region. Pruritus may be present or absent. Lesions are rarely considered to be painful, but can be associated with discomfort, burning, and pruritis.[111] A biopsy is rarely needed, but may be indicated for lesions that are atypical, recurrent, or resistant to treatment.

Treatment Thirty percent of AGW lesions will spontaneously regress.[112] There is a paucity of published randomized trials and there is no consensus on ideal treatment for AGWs, but surgical destruction or removal remains the treatment of choice.[110,113] Cryotherapy, trichloroacetic acid, podophyllin, and imiquimod appear to have similar efficacy, but cryotherapy may have more associated adverse events.[113] Imiquimod is advantageous because it offers the option of patient-applied therapy.[112]

REFERENCES

1. Brown J, Shriner DL, Schwartz RA, et al. Impetigo: an update. Int J Dermatol 2003;42:251–5.
2. Cole C, Gazewood J. Diagnosis and treatment of impetigo. Am Fam Physician 2007;75(6):859–64.
3. Feaster T, Singer JI. Topical therapies for impetigo. Pediatr Emerg Care 2010; 26(3):222–7 [quiz: 228–31].
4. Koning S, van der Sande R, Verhagen AP, et al. Interventions for impetigo. Cochrane Database Syst Rev 2012;(1):CD003261.
5. Stevens DL, Bisno AL, Chambers HF, et al. Practice guidelines for the diagnosis and management of skin and soft tissue infections: 2014 update by the Infectious Diseases Society of America. Clin Infect Dis 2014;59(2):e10–52.
6. Mancini AJ. Bacterial skin infections in children: the common and the not so common. Pediatr Ann 2000;29(1):26–35.
7. Swartz MN. Clinical practice. Cellulitis. N Engl J Med 2004;350(9):904–12.
8. Moran GJ, Krishnadasan A, Gorwitz RJ, et al, EMERGEncy ID Net Study Group. Methicillin-resistant *S. aureus* infections among patients in the emergency department. N Engl J Med 2006;355(7):666–74.
9. Parada JP, Maslow JN. Clinical syndromes associated with adult pneumococcal cellulitis. Scand J Infect Dis 2000;32:133–6.
10. Fisher MG, Goldsmith JF, Gilligan PH. Sneakers as a source of *Pseudomonas aeruginosa* in children with osteomyelitis following puncture wounds. J Pediatr 1983;106:607–9.
11. Keene WE, Markum AC, Samadpour M. Outbreak of *Pseudomonas aeruginosa* infections caused by commercial piercing of upper ear cartilage. JAMA 2004; 291:981–5.
12. Jenkins TC, Knepper BC, Sabel AL. Decreased antibiotic utilization after implementation of a guideline for inpatient cellulitis and cutaneous abscess. Arch Intern Med 2011;11:1072–9.
13. Corwin P, Toop L, McGeoch G, et al. Randomised controlled trial of intravenous antibiotic treatment for cellulitis at home compared with hospital. BMJ 2005; 330:129.
14. Weigelt J, Itani K, Stevens D, et al, Linezolid CSSTI Study Group. Linezolid versus vancomycin in treatment of complicated skin and soft tissue infections. Antimicrob Agents Chemother 2005;49:2260–6.

15. Daum RS. Clinical practice. Skin and soft-tissue infections caused by methicillin-resistant *Staphylococcus aureus*. N Engl J Med 2007;357(4):380–90 [Erratum appears in N Engl J Med 2007;357(13):1357].
16. Miller LG, Perdreau-Remington F, Bayer AS, et al. Clinical and epidemiologic characteristics cannot distinguish community-associated methicillin-resistant *Staphylococcus aureus* infection from methicillin-susceptible *S. aureus* infection: a prospective investigation. Clin Infect Dis 2007;44(4):471–82.
17. Naimi TS, LeDell KH, Como-Sabetti K, et al. Comparison of community- and health care-associated methicillin-resistant *Staphylococcus aureus* infection. JAMA 2003;290:2976–84.
18. Liu C, Bayer A, Cosgrove SE, et al. Clinical practice guidelines by the Infectious Diseases Society of America for the treatment of methicillin-resistant *Staphylococcus aureus* infections in adults and children. Clin Infect Dis 2011;52(3): e18–55.
19. Rodvold KA, McConeghy KW. Methicillin-resistant *Staphylococcus aureus* therapy: past, present, and future. Clin Infect Dis 2014;58(Suppl 1):S20–7.
20. Hauser A, Fogarasi S. Periorbital and orbital cellulitis. Pediatr Rev 2010;31(6): 242–9.
21. Ambati BK, Ambati J, Azar N, et al. Periorbital and orbital cellulitis before and after the advent of *Haemophilus influenzae* type B vaccination. Ophthalmology 2000;107:1450–3.
22. Liu IT, Kao SC, Wang AG, et al. Preseptal and orbital cellulitis: a 10-year review of hospitalized patients. J Chin Med Assoc 2006;69:415–22.
23. Blomquist PH. Methicillin-resistant *Staphylococcus aureus* infections of the eye and orbit. Trans Am Ophthalmol Soc 2006;104:322–45.
24. Prentiss KA, Dorfman DH. Pediatric ophthalmology in the emergency department. Emerg Med Clin North Am 2008;26(1):181–98.
25. Pereira FJ, Velasco e Cruz AA, Anselmo-Lima WT, et al. Computed tomographic patterns of orbital cellulitis due to sinusitis. Arq Bras Oftalmol 2006;69:513–8.
26. Al-Nammari S, Roberton B, Ferguson C. Should a child with preseptal periorbital cellulitis be treated with intravenous or oral antibiotics? Emerg Med J 2007;24: 128–9.
27. Howe L, Jones NS. Guidelines for the management of periorbital cellulitis/abscess. Clin Otolaryngol Allied Sci 2004;29(6):725–8.
28. Chaudhry IA, Shamsi FA, Elzaridi E, et al. Outcome of treated orbital cellulitis in a tertiary eye care center in the Middle East. Ophthalmology 2007;114:345–54.
29. Luelmo-Aguilar J, Santandreu MS. Folliculitis: recognition and management. Am J Clin Dermatol 2004;5(5):301–10.
30. Durdu M, Ilkit M. First step in the differential diagnosis of folliculitis: cytology. Crit Rev Microbiol 2013;39(1):9–25.
31. Kundu RV, Patterson S. Dermatologic conditions in skin of color: part II. Disorders occurring predominantly in skin of color. Am Fam Physician 2013;87(12): 859–65.
32. Stevens DL, Bisno AL, Chambers HF, et al, Infectious Diseases Society of America. Practice guidelines for the diagnosis and management of skin and soft-tissue infections. Clin Infect Dis 2005;41:1373–406.
33. Fridkin SK, Hageman JC, Morrison M, et al, Active Bacterial Core Surveillance Program of the Emerging Infections Program Network. Methicillin-resistant *Staphylococcus aureus* disease in three communities. N Engl J Med 2005; 352:1436–44.

34. Meislin HW, Lerner SA, Graves MH, et al. Cutaneous abscesses. Anaerobic and aerobic bacteriology and outpatient management. Ann Intern Med 1977;87: 145–9.
35. Gaspari RJ, Resop D, Mendoza M, et al. A randomized controlled trial of incision and drainage versus ultrasonographically guided needle aspiration for skin abscesses and the effect of methicillin-resistant *Staphylococcus aureus*. Ann Emerg Med 2011;57:483–91.
36. Morgan MS. Diagnosis and management of necrotising fasciitis: a multiparametric approach. J Hosp Infect 2010;75(4):249–57.
37. Wong CH, Khin LW, Heng KS, et al. The LRINEC (Laboratory Risk Indicator for Necrotizing Fasciitis) score: a tool for distinguishing necrotizing fasciitis from other soft tissue infections. Crit Care Med 2004;32:1535–41.
38. Bernal NP, Latenser BA, Born JM, et al. Trends in 393 necrotizing acute soft tissue infection patients 2000-2008. Burns 2012;38:252–60.
39. Vásquez-del-Mercado E, Arenas R, Padilla-Desgarenes C. Sporotrichosis. Clin Dermatol 2012;30(4):437–43.
40. Infectious Diseases Society of America (IDSA). Clinical practice guidelines for management of sporotrichosis: 2007 update by the IDSA. Clin Infect Dis 2007;45(10):1255–65.
41. Higgins EM, Fuller LC, Smith CH. Guidelines for the management of tinea capitis. British Association of Dermatologists. Br J Dermatol 2000;143:53–8.
42. Elewski BE. Tinea capitis: a current perspective. J Am Acad Dermatol 2000;42: 1–24.
43. Möhrenschlager M, Seidl HP, Ring J, et al. Pediatric tinea capitis: recognition and management. Am J Clin Dermatol 2005;6(4):203–13.
44. Pomeranz AJ, Sabnis SS. Tinea capitis: epidemiology, diagnosis, and management strategies. Paediatr Drugs 2002;4(12):779–83.
45. Ely JW, Rosenfeld S, Seabury Stone M. Diagnosis and management of tinea infections. Am Fam Physician 2014;90(10):702–10.
46. Moriarty B, Hay R, Morris-Jones R. The diagnosis and management of tinea. BMJ 2012;345:e4380.
47. Drake LA, Dinehart SM, Farmer ER, et al. Guidelines of care for superficial mycotic infections of the skin: tinea corporis, tinea cruris, tinea faciei, tinea manuum, and tinea pedis. Guidelines/Outcomes Committee. American Academy of Dermatology. J Am Acad Dermatol 1996;34:282–6.
48. Klenk AS, Martin AG, Heffernan MP. Yeast infections: candidiasis, pityriasis (tinea) versicolor. In: Freedberg IM, Eisen AZ, Wolff K, et al, editors. Dermatology in general medicine. New York: McGraw-Hill; 2003. p. 2006.
49. Jautová J, Baloghová J, Dorko E, et al. Cutaneous candidosis in immunosuppressed patients. Folia Microbiol (Praha) 2001;46:359.
50. Yaar M, Gilchrest BA. Aging of skin. In: Freedberg IM, Eisen AZ, Wolff K, et al, editors. Fitzpatrick's dermatology in general medicine. New York: McGraw-Hill; 2003. p. 1386.
51. Kalra MG, Higgins KE, Kinney BS. Intertrigo and secondary skin infections. Am Fam Physician 2014;89(7):569–73.
52. Sobera JO, Elewski BE. Fungal diseases. In: Bolognia JL, Jorizzo JL, Rapini RP, editors. Dermatology. London: Mosby; 2003. p. 1171.
53. Scherwitz C. Ultrastructure of human cutaneous candidosis. J Invest Dermatol 1982;78:200.
54. Mistiaen P, van Halm-Walters M. Prevention and treatment of intertrigo in large skin folds of adults: a systematic review. BMC Nurs 2010;9:12.

55. Guitart J, Woodley DT. Intertrigo: a practical approach. Compr Ther 1994;20: 402.
56. Hay RJ. The management of superficial candidiasis. J Am Acad Dermatol 1999; 40:S35.
57. Sundaram SV, Srinivas CR, Thirumurthy M. Candidal intertrigo; treatment with filter paper soaked in Castellani's paint. Indian J Dermatol Venereol Leprol 2006; 72:386.
58. Cramer DW, Liberman RF, Titus-Ernstoff L, et al. Gential talc exposure and risk of ovarian cancer. Int J Cancer 1999;81:351.
59. Gupta AK. Systemic antifungal agents. In: Wolverton SE, editor. Comprehensive dermatologic drug therapy. Philadelphia: W.B. Saunders; 2001. p. 55.
60. Pierard GE, Arrese JE, De Doncker P. Antifungal activity of terbinafine and itraconazole in human stratium corneum; a comparative study. J Am Acad Dermatol 1995;32:429.
61. Daning L, Dinguo Z, Wenwei S, et al. Extensive skin candidosis in an adult; effective treatment with itraconazole. Mycoses 1998;41:219.
62. Stengel F, Robles-Soto M, Galimberti R, et al. Fluconazole versus ketoconazole in the treatment of dermatophytoses and cutaneous candidiasis. Int J Dermatol 1994;33(10):726–9.
63. American Academy of Pediatrics. Antimicrobial agents and related therapy. In: Pickering LK, editor. Red book: 2009 report of the committee on infectious diseases. 28th edition. Elk Grove Village (IL): American Academy of Pediatrics; 2009. p. 73.
64. Available at: https://www.fda.gov/Drugs/DrugSafety/ucm500597.htm. Accessed February 16, 2018.
65. Friedlander SF, Rueda M, Chen BK, et al. Fungal, protozoal, and helminthic infections. In: Schachner LA, Hansen RC, editors. Pediatric dermatology. Edinburgh (Scotland): Mosby; 2003. p. 1093.
66. Klunk C, Domingues E, Wiss K. An update on diaper dermatitis. Clin Dermatol 2014;32:477.
67. Arnsmeier SL, Paller AS. Getting to the bottom of diaper dermatitis. Contemp Pediatr 1997;14:115.
68. Eichenfield LF, Bogen ML. Absorption and efficacy of miconazole nitrate 0.25% ointment in infants with diaper dermatitis. J Drugs Dermatol 2007;6:522.
69. Bonifaz A, Tirado-Sánchez A, Graniel MJ, et al. The efficacy and safety of sertaconazole cream (2%) in diaper dermatitis candidiasis. Mycopathologia 2013;175:249.
70. Gupta AK, Foley KA. Antifungal treatment for pityriasis versicolor. J Fungi (Basel) 2015;1(1):13–29.
71. Nenoff P1, Krüger C, Mayser P. Cutaneous *Malassezia* infections and *Malassezia* associated dermatoses: an update. Hautarzt 2015;66(6):465–84 [quiz: 485–6].
72. Gaitanis G, Velegraki A, Alexopoulos EC, et al. Distribution of *Malassezia* species in pityriasis versicolor and seborrhoeic dermatitis in Greece. Typing of the major pityriasis versicolor isolate *M. globosa*. Br J Dermatol 2006;154(5): 854–9.
73. Gupta AK, Batra R, Bluhm R, et al. Pityriasis versicolor. Dermatol Clin 2003; 21(3):413–29, v–vi.
74. Hu SW, Bigby M. Pityriasis versicolor: a systematic review of interventions. Arch Dermatol 2010;146(10):1132–40.

75. Glogau R, Hanna L, Jawetz E. Herpetic whitlow as part of genital virus infection. J Infect Dis 1977;136:689.
76. Freeman ML, Sheridan BS, Bonneau RH, et al. Psychological stress compromises CD8+ T cell control of latent herpes simplex virus type 1 infections. J Immunol 2007;179(1):322–8.
77. Walker LG, Simmons BP, Lovallo JL. Pediatric herpetic hand infections. J Hand Surg Am 1990;15:176.
78. Szinnai G, Schaad UB, Heininger U. Multiple herpetic Whitlow lesions in a 4 year old girl: case report and review of the literature. Eur J Pediatr 2001;160:528.
79. Corey L. Laboratory diagnosis of herpes simplex virus infections. Principles guiding the development of rapid diagnostic tests. Diagn Microbiol Infect Dis 1986;4:111S.
80. Workowski KA, Bolan GA. Centers for Disease Control and Prevention. Sexually transmitted diseases treatment guidelines, 2015. MMWR Recomm Rep 2015;64:1.
81. Heslop R, Roberts H, Flower D, et al. Interventions for men and women with their first episode of genital herpes. Cochrane Database Syst Rev 2016;(8):CD010684.
82. Chi C, Wang S, Delamere FM, et al. Interventions for prevention of herpes simplex labialis (cold sores on the lips). Cochrane Database Syst Rev 2015;(8):CD010095.
83. Rooney JF, Straus SE, Mannix ML, et al. Oral acyclovir to suppress frequently recurrent herpes labialis. A double-blind, placebo-controlled trial. Ann Intern Med 1993;118:268.
84. Baker D, Eisen D. Valacyclovir for prevention of recurrent herpes labialis: 2 double-blind, placebo-controlled studies. Cutis 2003;71(3):239–42.
85. Cassuto J. Topical local anaesthetics and herpes simplex. Lancet 1989;1(8629): 100–1.
86. Opstelten W, Neven AK, Eekhof J. Treatment and prevention of herpes labialis. Can Fam Physician 2008;54(12):1683–7.
87. Lopez AS1, Burnett-Hartman A, Nambiar R, et al. Transmission of a newly characterized strain of varicella-zoster virus from a patient with herpes zoster in a long-term-care facility, West Virginia, 2004. J Infect Dis 2008;197(5):646–53.
88. Heininger U, Seward JF. Varicella. Lancet 2006;368:1365.
89. Kesson AM, Grimwood K, Burgess MA, et al. Acyclovir for the prevention and treatment of varicella zoster in children, adolescents and pregnancy. J Paediatr Child Health 1996;32:211.
90. Wood MJ, Kay R, Dworkin RH, et al. Oral acyclovir therapy accelerates pain resolution in patients with herpes zoster: a meta-analysis of placebo-controlled trials. Clin Infect Dis 1996;22(2):341–7.
91. Miller GG, Dummer JS. Herpes simplex and varicella zoster viruses: forgotten but not gone. Am J Transplant 2007;7:741.
92. Dworkin RH, Johnson RW, Breur J, et al. Recommendations for the management of herpes zoster. Clin Infect Dis 2007;44(Suppl 1):S1.
93. Chen N, Li Q, Yang J, et al. Antiviral treatment for preventing postherpetic neuralgia. Cochrane Database Syst Rev 2014;(2):CD006866.
94. Sampathkumar P, Drage LA, Martin DP. Herpes zoster (shingles) and postherpetic neuralgia. Mayo Clin Proc 2009;84(3):274–80.
95. Lee EG, Lee HJ, Hyun DJ, et al. Efficacy of low dose gabapentin in acute herpes zoster for preventing postherpetic neuralgia: a prospective controlled study. Dermatol Ther 2016;29:184–90.

96. van der Wouden JC, van der Sande R, Kruithof EJ, et al. Interventions for cutaneous molluscum contagiosum. Cochrane Database Syst Rev 2017;(5):CD004767.
97. Dohil MA, Lin P, Lee J, et al. The epidemiology of molluscum contagiousum in children. J Am Acad Dermatol 2006;54:47.
98. Zhang Q1, Davis JC, Lamborn IT, et al. Combined immunodeficiency associated with DOCK8 mutations. N Engl J Med 2009;361(21):2046–55.
99. Braue A, Ross G, Varigos G, et al. Epidemiology and impact of childhood molluscum contagiosum: a case series and critical review of the literature. Pediatr Dermatol 2005;22:287.
100. Brown J, Janniger CK, Schwartz RA, et al. Childhood molluscum contagiousum. Int J Dermatol 2006;45:93.
101. Osio A, Deslandes E, Saada V, et al. Clinical characteristics of molluscum contagiosum in children in a private dermatology practice in the greater Paris area, France: a prospective study in 661 patients. Dermatology 2011;222:314.
102. Stock I. Molluscum contagiosum–a common but poorly understood "childhood disease" and sexually transmitted illness. Med Monatsschr Pharm 2013;36(8): 282–90.
103. Saguil A, Mercada M, Lauters R. Herpes zoster and postherpetic neuralgia: prevention and management. Am Fam Physician 2017;96(10):656–63.
104. Forbat E, Al-Niaimi F, Ali FR. Molluscum contagiosum: review and update on management. Pediatr Dermatol 2017;34(5):504–15.
105. Silverberg NB1, Sidbury R, Mancini AJ. Childhood molluscum contagiosum: experience with cantharidin therapy in 300 patients. J Am Acad Dermatol 2000;43(3):503–7.
106. Barbosa P. Plantar verrucae and HIV infection. Clin Podiatr Med Surg 1998;15: 317.
107. Bae JM, Kang H, Kim HO, et al. Differential diagnosis of plantar wart from corn, callus, and headed ward with the aid of dermoscopy. Br J Dermatol 2009;160: 220.
108. Sterling JC, Gibbs S, Haque Hussain SS, et al. British Association of Dermatologists' guidelines for the management of cutaneous warts 2014. Br J Dermatol 2014;171(4):696–712.
109. Kwok CS, Gibbs S, Bennett C, et al. Topical treatments for cutaneous warts. Cochrane Database Syst Rev 2012;(9):CD001781.
110. Mistrangelo M, Dal Conte I, Volpatto S, et al. Current treatments for anal condylomata acuminata. Minerva Chir 2018;73(1):100–6.
111. Yanofsky VR, Patel RV, Goldenberg G. Genital warts: a comprehensive review. J Clin Aesthet Dermatol 2012;5(6):25–36.
112. Grillo Ardila CF, Angel-Müller E, Salazar-Díaz LC, et al. Imiquimod for anogenital warts in non-immunocompromised adults. Cochrane Database Syst Rev 2014;(11):CD010389.
113. Bertolotti A, Dupin N, Bouscarat F, et al. Cryotherapy to treat anogenital warts in nonimmunocompromised adults: systematic review and meta-analysis. J Am Acad Dermatol 2017;77(3):518–26.

Urinary Tract Infection Antibiotic Resistance in the United States

Thomas A. Waller, MD*, Sally Ann L. Pantin, MD, Ashley L. Yenior, MD, George G.A. Pujalte, MD

KEYWORDS

- Urinary tract infection (UTI) • Antibiotic resistance
- Uropathogenic *Escherichia coli* (UPEC) • Recurrent UTI

KEY POINTS

- In the United States, there are more than 8 million office visits for urinary tract infection (UTI) each year.
- Patients often present with "classic symptoms" of dysuria and increased frequency, but many often present as asymptomatic or with a mixed picture.
- Antibiotic resistance is a worldwide problem that has developed due to some degree from overprescribing of the medications.
- Prescribers should be aware of the most common bacteria causing UTIs and their propensity for resistance.
- Antibiotic stewardship programs have been designed to help encourage proper recognition and treatment of infections.

INTRODUCTION

Urinary tract infection (UTI) is one of the most common conditions in both outpatient and inpatient settings worldwide, where it has been noted to affect 150 million people annually.[1] In the United States, there are more than 8 million office visits each year.[1–3] Although most patients suffer only with a varying range of painful and annoying symptoms, the Centers for Disease Control and Prevention (CDC) reports that UTIs contribute to 13,000 deaths every year.[4]

A UTI is commonly associated with women,[5] because as many as 50% will likely be affected in their lifetime, and they are approximately 6 times more likely to be affected than men.[6] Although most UTIs resolve with treatment, almost 30% of women will

Disclosure Statement: The authors have nothing to disclose.
Department of Family Medicine, Mayo Clinic Florida, 4500 San Pablo Road, Jacksonville, FL 32224, USA
* Corresponding author.
E-mail address: Waller.thomas@mayo.edu

Prim Care Clin Office Pract 45 (2018) 455–466
https://doi.org/10.1016/j.pop.2018.05.005

have a recurrence and more than 20% will suffer with multiple recurrences.[7] For hospitalized patients or those in long-term care facilities with any infection, the urinary tract is frequently the setting.[8]

Because they are so common, UTIs and their associated urinary symptoms are frequently recognized by patients, who have also learned that it often takes an antibiotic to resolve the condition. This has led to many patients seeking treatment at the presence of almost any urinary symptom. Although treatment is often necessary, this can contribute to an increased use of empiric treatment and sometimes overtreatment of symptoms. Nearly 15% of all prescribed antibiotics are for the treatment of UTI.[9]

It was almost the twentieth century before physicians realized that bacteria were causing UTIs.[10] Numerous chemotherapeutic agents were tried and were unsuccessful.[10] Although penicillin was discovered in 1928 and was effective for many infectious diseases, it was not active against *Escherichia coli*.[10] In 1953, nitrofurantoin became available and was the preferred treatment for *E coli* UTI for many years.[10] Later when amoxicillin and trimethoprim/sulfamethoxazole (TMP-SMZ) were released, their overuse led to bacterial resistance against them.[10]

Global antibiotic use for UTI has led to resistant bacteria in both outpatient clinics and inpatient hospitals.[11,12] There are many bacteria that can cause UTIs, but the most common include *E coli, Klebsiella pneumoniae, Enterococcus* sp., and *Staphylococcus saprophyticus*.[3] These bacteria are capable of developing resistance, and the ability to eliminate these bacteria with antibiotics has declined over time. The Food and Drug Administration has been seeking the development of new antibiotics to combat bacterial resistance.[4,12]

One of the first steps in helping to reduce antibiotic resistance is to accurately diagnose a UTI. Although Hippocrates may have had to drink urine to evaluate the body's status,[13] we have several more accurate tests available today; however, there are varying methods practitioners often use to reach the diagnosis of UTI. Frequently, a urine culture is not performed to identify the bacterial organism. Other times, patients are treated based simply on their report of classic UTI symptoms. Although this possibly may save time and money, this practice may be contributing to further resistance due to the susceptibility traits of the bacteria. More rapid antimicrobial susceptibility reporting would be helpful.[1]

Antibiotic resistance has led to significant challenges in treating UTI. There are more than 12,000 deaths per year from UTIs and, if the patient has bacteremia, the mortality rate can be more than 9%.[4] Short of death, patients can suffer with pyelonephritis, recurrent infections, renal disease in the young, preterm birth, and even *Clostridium difficile* colitis from antibiotic use.[14] At a minimum, it is a significant, painful illness, which can have an impact on a patient's daily life and the patient's ability to be productive in society.

URINARY TRACT INFECTION SYMPTOMS

UTIs can typically be categorized into upper or lower maladies based on symptoms alone. The lower UTIs, like cystitis, prostatitis, or urethritis, generally present with dysuria and increased urinary frequency, whereas fever and flank or costovertebral angle pain is associated with an upper UTI, like pyelonephritis.[15] Additional signs of UTI include gross hematuria, new or worsening incontinence, odiferous urine, and suprapubic pain.[16,17] Nonspecific symptoms can range from anorexia, change in mental status, fatigue, and weakness.[18] Of note, vaginal discharge lessens the likelihood of a diagnosis of UTI.[16,17]

Less classic symptoms of UTI may present particularly in unique populations. For example, poor appetite, inability to mount a fever, confusion, and fatigue may be seen in the elderly.[8] In addition, several risk factors may alter or increase the frequency of symptoms and their presentation, including a suppressed immune system, as in diabetes mellitus, recent sexual activity, use of a spermicide, antecedent antibiotic use, and conditions leading to restricted urinary outflow.[17]

TESTING

In the office, differentiating between asymptomatic bacteriuria, symptomatic UTI, recurrent UTI, or a UTI that will develop progress into urosepsis is critical.[18] This challenge is more difficult if the patient presents only with nonspecific symptoms, such as back pain or fever,[19] and the failure to properly delineate these patients can lead to prescribing inappropriately.

Table 1 outlines the currently available tests on the market. Urine dipstick analysis remains the test of choice at the point-of-care due to its ease of use and its ability to detect nitrites.[2] However, remember that the nitrites are converted from the naturally occurring urinary nitrates by enteric bacteria.[21] Thus, among the common uropathogens, it may miss the presence of *Candida*, *Pseudomonas* species, *Enterococci*, or *S saprophyticus*. The urine dipstick can also detect leukocyte esterase as an indirect test of pyuria.[20,21] However, the test can produce a false-positive result in the presence of bladder tumors, contamination of the urine sample with bacteria from the vagina, as well as chlamydia urethritis.[20]

In the setting of a primary care practice, the absence of leukocyte esterase and nitrites on the dipstick has been shown sensitive (up to 90%) to exclude the presence of UTI; however, due to the low specificity, a positive reaction for either or both should be confirmed with a culture.[23]

Table 1
Methods of testing available on the market

Test	Comments	Sensitivity[a] (95% CI)	Specificity[a] (95% CI)
Gram stain microscopy	Rapid detection	Bacteriuria is more sensitive than pyuria on urine dip stick[a]	Bacteriuria is more specific than pyuria on urine dip stick[a]
Urine dipstick analysis[b]	Quick Inexpensive		
NIT	Intensity of reagent color may diminish with proteinuria and glycosuria	0.48 (0.40–0.57)	0.93 (0.87–0.98)
LE		0.64 (0.56–0.74)	0.73 (0.63–0.85)
NIT and LE (one or both positive)		0.80 (0.76–0.86)	0.80 (0.76–0.84)
Urine analysis	Microscopic counts of:		
	Leukocytes	68.3%	87.8%
	Bacteria	78.8%	97.8%
Urine culture[c]	Gold standard Up to 48 h incubation needed Blood and MacConkey agar most common supplement	94%	50%–70%

Abbreviations: CI, confidence interval; LE, leukocyte esterase; NIT, nitrite.
[a] Particularly in the elderly and pregnant women.[2]
[b] Roche Diagnostics, Chemstrip-10 or Siemens Multistix 10.[20–23]
[c] Colony counts of 10^5 colony-forming units/mL.

Urine culture remains the gold standard for the diagnosis of UTI, despite the need for 2 to 3 days to allow for growth and susceptibility testing.[2]

Although urine microscopy is often overlooked, it allows for rapid detection of bacteria, fungi, and parasites.[4] It is more sensitive and specific in detecting a true infection than simply pyuria on urine dipstick, especially in the elderly and those who are pregnant.[2]

EMERGING TESTS

Several emerging tests could make bacterial identification a faster and simpler process.

- Polymerase chain reaction can rapidly amplify the nucleic material when dealing with multiple organisms and allow for quick DNA identification[20,22]
- Isothermal microcalorimetry can identify bacteria by recognizing the amount of heat they produce[22]
- Enzyme-linked immunosorbent assays evaluate for the presence of specific antigens[22]
- DNA biosensor-based detection for rapid identification of uropathogens[22]

DIAGNOSIS

Because of the high number of antibiotics dispensed for UTIs, it is essential to correctly diagnose the infection.[17] Using clinical findings only, UTIs are incorrectly diagnosed in a third of cases.[17] A recent review of prescribing patterns in primary care revealed that antibiotic use for UTI appeared to be appropriate only 75% of the time. For other common conditions, including gastroenteritis, cough, sore throat, and otitis media, even with prescribing guidelines available, antibiotic use appeared appropriate only 10% to 13% of the time.[24]

To diagnose a UTI, a patient should have 2 or more symptoms and a positive result on an objective test such as a urine culture or urine dipstick.[18] A urine culture is preferred because the amount of bacterial burden can be calculated.[17] Along with UTI symptoms, a positive nitrite on a urine dipstick, which has an estimated positive predictive value of more than 95%, can be used to begin empiric therapy.[15] If the patient is asymptomatic and a urine dipstick is negative, there is a low likelihood of a UTI.[18] Most asymptomatic patients with bacteriuria will not require treatment, as it is most often due to colonization only.[18]

There remains room for improvement in the diagnosis of UTI, as the combination of symptom assessment and objective testing have a less than ideal sensitivity and specificity. These clinical inconsistencies can often lead to inappropriately prescribed antibiotics[25]; however, there are several diagnostic modalities that are being researched[26] that could lead to the improved use of antibiotics,[27] and thus possibly prevent antibiotic resistance. For example, immunotherapy[26] and immune signaling[28] both may lead to the use of a patient's genome to diagnose and individualize UTI treatment.[28] Also, inflammasomes, which are part of our natural defense system and can lead to an infected cell's death, could be a potential way to detect and eliminate UTIs without the use of antibiotics altogether.[29]

PREVALENCE AND IDENTITY OF UROPATHOGENS

The microbes responsible for UTIs are similar across the world in both advanced and developing nations. Although both gram-positive and gram-negative organisms can produce UTIs, gram-negative bacteria are, by far, the most prevalent.

They include *E coli*, *Proteus mirabilis*, *Pseudomonas aeruginosa*, *K pneumoniae*, *Klebsiella oxytoca*, *Salmonella paratyphi*, *Citrobacter freundii*, *Vibrio cholera*, *Serratia marcescens*, and *Providencia stuartii*. Uropathogenic *E coli* (UPEC) are the source for more than 75% of all routine UTIs and catheter-associated UTIs.[4,5] These bacteria have developed unique methods of survival and resistance to persist in the urinary system. Unfortunately, UPEC continue to show increased resistance to fluoroquinolones and TMP-SMZ around the world, making these drugs less effective for empiric treatment.[9]

WHAT MAKES RESISTANCE HAPPEN?

Recent data suggest that the normal, healthy bladder is not always sterile, and a complete picture of the urinary microbiome is only recently emerging.[5] The bacterial community within the human body can be markedly affected by even brief exposure to antibiotics, and their use can give rise to resistant pathogens and even symbiotic organisms. Antibiotic resistance can lead to increased patient morbidity, treatment, hospitalization, and the use of broad-spectrum antibiotics.[30]

On average, it takes only approximately 3 years of use for antibiotic resistance to be detected. Antibiotics will generally produce a "fitness cost" on bacteria, such as slowing their growth rate, but the bacteria can quickly develop mechanisms to compensate. Although all bacteria are capable of developing resistance, further study has suggested that the antibiotic resistance can be reversed if the antibiotic is removed from the environment.[31] The resistant bacteria are often hard to identify by routine susceptibility tests and have exceptional potential to cause outbreaks.[1]

One of the most important causes of antibiotic-resistant UTIs is prior antibiotic use for any condition. A recent retrospective study of young children showed a higher risk of UTI with a resistant organism if they had taken amoxicillin in the preceding 30 or 60 days, although not in those who had not received amoxicillin in more than 60 days.[32]

Other ways bacteria adapt and resist antibiotics include the following: the active removal of the drug by effluence pumps, which lower the intracellular concentration; inactivation or degradation of the antibiotic; modification of the bacterial cell wall, which prevents the antibiotic from recognizing its target site; and biofilm formation in which a community of bacteria work together to develop resistance.[33] Many of these mechanisms of drug resistance in bacteria are still being studied.[1]

Resistance may also be due to genetic factors, such as changes in the bacterial genome, which can result from mutations to chromosomal target genes and acquisition of foreign resistance genes.[30] Also, many bacterial strains have plasmid material that can produce extended-spectrum beta-lactamases (ESBLs), which allow intrinsic resistance to antibiotics like trimethoprim, fluoroquinolones, cephalosporins, and aminoglycosides.[34] Although these ESBLs are able to hydrolyze antibiotics, like third-generation and fourth-generation cephalosporins, they are routinely inhibited by clavulanic acid, sulbactam, and tazobactam. The ESBLs represent a public health concern because of the high prevalence in *E coli* in the community. Notably, in the 2 past decades of the past century, ESBL-positive strains were mainly confined to the hospital setting where they were responsible for nosocomial outbreaks. Since 2000, these strains have become prevalent in the outpatient setting.[9]

It has been suggested that resistant bacteria can survive between the minimum inhibitory concentration (MIC) and the mutant prevention concentration of antibiotics, which are the levels needed to prevent growth or limit the development of resistant organisms, respectively.[35,36] To close this "gap," antibiotics with adequate urinary kinetics should be used. This means using drugs that exceed the MIC of uropathogens at the appropriate dose and for an appropriate duration.[37]

TREATMENT

Once it is determined that the patient has a UTI and if it is consistent with a complicated or uncomplicated cystitis or pyelonephritis, then an antibiotic can be selected.[38] It is imperative to be familiar with the local causative bacteria and local patterns of susceptibility when considering treatment.[39] The Infectious Diseases Society of America in collaboration with the European Society for Microbiology and Infectious Diseases has established treatment guidelines for nonpregnant, premenopausal women with uncomplicated cystitis, in the absence of other comorbid conditions and urologic abnormalities.[38] **Table 2** outlines the most commonly recommended treatment choices for uncomplicated cystitis and pyelonephritis.

Resistance to commonly used antibiotics, including fluoroquinolones, is now prevalent in many strains of *E coli*. Therefore, fluoroquinolones should not be used for empirical therapy of serious complicated UTIs (cUTIs), especially when patients have an increased risk of having resistant organisms, such as recent antibiotic use. For mild, lower cUTIs, nitrofurantoin and TMP-SMZ can still be used empirically, depending on local resistance patterns. Serious cUTIs should be treated empirically with broad-spectrum antibiotics, such as carbapenems or piperacillin-tazobactam. Once specific bacteria and their susceptibilities are known, treatment should be adjusted.[47]

RECURRENT URINARY TRACT INFECTIONS

There are few things more challenging in the clinic then recurrent UTIs, and they are diagnosed when patients suffer at least 3 infections in a year, or 2 in a 6-month period.[33,48] Often this condition results from the increasing number of resistant bacteria that are not completely eradicated with the typical antibiotic therapy.[29] In addition, it is common to find the same strains of bacteria (as per the susceptibility report) causing the recurrent cases as well.[48] Although premenopausal women can develop recurrent infections, most are found in the postmenopausal period mostly due to the lack of estrogen.[48]

It is vital to obtain a thorough history and physical examination. The importance of sitting and taking time to listen to these patients cannot be emphasized enough. Consider the number and timing of infections, menopausal status, sexual history, and recent antibiotic use.[49] The presentation is usually similar to any other UTI, but often the patients are able to recognize the symptoms earlier. A urine culture is recommended to not only properly identify the bacteria and its susceptibilities but to also feel confident that the patient is correctly able to identify its presence. Look for repeating susceptibility patterns and antibiotic choices should be chosen accordingly. A repeat urine culture after treatment can help to confirm clearance of the bacteria.[33]

If the urine is cleared, then the clinician should consider further steps to possibly prevent further recurrence. Make efforts to reduce risk factors such as vaginal atrophy or behavior modifications, including sexual practices, spermicide use, and possibly obesity.[49] The choice and frequency of antibiotic use should be individualized for each patient and include long-term prophylactic antibiotic regimens, postcoital prophylactic antibiotics, or patient-initiated antibiotics for reliable patients.[14,48–50] The patient-initiated approach can reduce office visits and overall cost, but it can lead to higher rates of resistance.[48] A 3-day course of antibiotics

Table 2
Antibiotics for uncomplicated cystitis and pyelonephritis

Drug	Dose	Resistance Notes	Notable Precautions
Nitrofurantoin	100 mg BID × 5 d for cystitis[40]	No increase in 10 y, up to 92.2% susceptibility.[41,42]	Risk for peripheral neuropathy in diabetic patients and renal impairment
Fosfomycin	3 g mixed in water, single dose for cystitis	Strong susceptibility remains worldwide, up to 98.9%.[42,43]	Use with caution in *Clostridium difficile*–susceptible patients
Trimethoprim-sulfamethoxazole	800 mg/160 mg twice daily for 3 d if uncomplicated cystitis or 14 d if acute pyelonephritis	Resistance has increased to >20% in United States. It should not be used empirically unless local resistance patterns are known, but still good if culture reveals susceptibility.[39,44]	Severe dermatologic reactions possible
Fluoroquinolones	Cipro 250 mg BID or Levaquin 500 mg daily for 3 d for cystitis; Cipro 500 mg BID for 7 d or Levaquin 750 mg for 5 d for pyelonephritis	Reserve for patients with no alternative choices. Resistance has increased to 11.8% and even higher in the inpatient setting.[44,45]	Tendon rupture
Amoxicillin-clavulanate	875 mg BID for 5–7 d for cystitis; 10–14 d for pyelonephritis	Although resistance is only approximately 4%, these medications should be used as second line due to reported treatment failures.[39,44]	Dose adjustments for renal disease
Cephalosporins	Ceftriaxone 1–2 g IV every 24 h for 7–14 d for pyelonephritis only	Although susceptibility is near 90%, considered second line as ESBL organisms developing significant resistance and the overall impact on the microbiome.[46]	Diarrhea and allergic reactions

Abbreviations: BID, twice a day; ESBL, extended-spectrum beta-lactamase; IV, intravenous.

has been shown to be effective.[48] Postcoital and continuous antibiotic recommendations are outlined in **Table 3**. Optimal antibiotic choice for either approach not conclusive.[51]

Due to increasing resistance rates, several nonantibiotic treatment options have been researched, but the evidence is limited.[50] Cranberry products at 500 mg twice

Table 3
Antibiotic prophylaxis for recurrent urinary tract infections

Antimicrobial Prophylaxis	Comments
Postcoital antimicrobial (single dose): • TMP-SMX single strength • Nitrofurantoin 50–100 mg	TMP-SMZ reduced incidence rate to 0.3.[51,52]
Daily antimicrobial: • TMP-SMX single strength • Nitrofurantoin 50–100 mg • Fosfomycin 3g every 10 d[53]	Start with 3–6 mo trial, then repeat culture; 95% reduced rates of infection.[51] Rates of resistance have been shown to increase after just 1 mo, but improve after cessation.[54]

Abbreviation: TMP-SMX, trimethoprim/sulfamethoxazole.

daily have been shown to reduce the recurrence in approximately one-third of patients, but the cranberry is inferior to TMP-SMZ 480 mg once daily.[55] Other treatments under investigation include intravaginal probiotics,[56,57] vaccinations, and D-mannose.[49] In pediatric patients with a history of recurrent UTI, daily use of cranberry juice was shown to reduce the rate of pediatric nonfebrile UTIs by 65%.[58]

BACTERIAL RESISTANCE IN HIGH-RISK POPULATIONS

Several groups of people are at higher risk of developing significant UTIs. Due to glucose increasing bacterial development,[4] diabetic patients may actually present with pyelonephritis or other complications of UTI.[59] All types of catheterized patients are at higher risk, but intermittent catheters have a reduced rate of UTI compared with long-term tubes placed after surgery.[60] Long-term care facility residents often have reduced mobility and the ability to communicate or recognize symptoms.[61] Renal transplant patients are often immunocompromised and may have other predisposing urinary outflow issues.[59] Patients with spinal cord injury often have neurogenic bladder with reduced function.[62,63]

Many of the classic symptoms of UTI may be not present in these individuals.[62] In most cases, immediate treatment with antibiotics for 7 to 14 days is likely the best approach, as opposed to a wait-and-see plan.[64] Although the latter will likely reduce complications, such as sepsis or long-term damage, it of course can contribute to the development of resistance.[63]

PROPHYLAXIS IN INFANTS

When having to make an informed decision about the use of antibiotic prophylaxis, particularly in infants younger than 24 months, with underling renal malformations, consider alternatives to amoxicillin, trimethoprim, and cephalosporins, as these have shown variable resistance in the most common isolate, *E coli*. Other bacteria found in positive infant urine cultures include *Klebsiella* sp, *Enterococcus* sp, *Proteus* sp, and *Pseudomonas* sp.[65]

PREGNANCY

In pregnancy, treatment with appropriate antibiotics of bacteriuria with a colony count $\geq$100,000 colony-forming units per milliliter is standard of care.[66] In the case of pregnant women with Group B streptococcal bacteriuria, treatment should be initiated at labor or rupture of membranes with intravenous antibiotics.

ANTIBIOTIC STEWARDSHIP

It is imperative that health care providers strive to make good choices with antibiotic selection and confirm patient compliance with the treatment regimen. As discussed previously, antibiotic use for many common conditions seen every day in primary care, even with prescribing algorithms or guidelines, has much room for improvement.[24] All physicians should seek out their local resistance patterns by accessing the antibiograms typically created by the local hospital. Although these reports are typically from inpatient data, they can provide an insight to local trends. One may also access the CDC Web site to review national trends in antibiotic resistance.

The goal of antimicrobial stewardship programs are to reduce multidrug-resistant bacteria by improving the awareness of the problem and helping clinicians make smart choices with antibiotic prescribing.[67] These programs promote the following[56]:

- Avoid screening asymptomatic patients, unless pregnant or preparing for urologic surgery
- Choose empiric treatment based on your local antibiogram resistance profiles
- Obtain urine cultures in cUTI, so that the treatment can be adjusted with antibiotic sensitivities
- Use shortened treatment duration for cystitis and those with nonrecurrent UTI
- For recurrent uncomplicated UTIs, avoid antibiotics if possible. First try preventive measures, such as behavioral modification, cranberry extract, topical estrogens for atrophic vaginitis, or probiotics that may benefit the urinary system

REFERENCES

1. Khoshnood S, Heidary M, Mirnejad R, et al. Drug-resistant gram-negative uropathogens: a review. Biomed Pharmacother 2017;94:982–94.
2. Chu CM, Lowder JL. Diagnosis and treatment of urinary tract infections across age groups. Am J Obstet Gynecol 2018. [Epub ahead of print].
3. Flores-Mireles AL, Walker JN, Caparon M, et al. Urinary tract infections: epidemiology, mechanisms of infection and treatment options. Nat Rev Microbiol 2015; 13(5):269–84.
4. Kumar MS, Das AP. Emerging nanotechnology based strategies for diagnosis and therapeutics of urinary tract infections: a review. Adv Colloid Interface Sci 2017;249:53–65.
5. McLellan LK, Hunstad DA. Urinary tract infection: pathogenesis and outlook. Trends Mol Med 2016;22(11):946–57.
6. Best J, Kitlowski AD, Ou D, et al. Diagnosis and management of urinary tract infections in the emergency department. Emerg Med Pract 2014;16(7):1–23 [quiz 23–4].
7. Flower A, Wang LQ, Lewith G, et al. Chinese herbal medicine for treating recurrent urinary tract infections in women. Cochrane Database Syst Rev 2015;(6):CD010446.
8. Matthews SJ, Lancaster JW. Urinary tract infections in the elderly population. Am J Geriatr Pharmacother 2011;9(5):286–309.
9. Mazzariol A, Bazaj A, Cornaglia G. Multi-drug-resistant gram-negative bacteria causing urinary tract infections: a review. J Chemother 2017;29(sup1):2–9.
10. Curtis N. Management of urinary tract infections: historical perspective and current strategies: part 1—before antibiotics. J Urol 2005;173(1):21–6.
11. Kullar R, Wagenlehner FM, Popejoy MW, et al. Does moderate renal impairment affect clinical outcomes in complicated intra-abdominal and complicated urinary

tract infections? Analysis of two randomized controlled trials with ceftolozane/tazobactam. J Antimicrob Chemother 2017;72(3):900–5.

12. Majeed A, Alarfaj S, Darouiche R, et al. An update on emerging therapies for urinary tract infections. Expert Opin Emerg Drugs 2017;22(1):53–62.
13. Kouba E, Wallen EM, Pruthi RS. Uroscopy by Hippocrates and Theophilus: prognosis versus diagnosis. J Urol 2007;177(1):50–2.
14. O'Brien VP, Hannan TJ, Nielsen HV, et al. Drug and vaccine development for the treatment and prevention of urinary tract infections. Microbiol Spectr 2016;4(1).
15. Masajtis-Zagajewska A, Nowicki M. New markers of urinary tract infection. Clin Chim Acta 2017;471:286–91.
16. Gupta K, Trautner B. In the clinic. Urinary tract infection. Ann Intern Med 2012; 156(5). ITC3-1-ITC3-15.
17. Schmiemann G, Kniehl E, Gebhardt K, et al. The diagnosis of urinary tract infection: a systematic review. Dtsch Arztebl Int 2010;107(21):361–7.
18. Mody L, Juthani-Mehta M. Urinary tract infections in older women: a clinical review. JAMA 2014;311(8):844–54.
19. Cortes-Penfield NW, Trautner BW, Jump RLP. Urinary tract infection and asymptomatic bacteriuria in older adults. Infect Dis Clin North Am 2017;31(4):673–88.
20. Mambatta AK, Jayarajan J, Rashme VL, et al. Reliability of dipstick assay in predicting urinary tract infection. J Family Med Prim Care 2015;4(2):265–8.
21. Semeniuk H, Church D. Evaluation of the leukocyte esterase and nitrite urine dipstick screening tests for detection of bacteriuria in women with suspected uncomplicated urinary tract infections. J Clin Microbiol 1999;37(9):3051–2.
22. Kumar MS, Ghosh S, Nayak S, et al. Recent advances in biosensor based diagnosis of urinary tract infection. Biosens Bioelectron 2016;80:497–510.
23. Deville WL, Yzermans JC, van Duijn NP, et al. The urine dipstick test useful to rule out infections. A meta-analysis of the accuracy. BMC Urol 2004;4:4.
24. Smith DRM, Dolk FCK, Pouwels KB, et al. Defining the appropriateness and inappropriateness of antibiotic prescribing in primary care. J Antimicrob Chemother 2018;73(suppl_2):ii11–8.
25. Holm A, Cordoba G, Sørensen TM, et al. Point of care susceptibility testing in primary care—does it lead to a more appropriate prescription of antibiotics in patients with uncomplicated urinary tract infections? Protocol for a randomized controlled trial. BMC Fam Pract 2015;16:106.
26. Godaly G, Ambite I, Puthia M, et al. Urinary tract infection molecular mechanisms and clinical translation. Pathogens 2016;5(1) [pii:E24].
27. Tchesnokova V, Avagyan H, Rechkina E, et al. Bacterial clonal diagnostics as a tool for evidence-based empiric antibiotic selection. PLoS One 2017;12(3): e0174132.
28. Godaly G, Ambite I, Svanborg C. Innate immunity and genetic determinants of urinary tract infection susceptibility. Curr Opin Infect Dis 2015;28(1):88–96.
29. Hamilton C, Tan L, Miethke T, et al. Immunity to uropathogens: the emerging roles of inflammasomes. Nat Rev Urol 2017;14(5):284–95.
30. Moura A, Nicolau A, Hooton T, et al. Antibiotherapy and pathogenesis of uncomplicated UTI: difficult relationships. J Appl Microbiol 2009;106(6):1779–91.
31. Foxman B, Cronenwett AE, Spino C, et al. Cranberry juice capsules and urinary tract infection after surgery: results of a randomized trial. Am J Obstet Gynecol 2015;213(2):194.e1-8.
32. Paschke AA, Zaoutis T, Conway PH, et al. Previous antimicrobial exposure is associated with drug-resistant urinary tract infections in children. Pediatrics 2010;125(4):664–72.

33. Peri L. Fighting urinary tract infections with antibiotic and non-antibiotic therapies. Urologia 2016;(83 Suppl 1):5–10.
34. Pallett A, Hand K. Complicated urinary tract infections: practical solutions for the treatment of multiresistant gram-negative bacteria. J Antimicrob Chemother 2010;(65 Suppl 3):iii25–33.
35. Strukova EN, Portnoy YA, Zinner SH, et al. Predictors of bacterial resistance using in vitro dynamic models: area under the concentration-time curve related to either the minimum inhibitory or mutant prevention antibiotic concentration. J Antimicrob Chemother 2016;71(3):678–84.
36. Strukova EN, Portnoy YA, Romanov AV, et al. Searching for the optimal predictor of ciprofloxacin resistance in *Klebsiella pneumoniae* by using in vitro dynamic models. Antimicrob Agents Chemother 2015;60(3):1208–15.
37. Novelli A, Rosi E. Pharmacological properties of oral antibiotics for the treatment of uncomplicated urinary tract infections. J Chemother 2017;29(sup1):10–8.
38. Gupta K, Hooton TM, Naber KG, et al. International clinical practice guidelines for the treatment of acute uncomplicated cystitis and pyelonephritis in women: a 2010 update by the Infectious Diseases Society of America and the European Society for Microbiology and Infectious Diseases. Clin Infect Dis 2011;52(5): e103–20.
39. Bader MS, Loeb M, Brooks AA. An update on the management of urinary tract infections in the era of antimicrobial resistance. Postgrad Med 2017;129(2): 242–58.
40. Gupta K, Hooton TM, Roberts PL, et al. Short-course nitrofurantoin for the treatment of acute uncomplicated cystitis in women. Arch Intern Med 2007;167(20): 2207–12.
41. Stapleton PJ, Lundon DJ, McWade R, et al. Antibiotic resistance patterns of *Escherichia coli* urinary isolates and comparison with antibiotic consumption data over 10 years, 2005-2014. Ir J Med Sci 2017;186(3):733–41.
42. Chlabicz S, Leszczynska K, Lukas W, et al. Uncomplicated lower urinary tract infections in females–clinical aspects, aetiology and antimicrobial resistance epidemiology. Results of the ARESC (antimicrobial resistance epidemiological survey on cystitis) study in Poland and their implications for empiric therapy. Przegl Epidemiol 2011;65(2):345–51 [in Polish].
43. Banerjee S, Sengupta M, Sarker TK. Fosfomycin susceptibility among multidrug-resistant, extended-spectrum beta-lactamase-producing, carbapenem-resistant uropathogens. Indian J Urol 2017;33(2):149–54.
44. Sanchez GV, Babiker A, Master RN, et al. Antibiotic resistance among urinary isolates from female outpatients in the United States in 2003 and 2012. Antimicrob Agents Chemother 2016;60(5):2680–3.
45. Khawcharoenporn T, Vasoo S, Ward E, et al. High rates of quinolone resistance among urinary tract infections in the ED. Am J Emerg Med 2012;30(1):68–74.
46. Kranz J, Schmidt S, Lebert C, et al. The 2017 update of the German clinical guideline on epidemiology, diagnostics, therapy, prevention, and management of uncomplicated urinary tract infections in adult patients. Part II: therapy and prevention. Urol Int 2018;100(3):271–8.
47. Bader MS, Hawboldt J, Brooks A. Management of complicated urinary tract infections in the era of antimicrobial resistance. Postgrad Med 2010;122(6):7–15.
48. Arnold JJ, Hehn LE, Klein DA. Common questions about recurrent urinary tract infections in women. Am Fam Physician 2016;93(7):560–9.
49. Aydin A, Ahmed K, Zaman I, et al. Recurrent urinary tract infections in women. Int Urogynecol J 2015;26(6):795–804.

50. Geerlings SE, Beerepoot MA, Prins JM. Prevention of recurrent urinary tract infections in women: antimicrobial and nonantimicrobial strategies. Infect Dis Clin North Am 2014;28(1):135–47.
51. Bergamin PA, Kiosoglous AJ. Non-surgical management of recurrent urinary tract infections in women. Transl Androl Urol 2017;6(Suppl 2):S142–52.
52. Wagenlehner FM, Vahlensieck W, Bauer HW, et al. Prevention of recurrent urinary tract infections. Minerva Urol Nefrol 2013;65(1):9–20.
53. Hooton TM. Clinical practice. Uncomplicated urinary tract infection. N Engl J Med 2012;366(11):1028–37.
54. Ahmed H, Davies F, Francis N, et al. Long-term antibiotics for prevention of recurrent urinary tract infection in older adults: systematic review and meta-analysis of randomised trials. BMJ Open 2017;7(5):e015233.
55. Beerepoot MA, ter Riet G, Nys S, et al. Cranberries vs antibiotics to prevent urinary tract infections: a randomized double-blind noninferiority trial in premenopausal women. Arch Intern Med 2011;171(14):1270–8.
56. Beerepoot M, Geerlings S. Non-antibiotic prophylaxis for urinary tract infections. Pathogens 2016;5(2) [pii:E36].
57. Chisholm AH. Probiotics in preventing recurrent urinary tract infections in women: a literature review. Urol Nurs 2015;35(1):18–21, 29.
58. Afshar K, Stothers L, Scott H, et al. Cranberry juice for the prevention of pediatric urinary tract infection: a randomized controlled trial. J Urol 2012;188(4 Suppl):1584–7.
59. Nicolle LE. Urinary tract infections in special populations: diabetes, renal transplant, HIV infection, and spinal cord injury. Infect Dis Clin North Am 2014;28(1):91–104.
60. Han CS, Kim S, Radadia KD, et al. Comparison of urinary tract infection rates associated with transurethral catheterization, suprapubic tube and clean intermittent catheterization in the postoperative setting: a network meta-analysis. J Urol 2017;198(6):1353–8.
61. Caljouw MA, van den Hout WB, Putter H, et al. Effectiveness of cranberry capsules to prevent urinary tract infections in vulnerable older persons: a double-blind randomized placebo-controlled trial in long-term care facilities. J Am Geriatr Soc 2014;62(1):103–10.
62. Hibbing ME, Conover MS, Hultgren SJ. The unexplored relationship between urinary tract infections and the autonomic nervous system. Auton Neurosci 2016;200:29–34.
63. McKibben MJ, Seed P, Ross SS, et al. Urinary tract infection and neurogenic bladder. Urol Clin North Am 2015;42(4):527–36.
64. Grigoryan L, Trautner BW, Gupta K. Diagnosis and management of urinary tract infections in the outpatient setting: a review. JAMA 2014;312(16):1677–84.
65. Alberici I, Bayazit AK, Drozdz D, et al. Pathogens causing urinary tract infections in infants: a European overview by the ESCAPE study group. Eur J Pediatr 2015;174(6):783–90.
66. Allen VM, Yudin MH, Infectious Diseases Committee. Management of group B streptococcal bacteriuria in pregnancy. J Obstet Gynaecol Can 2012;34(5):482–6.
67. Abbo LM, Hooton TM. Antimicrobial stewardship and urinary tract infections. Antibiotics (Basel) 2014;3(2):174–92.

Emergence of Global Antibiotic Resistance

Martha Shawn Morehead, MD, MPH[a,b,c], Catherine Scarbrough, MD, MSc[d,*]

KEYWORDS

- Antibiotic resistance • Global health • Antibiotic stewardship • CDC bacterial threats
- Gram-positive bacteria • Gram-negative bacteria • WHO global action plan

KEY POINTS

- Antibiotic resistance is a worldwide phenomenon and a global public health crisis.
- The overuse and misuse of antibiotics in the human sector as well as the animal, food, and agricultural arenas have contributed to the current dilemma.
- Both gram-positive and gram-negative resistant bacteria have been deemed serious and urgent threats by the Centers for Disease Control and Prevention.
- The World Health Organization has created a 5-objective global action plan to address antimicrobial resistance and to coordinate numerous international sectors.
- Antibiotic resistance affects both this generation and the next; thus, related ethical challenges such as patient autonomy and justice have yet to be fully understood.

INTRODUCTION

The World Health Organization (WHO) has warned that unless the issue of antibiotic resistance is effectively addressed and contained, the phenomenon has the capacity to fundamentally change health care systems as we know them. The potential for a multiplicity of infectious diseases to have no viable antibiotic therapy is an imposing and impending reality. The complexity of the resistance problem must be confronted on multiple levels, from individual practitioners and patients, to community and national hospital systems, from local to global public health organizations, and via global surveillance and collaboration structures. Only a comprehensive paradigm shift, from

---

Disclosure Statement: The authors have nothing to disclose.
[a] St. Vincent's East Family Medicine Residency, Christ Health Center, 2152 Old Springville Road, Birmingham, AL 35215, USA; [b] Department of Family and Community Medicine, The University of Alabama at Birmingham School of Medicine, Community Health Services Building - 20th Street, 930 20th Street South, Suite 201, Birmingham, AL, 35294, USA; [c] Department of Family Medicine, Alabama College of Osteopathic Medicine, 445 Health Sciences Boulevard, Dothan, AL 36303, USA; [d] Department of Family, Internal, and Rural Medicine, College of Community Health Sciences, The University of Alabama Family Medicine Residency, 850 Peter Bryce Boulevard, Tuscaloosa, AL 35401, USA
* Corresponding author. 850 Peter Bryce Boulevard, Tuscaloosa, AL 35401.
E-mail address: cpscarbrough@ua.edu

Prim Care Clin Office Pract 45 (2018) 467–484
https://doi.org/10.1016/j.pop.2018.05.006
primarycare.theclinics.com

both public and private sectors, can stem the advancing tide of antimicrobial resistance (AMR) and its consequences for current and future generations.[1]

EPIDEMIOLOGY: ANTIBIOTIC USE AND RESISTANCE

- The Centers for Disease Control and Prevention (CDC) estimates 30% to 50% of all antibiotics prescribed in outpatient clinics are unnecessary.[2]
- Approximately 269 million antibiotic prescriptions were dispensed in the United States in 2015, enough for 5 of every 6 people to receive 1 antibiotic prescription.[2]
- Excess prescriptions put patients at risk for drug reactions or other complications, including *Clostridium difficile.*
- One-third of the ~500,000 *C difficile* infections in the United States in 2011 were community-associated.[2]
- Approximately 250,000 people each year require hospitalization for *C difficile* infections.[3]
- In the United States, ≥14,000 people die each year from *C difficile* infections, many preventable.[3]
- Eleven percent of nursing home residents take antibiotics on any single day, according to a small CDC study, yet many of these prescriptions were for the wrong drug, dose, or duration.[2]
- Overall rates of antibiotic use in US hospitals were stable in 2006 to 2012, but use of high-powered antibiotics increased by ~40% for carbapenems and 30% for vancomycin.[3]
- The CDC estimates ~30% of antibiotics used in hospitals are unnecessary or prescribed incorrectly.[2]
- The CDC estimates antibiotic-resistant bacteria cause more than 2 million illnesses and 23,000 deaths per year in the United States.[3]
- The European Center for Disease Prevention and Control estimates antibiotic-resistant bacteria cause ~25,000 deaths and €1.5 billion in health expenditures per year in Europe.[4]

Antibiotic resistance is a threat to individuals, health care and veterinary systems, and agricultural industries. The total economic cost of antibiotic resistance could be as high as $20 billion in excess of direct health care costs, with additional costs for lost productivity of $35 billion.[3] Estimates from the UK government project the cost of drug resistance to be US $100 trillion worldwide by 2050, with a death toll up to 10 million per year.[5]

BACKGROUND: HISTORY OF ANTIBIOTIC DEVELOPMENT AND RESISTANCE

The emergence of antibiotic resistance is a complex, multifactorial issue.[6] Soon after antibiotic discovery, the identification of resistance was not far behind (**Table 1**). *Staphylococcus* resistance to penicillin was identified even before widespread production of the first antibiotic in 1943.[6] Research shows that the genetic diversity required for this type of resistance to develop could not have come about in the time frame since the introduction of penicillin. This discovery indicates that bacteria likely have an intrinsic predilection for resistance stored within their genome that has been advancing over thousands of years.[6] The development of bacterial resistance to antibiotics is therefore a natural process and would exist with or without human intervention.[7]

However, since the introduction of penicillin, selection pressure from the use of antibiotics allows these bacterial adaptive mechanisms to further accelerate the selection of naturally resistant or more virulent bacteria. The inappropriate use of antibiotics

Table 1
Timeline of antibiotic development, resistance, and global response

1928	Alexander Fleming discovers penicillin
1930s	Prontosil, a sulfonamide, is first commercially available antibacterial
1940	Penicillin-R *Staphylococcus* identified
1943	Florey and Chain efficiently purify and scale-up production of penicillin
1940–1962	Golden age of antibiotic discovery and production
1950	Tetracycline introduced
1953	Erythromycin introduced
1955	Penicillin use is restricted to prescription only due to widespread misuse
1959	Tetracycline-R *Shigella* identified
1960	Methicillin introduced
1962	Methicillin-R *Staphylococcus* identified
1962	Nalidixic acid introduced (predecessor to fluoroquinolones)
1965	Penicillin-R pneumococcus identified
1967	Gentamicin introduced
1968	Erythromycin-R *Streptococcus* identified
1972	Vancomycin introduced
1979	Gentamicin-R *Enterococcus* identified
1985	Imipenem and ceftazidime introduced
1987	Ceftazidime-R Enterobacteriaceae identified
1988	Vancomycin-R *Enterococcus* identified
1996	Levofloxacin introduced
1996	Levofloxacin-R pneumococcus identified
1998	Imipenem-R Enterobacteriaceae identified
2000	Linezolid introduced
2000	XDR tuberculosis identified
2001	Linezolid-R *Staphylococcus* identified
2001	WHO launches Global Strategy for Containment of Antimicrobial Resistance
2002	Vancomycin-R *Staphylococcus* identified
2003	Daptomycin introduced
2004/5	PDR-*Acinetobacter* and *Pseudomonas* identified
2008	NDM-1, the New Delhi metallo-carbapenemase, observed in Enterobacteriaceae
2009	Ceftriaxone-R *Neisseria gonorrhoeae* and PDR-Enterobacteriaceae identified
2010	Ceftaroline introduced
2011	Ceftaroline-R *Staphylococcus* identified
2013	CDC Report on Antibiotic Resistance Threats in the United States
2014	WHO releases Antimicrobial Resistance: Global Report on Surveillance
2015	WHO releases Antibiotic Resistance: Multi-Country Public Awareness Survey
2015	WHO launches Global Action Plan on Antimicrobial Resistance

Dates are based on early reports of resistance in the literature. In the case of PDR-*Acinetobacter* and *Pseudomonas*, the date is based on reports of health care transmission or outbreaks.

Abbreviations: CDC, Centers for Disease Control and Prevention; PDR, pan drug-resistant; R: resistant; WHO, World Health Organization; XDR, extensively drug-resistant.

Adapted from Centers for Disease Control and Prevention. Antibiotic resistance threats in the United States. 2013. Available at: https://www.cdc.gov/drugresistance/threat-report-2013/pdf/ar-threats-2013-508.pdf. Accessed January 10, 2018.

in multiple arenas, from humans to animals to agriculture, has rapidly exacerbated the resistance issue.[6]

FACTORS LEADING TO THE RISE OF ANTIBIOTIC RESISTANCE

Antibiotic resistance is present throughout the world. Effective antibiotics are a necessity for both prevention and cure of communicable illness[8]; however, few new, novel, and innovative antibiotics are being developed within the pharmaceutical industry. Finally, issues of both access and excess are playing key roles in the global resistance dilemma.

The decline in research and development of newer antibiotics is a multifactorial issue.[7] Many of the largest pharmaceutical companies have reduced or eliminated their antibiotic divisions due to lack of profitability.[7] Short-course and reserved usage, increased regulatory costs, generic competition, and inevitable resistance leading to further decline in drug utilization, have all led to a negative risk-to-reward ratio.[7] Ultimately, since 2013, only 4 multinational pharmaceutical companies still maintain antibiotic development divisions.[7] Consequently, both US and international organizations have enacted policies to incentivize corporations to promote antibiotic development.[7]

ANTIBIOTIC OVERUSE/MISUSE IN HUMANS

Overuse, as well as inappropriate use (in choice, dose, patient adherence), of antibiotics contributes to the emergence of bacterial resistance. In the developing world, the unregulated availability of antibiotics in a community frequently leads to ill-advised self-medication. In certain countries of Africa, almost all antibiotic use is without a prescription.[9] Such self-treatment is fraught with inadequate dosing and duration of use as well as unnecessary consumption.[10] In the developed world, indiscriminate prescribing due to patient expectations and uncertain diagnoses also equates to mounting AMR.[9]

In the inpatient setting, prolonged use of multiple antibiotics in highly susceptible, immunocompromised patients is the main factor leading to antibacterial resistance. Patient-to-patient spread of highly resistant bacteria further intensifies nosocomial pressures, promoting further dissemination of difficult-to-treat microbes.[10] Mortality from resistant organisms is much higher than susceptible counterparts, not necessarily from increased virulence but due to delayed or inappropriate antibiotic therapy.[7]

ANTIBIOTIC OVERUSE/MISUSE IN THE FOOD/VETERINARY INDUSTRY

The food and animal industries also have contributed to the realm of antibiotic resistance.[11] Before 2003, antibiotics were used not only for animal disease treatment, but more significantly for prevention and growth promotion, both in the United States and in Europe. The European Union banned antibiotic use completely for animal growth promotion in 2006, with the United States curtailing veterinary antibiotic use without a prescription in 2012.[7] In the lesser developed world, the same practice continues unabated. Other environmental donors to the antibiotic resistance predicament include waste runoff from large farms, municipal wastewater containing partially metabolized or discarded medications, industrial agricultural plants with water and ground dissemination of drugs, and naturally occurring pathogenic bacteria found in waterways and soil.[7] In the United States, approximately 80% of all antibiotic use is found in agriculture and aquaculture.[6]

EMERGING BACTERIAL THREATS: GRAM-POSITIVE BACTERIA

Key Facts

- 20%: proportion of people who are persistent carriers of *Staphylococcus aureus*[7]
- 19,000: deaths per year due to methicillin-resistant *S aureus* (MRSA) in the United States[7]
- 61%: vancomycin-resistance rate of *Enterococcus faecium* in the United States[7]
- 40%: *Streptococcus pneumoniae* strains resistant to penicillin[7]
- 1.7 million: worldwide deaths caused by tuberculosis (TB) per year[7]
- 50%: chance of contracting *C difficile* if one spends more than 4 weeks in the hospital[7]
- See **Figs. 1** and **2**

Staphylococcus aureus

The resistance story of *Staphylococcus aureus* remains a prototype historical example. *S aureus* rapidly became multidrug resistant (MDR) over several decades, beginning with penicillinase production and penicillin resistance in the 1940s, then macrolide and tetracycline resistance in the 1950s, and finally methicillin resistance (MRSA) in the early 1960s. Multidrug resistance subsequently developed and is now worldwide.[12]

S aureus is a gram-positive, facultative aerobe with both community-acquired and hospital-acquired strains. The CDC estimates that 7% of people are colonized (via nares) in the United States with this bacterium.[3] Community-acquired MRSA infections most frequently involve the skin but also may be causative in serious necrotizing pneumonia and fasciitis.[10] Nosocomially acquired MRSA is a key pathogen in almost all arenas of hospital-acquired infections, including bacteremia, endocarditis, osteomyelitis, cellulitis, and pneumonia. It is also the leading cause of chronic infections

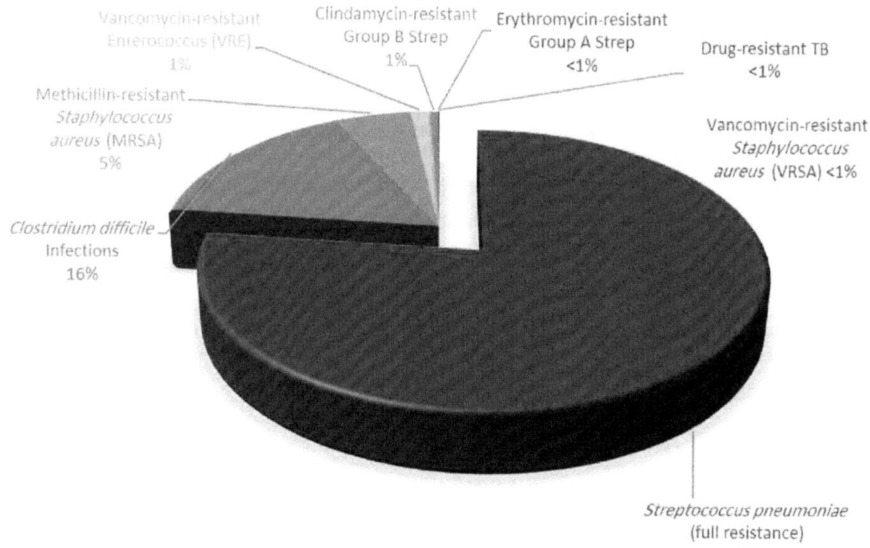

Fig. 1. Estimated annual number of cases in the United States: gram-positive antibiotic-resistant bacteria. Strep, *Streptococcus*. (*Adapted from* Centers for Disease Control and Prevention. Antibiotic resistance threats in the United States. 2013. Available at: https://www.cdc.gov/drugresistance/threat-report-2013/pdf/ar-threats-2013-508.pdf. Accessed January 10, 2018.)

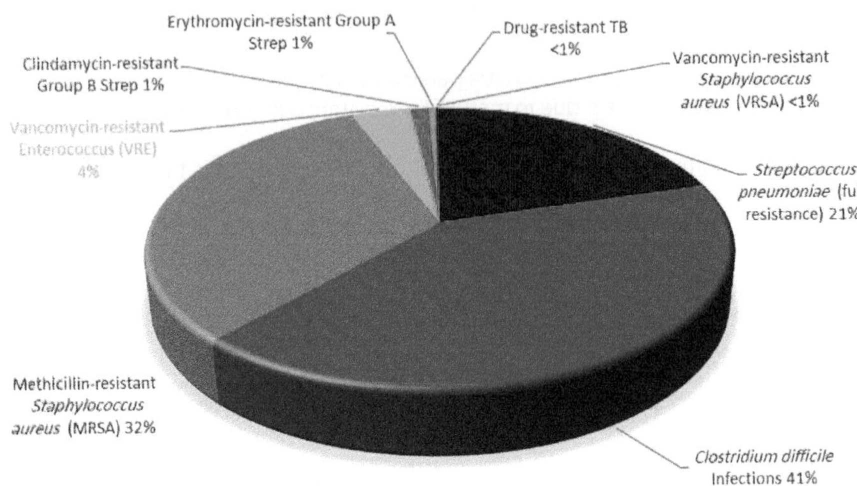

Fig. 2. Estimated annual number of deaths in the United States: gram-positive antibiotic-resistant bacteria. Strep, *Streptococcus*. (*Adapted from* Centers for Disease Control and Prevention. Antibiotic resistance threats in the United States. 2013. Available at: https://www.cdc.gov/drugresistance/threat-report-2013/pdf/ar-threats-2013-508.pdf. Accessed January 10, 2018.)

in indwelling medical devices.[13] Thankfully, more recent data noted a significant decrease in invasive, hospital-acquired MRSA infections.[3] Community-acquired MRSA rates, however, have swelled over the past decade, only recently beginning to plateau. Globally, MRSA rates still vary from 20% to 80% worldwide, inversely proportional from greater to lesser developed areas.[10,14,15]

Despite MRSA being one of the leading causative agents of all the antibiotic-resistant infections, the CDC has categorized it as a *serious threat* (rather than an urgent threat) based on: (1) the declining number of invasive infections and (2) existence of multiple effective antibiotics for treatment[3] (**Table 2**). However, MRSA treatment requires either newer antibiotic options that are expensive, like daptomycin (not for pneumonia) or linezolid (more recently approved in this category in **Table 3**) or vancomycin, the mainstay for hospital-treated infections, that requires significant monitoring. Each of the aforementioned drugs have elevated risks of adverse reactions.[10] In the past several years, Ceftaroline, the only beta-lactam antibiotic with MRSA and vancomycin-resistant *S aureus* activity, has been approved for use in acute bacterial skin and skin structure infections (ABSSIs) and community-acquired pneumonia, adding another treatment option.[15]

Resistant Enterococci

Enterococci are considered normal gastrointestinal flora but may become resistant colonizers when exposed to antibiotics. *Enterococcus faecalis* and *Enterococcus faecium* are the 2 most important species of resistant Enterococci, both being potentially pathogenic, gram-positive organisms. Both groups are highly resistant to aminoglycosides (30%–50%), ampicillin, and vancomycin.[15] *E faecium* has become a CDC-categorized *serious threat* due to its inherent beta-lactam resistance coupled with its propensity to become vancomycin-resistant Enterococci (VRE), doing so at a much higher rate than its counterpart, *E faecalis* (77% vs 9%).[3,7]

Table 2
Centers for Disease Control and Prevention assessment of antibiotic-resistance threats

Threat Level	Bacteria	Comments
Urgent	*Clostridium difficile* Carbapenem-R Enterobacteriaceae (CRE) Drug-resistant *Neisseria gonorrhoeae*	High-consequence antibiotic-resistant threats due to significant risks. May not be currently widespread but have potential and require urgent public health attention to identify infections and to limit transmission.
Serious	MDR *Acinetobacter* Drug-resistant *Campylobacter* Extended-spectrum β-lactamase producing Enterobacteriaceae (ESBLs) Vancomycin-R *Enterococcus* (VRE) MDR *Pseudomonas aeruginosa* Drug-resistant non-typhoidal *Salmonella* Drug-resistant *Salmonella typhi* Drug-resistant *Shigella* Methicillin-resistant *Staphylococcus aureus* (MRSA) Drug-resistant *Streptococcus pneumoniae* Drug-resistant tuberculosis	Significant antibiotic-resistant threats. Not considered urgent due to low or declining domestic incidence or reasonable availability of therapeutic agents, but these threats will worsen and may become urgent without ongoing public health monitoring and prevention activities.
Concerning	Vancomycin-R *S aureus* (VRSA) Erythromycin-R Group A *Streptococcus* Clindamycin-R Group B *Streptococcus*	Bacteria for which the threat of antibiotic resistance is low, and/or there are multiple therapeutic options for resistant infections. Cause severe illness and require monitoring and in some cases rapid incident or outbreak response.

Abbreviations: MDR, multidrug-resistant; R, resistant.

Adapted from Centers for Disease Control and Prevention. Antibiotic resistance threats in the United States. 2013. Available at: https://www.cdc.gov/drugresistance/threat-report-2013/pdf/ar-threats-2013-508.pdf. Accessed January 10, 2018.

VRE infections are common culprits essentially only for hospital-acquired infection, especially in colonization of indwelling medical devices.[7] It is important to distinguish between colonization and true infection with VRE that requires treatment.[15] Frequent sites of VRE infection include intra-abdominal, skin and soft tissues, bloodstream, heart valves, and urinary tract. Treatment options for VRE infections are noted in **Table 2**. Unresponsive VRE disease may require daptomycin in combination with a beta-lactam or linezolid, depending on specific local resistance patterns.[15]

Streptococcus pneumoniae

S pneumoniae is the leading cause of bacterial pneumonia for all age groups, both in community and hospital settings, although the very young and the elderly are disproportionately affected. *S pneumoniae* is also frequently implicated in otitis media, sinusitis,

Table 3
Drug therapies for nosocomial resistant gram-positive infections

Medication	Target	Comments
Glycopeptide, lipopeptide, and lipoglycopeptides		
Vancomycin	MRSA	Consider an alternative agent for MRSA with a MIC >2 μg/mL. Nephrotoxic.
Daptomycin	MRSA, VRE	Not for pneumonia; inactivated by pulmonary surfactant. Monitor CPK with concomitant statin use.
Dalbavancin	MRSA	—
Oritavancin	MRSA	Can cause false elevations in coags after administration.
Telavancin	MRSA	Black box for nephrotoxicity; avoid use in pregnancy.
Oxazolidinones		
Linezolid	MRSA, VRE	Bone marrow suppression when used >14 d.
Tedizolid	MRSA	Similar to above.
Beta-lactams		
Ceftaroline	MRSA	—
Ampicillin (+/− gentamicin)	Susceptible VRE only	90% *Enterococcus faecium* are resistant.
Miscellaneous		
Quinupristin/dalfopristin	MRSA, VRE (*E faecium* only)	Salvage therapy only. Causes significant arthralgias/myalgias.
Tigecycline	CA-MRSA, VRE	Black box for increased mortality. Hepatotoxic. Cross-reactivity with tetracycline allergy.
Fosfomycin	VRE (urine only)	Limited data in complicated UTI. Must request susceptibility testing.
Nitrofurantoin	VRE (urine only)	Contraindicated in CrCl <30 mL/min.

Abbreviations: CA-MRSA, community-associated MRSA; CPK, creatine phoshokinase; coags, coagulation panel; CrCl, creatinine clearance; MIC, minimum inhibitory concentration; MRSA, methicillin-resistant *Staphylococcus aureus*; UTI, urinary tract infection; VRE, vancomycin-resistant Enterococci.

Adapted from Wiskirchen DE, Wu U, Summa M, et al. Inpatient antibiotic resistance: everyone's problem. J Fam Pract 2018;67(2):E11; with permission.

and meningitis. Resistance of this bacteria to penicillin has grown to approximately 40%, with correlating resistance to macrolides, sulfonamides, tetracyclines, and earlier cephalosporins.[7] *S pneumoniae* resistance also has been seen with levofloxacin.[7]

The advent and utilization of pneumococcal conjugate vaccine (PCV)7 (2000–2009), followed by PCV 13 (2010–today), has not only reduced pneumococcal infection and invasive disease, but has decreased antibiotic resistance by blocking transmission of resistant *S pneumoniae* strains.[3] The CDC rates *S pneumoniae* as a *serious threat* responsible for 1.2 million infections per year, but this organism bears close monitoring due to its wide range of pathogenicity.[3]

Clostridium difficile

C difficile, the gram-positive spore-forming, obligate anaerobe, is best known for antibiotic-associated diarrhea, or *C difficile* colitis. The spores formed by *C difficile* are highly environmentally tolerant, resisting heat, pH change, and alcohol-based cleaners, making them difficult to eradicate without special cleaning protocols.[7] *C difficile* is both community-acquired and hospital-acquired with a high rate of acquisition during prolonged hospitalizations approaching 50% for a 4-week hospital stay.[7] Consequently, *C difficile* mortality is most prominent in the geriatric population, with more than 90% of deaths occurring in patients older than 65.[3]

C difficile produces 2 toxins, an enterotoxin (toxin A) and a cytotoxin (toxin B) that lead to the symptoms of colitis, as well as its life-threatening complications.[7] The CDC has designated *C difficile* as an *urgent threat*, the highest level, due to its ease of acquisition, increasing incidence and mortality rates, and its expanding costs to the health care sector, totaling more than $1,000,000,000 in excess medical costs.[3] Resistance patterns with *C difficile* are fortunately rare. Thus, this antibiotic-driven, disease-producer requires the judicious use and the elimination of unnecessary antibiotics. Multiple health care systems in the United States are developing antibiotic surveillance systems to successfully reduce *C difficile* infection rates.[2]

EMERGING BACTERIAL THREATS: GRAM-NEGATIVE BACTERIA

Key Facts

- 30%: increase in carbapenem-resistant *Acinetobacter baumannii* strains from 1995 to 2004[7]
- 30%: quinolone resistance rate for *Enterobacter*[7]
- 460,000: *Neisseria gonorrhoeae* infections in the United States per year[7]
- 15.5%: hospital-acquired infection incidence rate in developing countries[7]
- See **Figs. 3** and **4**

The advent and ease of global movement and travel has facilitated the spread of MDR gram-negative bacteria. People carry their gastrointestinal flora with them, exposing other populations around the world to their colonized and pathogenic

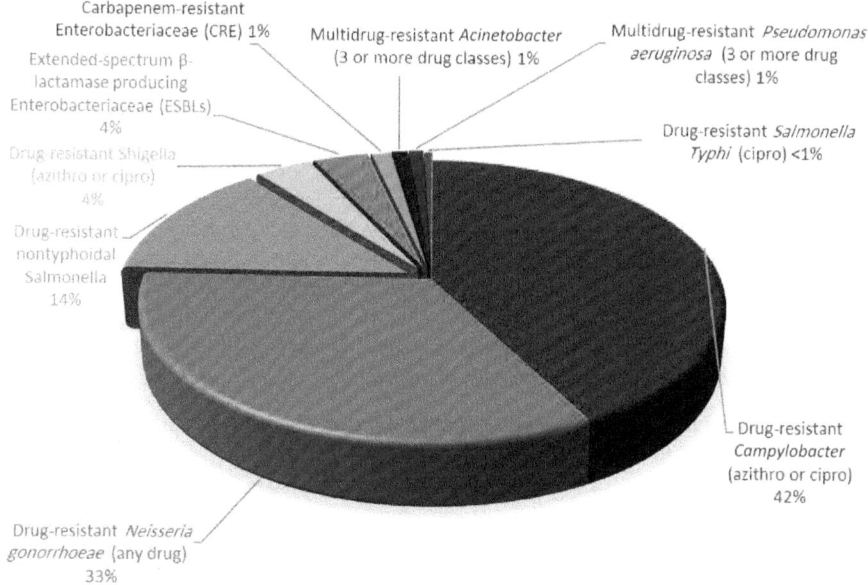

Fig. 3. Estimated annual number of cases in the United States: gram-negative antibiotic-resistant bacteria. (*Adapted from* Centers for Disease Control and Prevention. Antibiotic resistance threats in the United States. 2013. Available at: https://www.cdc.gov/drugresistance/threat-report-2013/pdf/ar-threats-2013-508.pdf. Accessed January 10, 2018.)

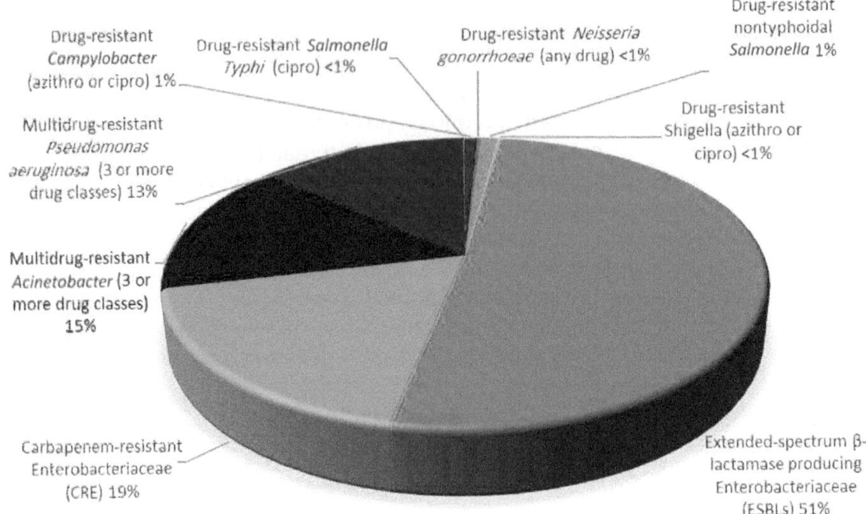

Fig. 4. Estimated annual number of deaths in the United States: gram-negative antibiotic-resistant bacteria. (*Adapted from* Centers for Disease Control and Prevention. Antibiotic resistance threats in the United States. 2013. Available at: https://www.cdc.gov/drugresistance/threat-report-2013/pdf/ar-threats-2013-508.pdf. Accessed January 10, 2018.)

digestive contents.[16] Of particular importance in these gastrointestinal transfers are *Escherichia coli* and *Klebsiella* species, part of the Enterobacteriaceae group.[3] These bacteria have a highly fluid genome, mediated by plasmids that contain antibiotic resistance and pathogenicity genes facilitating resistance from environment to animals and humans.[16]

Extended-Spectrum Beta-Lactamases

One of the most important resistance issues in the past 20 years relates to the rapidity of emergence of extended-spectrum beta-lactamases (ESBLs), first noted in the late 1990s.[16] The swift spread of ESBLs relates to many factors, including poor sanitation and hygiene, as well as lack of clean drinking water in emerging contexts.[16] However, even high-quality sewage treatment does not fully remove antibiotic resistance-genes producing *E coli*. Studies have revealed that in these circumstances, bacteria may still be acquired by humans (and livestock) during water activities from clean river sources.[16] Finally, the abundance of antibiotic use in the global contexts of agriculture, fish farming, and livestock-raising breed concerns for further multiplication of the effect of ESBLs on disease and antibiotic resistance.

Enterobacteriaceae (Extended-Spectrum Beta-Lactamase and Carbapenem-Resistant)

The 2 main threats in this category relate to *E coli* and *Klebsiella* species. These bacteria are resistant to nearly all penicillins and cephalosporins, with the only remaining treatment options being carbapenems.[14] ESBL-producing Enterobacteriaceae account for ~19% of hospital-acquired *E coli* and *Klebsiella* species infections, with more than twice the mortality of non-ESBL producers.[15] ESBL-producing Enterobacteriaceae are deemed a *serious threat* per the CDC.[3] Drug-resistant *E coli* is especially concerning, being the most common gram-negative bacterial infection in humans. ESBL and non-ESBL strains have a high cross-resistance to fluoroquinolones (>80%) as well as aminoglycosides. *E coli* resistance patterns continue to expand with the acquisition of carbapenemases, leading to carbapenem resistance (CRE) as well.[7]

As noted previously, the issue of increasing ESBL-producing bacteria leads to expanding use of carbapenem antibiotics, a drug group of last resort.[15] The escalation of carbapenem usage has rapidly led to resistance in the Enterobacteriaceae organisms noted as CRE in the literature.[15] These infections, denoted as *urgent threats* per the CDC, have become resistant to almost all antibiotics, with a >50% mortality for patients who become bacteremic.[3] Current potential treatments are noted in **Table 4**.

Table 4
Drug therapies for nosocomial resistant gram-negative infections

Medication	Target	Comments
Cephalosporins		
Ceftazidime Cefepime	Some *Pseudomonas* spp *Pseudomonas* spp	Subject to inoculum effect with ESBL producers. Dose requires renal adjustment. Some infections require high-dose, prolonged regimens.
Carbapenems		
Ertapenems Imipenem/cilastatin Merpenem Doripenem	ESBL-producing organisms ESBL-producing organisms, ampC-producers, *Pseudomonas* spp, some *Acinetobacter* species	Dose requires renal adjustment. Some infections require high-dose, prolonged regimens.
Beta-lactam/beta-lactam inhibitor combination		
Ampicillin/sulbactam	*Acinetobacter baumannii*	Dose requires renal adjustment. May need >6 g of sulbactam per day for some infections.
Piperacillin/tazobactam	*Pseudomonas* spp	Subject to inoculum effect with ESBL producers. Dose requires renal adjustment. Some infections require high-dose, prolonged regimens.
Ceftolozane/tazobactam	ESBL-producing organisms, *Pseudomonas* spp	Dose requires renal adjustment.
Ceftolozane/avibactam	ESBL-producing and KPC-producing organisms, *Pseudomonas* spp	Dose requires renal adjustment.
Aminoglycosides		
Gentamicin Tobramycin Amikacin	ESBL-producing organisms, CRE, *Pseudomonas* spp, some *Acinetobacter* spp	Used as combination therapy. Ototoxic; nephrotoxic. Dose requires renal adjustment.
Miscellaneous		
Polymixins	ESBL-producing organisms, CRE, *Pseudomonas* spp, some *Acinetobacter* spp	Nephrotoxic. Dose requires renal adjustment. Reserve for MDR gram-negative infections.
Fosfomycin	ESBL-producing organisms and CRE (urine only)	Limited data in complicated UTI. Must request susceptibility testing.
Tigecycline	ESBL-producing organisms and CRE (urine only)	Black box for increased mortality. Hepatotoxic. Cross-reactivity with tetracycline allergy.

Abbreviations: CRE, carbapenem-resistant Enterobacteriaceae; ESBL, extended-spectrum beta-lactamase; KPC, *Klebsiella pneumoniae* Carbapenemase; MDR, multidrug resistant; UTI, urinary tract infection.

Adapted from Wiskirchen DE, Wu U, Summa M, et al. Inpatient antibiotic resistance: everyone's problem. J Fam Pract 2018;67(2):E11; with permission.

Neisseria gonorrhoeae

Unlike most of its *urgent threat* (per CDC) counterparts, *N gonorrhoeae* is not a life-threatening illness.[3] Gonorrhea, once thought an easily treated sexually transmitted disease (STD), has become a broadly resistant pathogen with some resistance to almost all oral antibiotics, including beta-lactams, quinolones, tetracyclines, macrolides, and even ceftriaxone, the current mainstay of treatment (injectable cephalosporin).[7] The CDC now *only* recommends ceftriaxone *plus* azithromycin as first-line treatment. Ceftriaxone plus doxycycline is only indicated in azithromycin allergic/intolerant patients and for proctitis/epididymitis caused by *N gonorrhoeae*.[7] In all cases, an increase in dose of ceftriaxone to 250 mg from 125 mg and the addition of second agent in combination is a major departure in treatment guidelines. The rationale for these changes is to (1) ensure clinical cure and (2) reduce development of resistance.[17,18] With resistance to ceftriaxone growing, efforts at controlling the spread of this common STD pathogen will be hindered, resulting in an increase in reproductive and genitourinary complications and further expansion of other STDs.[15]

Diarrheal Pathogens: Campylobacter, Salmonella, Shigella

The CDC places drug-resistant *Campylobacter*, *Shigella*, and *Salmonella* all in the *serious threat* category for antibiotic resistance.[3] The pathogenicity of *Campylobacter* is most concerning for its association with development of Guillain-Barre syndrome in 1 of 1000 patients.[19] These pathogens, apart from *Salmonella typhi*, have similar clinical presentations, including diarrhea (sometimes bloody), fever, abdominal pain, and a self-limited course in immune-competent persons. Mild-moderate gastrointestinal illnesses with these agents should not be treated with antibiotics, left to resolve spontaneously usually within a 7-day time frame. Only severe or complicated infections should prompt treatment with antibiotics.[20]

These diarrheal illnesses are similar epidemiologically and clinically, occurring via contaminated food and water sources or through direct contact with feces or infected animals. Of this group, non-typhoidal *Salmonella* (NTS) is the most common and widely distributed with more than 1500 serotypes.[10] The worldwide incidence of NTS is growing with more than 1.2 million cases in the United States. MDR NTS has been associated with a higher risk of invasive infection, greater frequency and duration of hospitalization, and increased mortality compared with infections caused by susceptible strains.[10] Five percent of NTS strains are deemed MDR, defined as resistance to 5 or more drugs.[3] Therefore, prevention by frequent handwashing, good hygiene, and avoidance of contaminated sources, usually undercooked chicken and unpasteurized milk, is of paramount importance.[3]

The outlier of the diarrheal pathogen group is *S typhi*, the origin of typhoid fever, a potentially life-threatening illness. Typhoid fever is characterized by high fever, abdominal pain, severe headache, and relative bradycardia. In its severest form, typhoid fever can lead to bowel perforation, peritonitis, shock, and death. Worldwide, *S typhi* is responsible for more than 21 million infections.[21] The CDC notes that ~67% of all *S typhi* has at least partial resistance to ciprofloxacin, rendering quinolones unusable.[21] Unlike the other drug-resistant diarrheal pathogens, there is a vaccination, both oral and injectable, for *S typhi*.[21]

Among the drug-resistant diarrheal microbes, all are showing resistance to ciprofloxacin and azithromycin, with both forms of *Salmonella* (NTS and *S typhi*) showing ceftriaxone resistance as well.[3,10,21] Overuse and inappropriate use of antibiotics for mild infections and those encountered via other contaminated sources (animals, food, water) are definitively causal in the antibiotic resistance noted in these diarrheal infections.

Multidrug-Resistant Acinetobacter

MDR *Acinetobacter*, another gram-negative bacterium in the *serious threat* CDC category, is a highly virulent source of pneumonia and bacteremia in hospitalized, critically ill patients.[3] *Acinetobacter baumannii*, the most common species, is especially prevalent in mechanically ventilated patients.[15] Unlike its highly resistant counterpart, *Pseudomonas aeruginosa,* whose resistance pattern has become more stabilized in the United States, *Acinetobacter* resistance continues to rise.[7] Additionally, death rates for MDR *Acinetobacter* infection are also proportionately higher than *Pseudomonas*.[7]

Acinetobacter baumannii rapidly emerged in wounded soldiers during the Iraq war, being dubbed "Iraqibacter" at that time. The ability of *Acinetobacter* to develop resistance relates to its environmental resilience secondary to its thick walls, shielding it from dry settings, extreme temperatures, and unstable pH conditions, explaining its appearance onto the wartime landscape in Iraq.[7,15] It is capable of survival for many months in various locations, including inanimate objects, giving it a pronounced pathogenic selective advantage.[7]

The CDC Antimicrobial Resistance Report found *A baumannii* to have a 63% MDR rate. Some of its highest resistance is to both carbapenems and aminoglycosides, defining this pathogen as one of the most difficult-to-treat health care–acquired infections.[3] The resistance mechanisms of these organisms have 2 main modes: (1) efflux pumps, promoting resistance to ammonia-based disinfectants, and (2) beta-lactamases, including ESBLs and carbapenemases.[7] These mechanisms, in conjunction with its naturally thick cell wall, have produced *A baumannii* strains with resistance to *all* known antibiotics.[7] MDR *Acinetobacter* has emerged so quickly and has become so dangerous that hospital outbreaks have resulted in ward closures in efforts to reduce further mortality.[7] Appropriate and effective treatment for *A baumannii* is increasingly difficult. For susceptible strains, carbapenems or quinolones can be used. In more than 60% of resistant strains, meropenem plus polymyxin B is preferred.[20]

Multidrug-Resistant Pseudomonas

P aeruginosa is another lethal, opportunistic gram-negative pathogen. In many ways, it appears to be the mentor of *A baumannii* in terms of natural and acquired resistance patterns. *P aeruginosa* is a nosocomial infection with frequent occurrence in patients in the intensive care unit and who are ventilator-dependent. It is the most common lung infection in patients with cystic fibrosis, whose pseudomonal infections include strains resistant to all antibiotics, save polymixins.[7]

P aeruginosa has been deemed a *serious threat* by the CDC, accounting for greater than 50,000 infections per year and ~8% of all hospital-acquired infections.[3] Approximately 13% of these infections are MDR. Resistance is generated through similar mechanisms to *A baumannii,* including efflux pump systems, beta-lactamases (ESBLs, metallo-beta-lactamases), and carbapenemases. *Pseudomonas* has innately high environmental tolerance, an almost impenetrable outer membrane, and a high propensity to form biofilms, further increasing its resistance to many antibiotics.[7]

Treatment of MDR *P aeruginosa* has followed the Infectious Diseases Society of America (IDSA) 2016 guidelines, advocating combination therapy with 2 antibiotics from different classes.[15] This dual therapy is used per the IDSA for both empiric and specific therapy, involving suspected and identified pseudomonal infection. It is inferred per the IDSA recommendations that combination treatment *empirically* for MDR strains will

- Increase the likelihood that at least 1 of the 2 drugs will be effective
- Decrease risk of resistant subpopulation selection
- Promote additive or synergistic antibacterial activity[22]

Possible benefits of combined drugs for *specific* therapy may lead to the following:

- Faster reduction of bacterial load
- Less dependence on pharmacokinetic/pharmacodynamic optimization
- Decreased risk of resistance selection
- Potential reduction in mortality[15]

Despite IDSA assertions, other specialty groups remain conflicted on the efficacy of dual treatment, high treatment cost, and undesirable toxic side effects and complications.[22,23] Therefore, given the lack of definitive evidence, antibiotic selection should be based on patient-specific factors, including site of infection, drug sensitivity data, and local resistance patterns.

A CATEGORY UNTO ITSELF: TUBERCULOSIS

Mycobacterium tuberculosis is a highly aerobic, pathogenic bacterium that is the primary cause of tuberculosis (TB). *Mycobacterium* do not Gram stain.[7] However, because of the lack of an outer membrane in gram-negative bacteria, TB is often categorized as a gram-positive organism. The atypical cell wall of TB gives it inherent antibiotic resistance by protecting it from digestion via macrophages.[7]

It is estimated that one-third of the world's population is infected with latent TB, among the most common infectious diseases and causes of death.[24] Consequently, the development and spread of MDR-TB is considered one of the greatest obstacles to disease control on a global scale. MDR-TB, by definition, is resistant to at least 2 of the 3 drugs considered first-line combination therapy, isoniazid (INH) and rifampin. Some TB strains develop further resistance to become XDR-TB, defined as MDR-TB plus resistance to any fluoroquinolone and any of the injectable second-line drugs, including amikacin, kanamycin, and capreomycin.[7] Globally, 4% of new TB cases are MDR-TB; 10% of MDR-TB cases are actually XDR-TB. XDR-TB has now been reported in 92 countries, with Russia, India, and South Africa harboring the highest number of cases.[24]

The main contributors to TB resistance have been incorrect diagnoses and treatment, poor patient compliance, unavailable/low-quality TB medications, or inappropriate duration/dosing of treatment or combination of drugs.[10] The only means for reduction in XDR-TB cases is to effectively treat the MDR-TB patient population.[10] XDR-TB may require up to a 2-year course of antibiotics at a cost approaching $500,000, without assurance of recovery.[7,24,25] Thus, the need for new and effective drugs in the TB armamentarium.

THE PROBLEM ADDRESSED

In May 2014, the World Health Assembly developed a global action plan due to an international consensus that AMR posed a profound threat to human health.[14] The WHO global report on surveillance of AMR provided a first-time picture of the magnitude of the issue, the lack of adequate surveillance in many areas of the world, and large gaps in information on bacteria of major public health importance.[14] The WHO global action plan sets out 5 strategic objectives:

1. To improve awareness and understanding of AMR
2. To strengthen knowledge through surveillance and research
3. To reduce the incidence of infection
4. To optimize the use of antimicrobial agents
5. To ensure sustainable investment in countering AMR[8]

The WHO global action plan also provides the framework for individual national action plans using an incremental approach over the next 5 to 10 years. The strategy involves the following changes:

- Patients must be educated on the safe and appropriate use of antibiotics.[8]
- Health care workers must act as stewards of the dwindling effective antibiotic supply.[8]
- In the realms of agricultural and veterinary medicine, development of antibiotic-prescribing databases and new diagnostic and clinical decision tools will assist with evidence-based dispensing to decrease inappropriate or unregulated use of antimicrobial agents.[8]
- Political groups must be willing to adopt and enforce new policies controlling use of antibiotics in humans, animals, and food production.[8]
- Developing countries will need financial and technical support to combat AMR.[8]
- The private-sector pharmaceutical industry must contribute by development of new therapies.[8]

In the United States, the CDC has spearheaded the country's specific action plan in response to the WHO global action plan. The CDC's 4 core actions include the following:

- Preventing infections and the spread of resistance
- Tracking resistant bacteria
- Improving the use of current antibiotics
- Promoting the development of new antibiotics and diagnostic tests for resistant bacteria[3]

The CDC has developed programs to prevent infection and the spread of resistance, including the following:

- Get Smart Program: national campaign to improve antibiotic prescribing.[3]
- Contact Tracing: strategy that traces contacts of infected patients to ensure those needing treatment, prophylaxis, or temporary isolation are identified and managed appropriately, which is critical for tuberculosis, gonorrhea, and meningococcus.[3]
- Vaccination Guidelines and Education: *S pneumoniae* vaccine is proof that an effective vaccine can reduce resistance rates. Conjugate pneumococcal vaccines, PCV7 introduced in 2000 followed by PCV13 (2010–present), with the addition of serotype 19A, are responsible for cutting invasive pneumococcal infection cases in half and reducing resistant infections by 25%.[3]
- Treatment Guidelines: guidelines are based on up-to-date resistance patterns to limit progression and spread of resistant bacteria.[3]
- Promotion of Safe Sex: due to the challenges of drug-resistant *N gonorrhoeae*, the CDC promotes abstinence, mutual monogamy, and condom use.[3]

Additionally, the CDC has several means of tracking antibacterial resistance via various entities, as outlined in **Table 5**. Coupled with effective stewardship programs both locally and nationally, the goal of maximum benefit from antibiotics, avoidance of unnecessary harm, and preservation of future life-saving potential of these drugs is achievable. Moreover, these efforts have shown to improve outcomes and decrease costs.[3]

THE ETHICAL CHALLENGES OF ANTIBIOTIC RESISTANCE

Ethical concerns have come to the forefront of antibiotic resistance issues because of the complexity of this challenge. Individual patient autonomy versus the rights of larger

Table 5
Centers for Disease Control and Prevention antibiotic resistance tracking networks

Tracking Networks	Resistant Bacteria
EIP: Emerging Infections Program	
ABCs: Active Bacterial Core surveillance	*Streptococcus pneumoniae* Groups A and B *Streptococcus* MRSA
HAIC: Healthcare-Associated Infections-Community Interface	*Clostridium difficile* Carbapenem-R Enterobacteriaceae MDR *Acinetobacter*
FoodNet: Foodborne Diseases Active Surveillance Network	*Salmonella* *Campylobacter* *Shigella*
NARMS: National Antimicrobial Resistance Monitoring System	*Salmonella* *Campylobacter* *Shigella*
NHSN: National Healthcare Safety Network	*Staphylococcus aureus* *Enterococcus* Enterobacteriaceae *Acinetobacter* *Pseudomonas aeruginosa*
GISP: Gonococcal Isolate Surveillance Program	*Neisseria gonorrhoeae*
NTSS: National Tuberculosis Surveillance System	*Mycobacterium tuberculosis*

Abbreviations: MDR, multidrug-resistant; R, resistant.

Adapted from Center for Disease Control and Prevention. Antibiotic resistance threats in the United States. 2013. Available at: https://www.cdc.gov/drugresistance/threat-report-2013/pdf/ar-threats-2013-508.pdf. Accessed January 10, 2018.

society remains a controversy surrounding mandatory reporting of infections. Increasing costs and longer hospital stays needed to treat resistant forms of disease pose further questions on personal autonomy versus health care rights and responsibilities relating to dwindling resources.[26]

Another ethical challenge involves the use of antibiotics in veterinary medicine and food industry practices. Half of the world's total antibiotics are used in the veterinary world. An open discussion of animal welfare standards in food production, where prophylactic antibiotics are used to compensate for overcrowded conditions, is essential.[26]

Finally, there are ethical uncertainties related to justice. The global burden of antibiotic resistance disproportionately affects low-income and middle-income countries. Objective 5 of the WHO global action plan addresses this issue.[8] More people die from *lack of access* to high-quality antibiotics in low-income countries than die from antibiotic resistance in high-income countries.[26] Therefore, success of the WHO plan will require an ethical policy response toward resource-poor health care systems.

With increasing antibiotic resistance, a dwindling production pipeline, and a sluggish response to this global crisis on the world stage, the current question is whether antibiotics should be classified as a nonrenewable resource on the same level as fossil fuels.[26] If so, then justice plays an even larger role in the allocation of this scarce resource. Consequently, the goal of any plan to reduce antibiotic resistance also includes preserving the effectiveness of antibiotics via implementation of antibiotic stewardship programs and rational prescribing guidelines. Future generations will face similar, and potentially more complicated, struggles with an even greater need for effective disease responses.[26] Disease X is looming. Will we have a cure?[27]

REFERENCES

1. Tomson G, Vlad I. The need to look at antibiotic resistance from a health systems perspective. Ups J Med Sci 2014;119(2):117–24.
2. Centers for Disease Control and Prevention. Antibiotic use in the United States: progress and opportunities. 2017. Available at: https://www.cdc.gov/antibiotic-use/stewardship-report/pdf/stewardship-report.pdf. Accessed February 5, 2018.
3. Centers for Disease Control and Prevention. Antibiotic resistance threats in the United States. 2013. Available at: https://www.cdc.gov/drugresistance/threat-report-2013/pdf/ar-threats-2013-508.pdf. Accessed January 10, 2018.
4. European Centre for Disease Prevention and Control (ECDC). Antimicrobial resistance in focus. Available at: https://ecdc.europa.eu/en/antimicrobial-resistance. Accessed March 12, 2018.
5. O'Neill J. Antimicrobial resistance: tackling a crisis for the health and wealth of nations. London: The Review on Antimicrobial Resistance; 2014.
6. Hwang AY, Gums JG. The emergence and evolution of antimicrobial resistance: Impact on a global scale. Bioorg Med Chem 2016;24(24):6440–5.
7. Fair RJ, Tor Y. Antibiotics and bacterial resistance in the 21st century. Perspect Med Chem 2014;6:25–64.
8. World Health Organization. Global action plan on antimicrobial resistance. 2015. Available at: http://www.who.int/antimicrobial-resistance/publications/global-action-plan/en/. Accessed January 10, 2018.
9. Morgan DJ, Okeke IN, Laxminarayan R, et al. Non-prescription antimicrobial use worldwide: a systematic review. Lancet Infect Dis 2011;11(9):692–701.
10. Prestinaci F, Pezzotti P, Pantosti A. Antimicrobial resistance: a global multifaceted phenomenon. Pathog Glob Health 2015;109(7):309–18.
11. Marshall BM, Levy SB. Food animals and antimicrobials: impacts on human health. Clin Microbiol Rev 2011;24(4):718–33.
12. Enright MC, Robinson DA, Randle G, et al. The evolutionary history of methicillin-resistant *Staphylococcus aureus* (MRSA). Proc Natl Acad Sci U S A 2002;99: 7687–92.
13. Klevens RM, Morrison MA, Nadle J, et al. Invasive methicillin-resistant *Staphylococcus aureus* infections in the United States. JAMA 2007;298(15):1763–71.
14. World Health Organization. Antimicrobial resistance: global report on surveillance. 2014. Available at: http://apps.who.int/iris/bitstream/10665/112642/1/9789241564748_eng.pdf. Accessed January 10, 2018.
15. Wiskirchen DE, Wu U, Summa M, et al. Inpatient antibiotic resistance: everyone's problem. J Fam Pract 2018;67(2):E11.
16. Hawkey PM. Multidrug-resistant gram-negative bacteria: a product of globalization. J Hosp Infect 2015;89(4):241–7.
17. Workowski KA, Berman SM, Douglas JM. Emerging antimicrobial resistance in *Neisseria gonorrhoeae*: urgent need to strengthen prevention strategies. Ann Intern Med 2008;148:606.
18. Workowski KA, Bolan GA, Centers for Disease Control and Prevention. Sexually transmitted diseases treatment guidelines, 2015. MMWR Recomm Rep 2015; 64:1.
19. Centers for Disease Control and Prevention Web site: Campylobacter. Available at: http://www.cdc.gov/nczved/divisions/dfbmd/diseases/campylobacter/. Accessed March 14, 2018.
20. Gilbert DN, Chambers HF, Eliopoulos GM, et al. Sanford guide to antimicrobial therapy. 48th edition. Sperryville (VA): Antimicrobial Therapy, Inc; 2018.

21. Centers for Disease Control and Prevention Web site: Typhoid fever. Available at: https://www.cdc.gov/typhoid-fever/index.html. Accessed March 12, 2018.
22. Vazquez-Grande G, Kumar A. Optimizing antimicrobial therapy of sepsis and septic shock: focus on antibiotic combination therapy. Semin Respir Crit Care Med 2015;36(01):154–66.
23. Kalil A. Antibiotic combination therapy for patients with gram-negative septic shock. Crit Care Med 2017;45(11):1933–6.
24. World Health Organization Web site: Tuberculosis. Available at: http://www.who.int/tb/en/. Accessed March 12, 2018.
25. Centers for Disease Control and Prevention. World health day: media fact sheet. Available at: http://www.cdc.gov/media/releases/2011/f0407_antimicrobialresistance.pdf. Accessed March 12, 2018.
26. Littmann J, Buyx A, Cars O. Antibiotic resistance: an ethical challenge. Int J Antimicrob Agents 2015;46(4):359–61.
27. World Health Organization Web site: List of blueprint priority diseases, 2018. Available at: http://www.who.int/blueprint/priority-diseases/en/. Accessed March 12, 2018.

Guidelines for the Evaluation and Treatment of Pneumonia

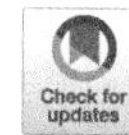

Samuel N. Grief, MD, FCFP[a,*], Julie K. Loza, MD[b]

KEYWORDS

- Pneumonia • Ventilator-associated • Community-acquired • Pediatric
- Antibiotic resistance • Microbial pathogens

KEY POINTS

- Pneumonia is a common respiratory infection and warrants careful consideration of antibiotic initiation and choice, along with knowledge of local antibiotic resistance patterns.
- Community-acquired pneumonia afflicts all age groups and although not always bacterial in origin, is clinically versatile, depending on its cause.
- Nonresolving pneumonia may be because of less common pathogens, or feature other conditions, and requires more detailed investigation.
- Pediatric pneumonia is also common, and first-line treatment is still amoxicillin, followed closely by cephalosporins or macrolides.
- Other categories of pneumonia, including mechanically induced (ventilator) or travel/geriatric pneumonia, benefit from astute clinical acumen, proper history and physical examination, and knowledge of microbial causes.

INTRODUCTION

Pneumonia is a leading cause of hospitalization among both adults and children in the United States, accounting for more than 800,000 hospitalizations and more than 400,000 emergency department visits in 2014.[1,2] It is among the most expensive conditions treated in US hospitals with national aggregate costs of $9.5 billion in 2013.[3]

A causal pathogen is often not identified. A 2015 prospective, multi-center study by the Centers for Disease Control and Prevention identified a responsible pathogen in only 38% of cases of community-acquired pneumonia (CAP) in adults requiring hospitalization.[4] CAP is an infection of the lung parenchyma that is acquired outside of

Disclosure Statement: The authors have nothing to disclose.
[a] Clinical Family Medicine, Department of Family Medicine, University of Illinois at Chicago, 1919 West Taylor Street, Suite 143, Chicago, IL 60612, USA; [b] Department of Family Medicine, University of Illinois at Chicago, 1919 West Taylor Street, Chicago, IL 60612, USA
* Corresponding author.
E-mail address: sgrief@uic.edu

Prim Care Clin Office Pract 45 (2018) 485–503
https://doi.org/10.1016/j.pop.2018.04.001
0095-4543/18/

hospitals or extended-care facilities.[5] Viral pathogens were identified in 27% of cases and bacterial pathogens in 14% of cases.[5] In adults of all ages, human rhinovirus and influenza were the most frequently identified viruses.[5] *Streptococcus pneumoniae* is the most common causal bacterium. *Staphylococcus aureus* and *Enterobacteriaceae* were significantly more common among patients requiring intensive care unit (ICU) level care.[4] Other bacteria identified in CAP include *Mycoplasma pneumoniae*, *Chlamydophila pneumoniae*, and *Haemophilus influenzae*.[5] Less common bacterial causes include *Mycobacterium tuberculosis*, *Legionella* sp, and *Pseudomonas aeruginosa*. These and other bacteria may be considered more likely in patients with certain risk factors (**Table 1**).[6]

DIAGNOSIS

A diagnosis of pneumonia should be considered in patients presenting with acute onset fever or chills and cough. The cough may be described as productive. Additional symptoms frequently seen include fatigue, anorexia, and pleuritic chest pain. Important components of a history include recent travel, history of underlying lung disease,

Table 1
Risk factors and infectious causes in community-acquired pneumonia

Risk Factor	Infectious
Agricultural animals	*Coxiella burnetii* (Q fever)
AIDS	*Aspergillus* and *Cryptococcus* species, *Histoplasma capsulatum*, *Haemophilus influenzae*, *Nocardia* species, nontuberculous mycobacteria, *Pneumocystis jiroveci*
Alcoholism (aspiration)	Anaerobic oral flora, *Klebsiella pneumoniae*, *Mycobacterium tuberculosis*, *Streptococcus pneumoniae*
Avian fecal matter	*H. capsulatum*
Chronic obstructive pulmonary disease	*Chlamydophila pneumoniae*, *H. influenzae*, *Legionella* species, *Moraxella catarrhalis*, *Pseudomonas aeruginosa* or other gram-negative rods, *S. pneumoniae*
HIV infection	*H. influenzae*, *M. tuberculosis*, *S. pneumoniae*
Hotel or cruise ship travel (recent)	*Legionella* species
Influenza	*H. influenzae*, influenza and other respiratory viruses, *S. pneumoniae*, *Staphylococcus aureus* (including MRSA)
Intravenous drug use	Anaerobes, *M. tuberculosis*, *S aureus* (including MRSA), *S. pneumoniae*
Pulmonary abscess	Anaerobic oral flora, *M. tuberculosis*, nontuberculous mycobacteria, *S. aureus* (including MRSA)
Travel (national/international)	*Blastomyces dermatitidis*, *Coccidioides* species, *Hantavirus* species Middle East respiratory syndrome, Avian influenza, inter alia

Abbreviations: AIDS, acquired immunodeficiency syndrome; HIV, human immunodeficiency virus; MRSA, methicillin-resistant staphylococcus aureus.

Adapted from Kaysin A, Viera AJ. Community-acquired pneumonia in adults: diagnosis and management. Am Fam Physician 2016;94(9):699; with permission.

and smoking history.[4,6] A study by Diehr and colleagues[7] found that history of alcoholism or bloody sputum have relative risk of 1, so the presence of these findings is not predictive of pneumonia. Physical examination findings frequently appreciated in patients with pneumonia include decreased breath sounds, rales, tactile fremitus, and crackles.[4,8] Tachypnea and hypotension are more worrisome symptoms that may also be seen and require urgent evaluation.[4] It is imperative to maintain a high level of suspicion in immunocompromised or elderly and nursing home patients, because they frequently display fewer overt symptoms of pneumonia when compared with the general population.[8,9]

No individual component of the history or physical examination is useful in diagnosing pneumonia, but the presence of multiple findings is required (**Table 2**). In adults presenting with acute cough, the baseline probability of pneumonia is only 5%. Absence of any vital sign abnormality (blood pressure, heart rate, respiratory rate) reduces the predicted probability of pneumonia to 1%.[8] A chest radiograph should be ordered for any patient with abnormal vital signs defined as temperature higher than 100°F, heart rate higher than 100 bpm, or respiratory rate higher than 20 bpm. Imaging should also be obtained for physical examination abnormalities of crackles or decreased breath sounds in a patient without asthma.[10] Infectious Disease Society of America 2016 Guidelines recommend imaging with a demonstrable infiltrate to confirm the diagnosis of pneumonia and to exclude other causes of cough and fever such as acute bronchitis.[11] Although X-ray imaging is a mainstay of diagnosis of pneumonia, the British Thoracic Society recommends the entire clinical picture should be considered when making a decision to treat.[12] A systematic review found that among patients who are sick enough to be admitted with a clinical diagnosis of CAP but have a normal initial chest radiograph, approximately 1 in 10 will develop radiographic evidence of pneumonia within 72 hours.[8] In such cases, it is appropriate to treat the patient empirically for pneumonia and repeat imaging in 24 to 48 hours.[11] Community resources and access to imaging may also affect decision to treat without imaging.

Routine blood and sputum culture testing is costly and often low-yield.[13] However, more extensive diagnostic testing should be considered in patients who are at risk for infection with unusual pathogens, who are not responding to treatment, or when additional testing is likely to change antibiotic management (**Table 3**).[11,12]

It is reasonable to consider respiratory viral polymerase chain reaction (PCR) to determine viral causes of symptoms, so that inappropriate antibiotic use can be limited. Additional testing for *M. tuberculosis* should be considered in a patient presenting with persistent cough, particularly in the setting of weight loss, malaise, night sweats, or hemoptysis. Additional risk factors for tuberculosis (TB) include

Table 2
Predictors of adult pneumonia

Score	Likelihood Ratio
≥3	14
≥1	5
≥−1	1.5
<−1	0.22

Add or subtract points as follows: rhinorrhea = −2, sore throat = −1, night sweats = 1, myalgias = 1, sputum all day = 1, respiratory rate >25/min = 2, temperature ≥37.8°C (100°F) = 2.

Adapted from Simel DL, Rennie D. Pneumonia, adult, community-acquired. In: Simel DL, Rennie D, editors. The rational clinical examination: evidence-based clinical diagnosis. New York: McGraw-Hill; 2009; with permission.

Table 3
Indications for further testing

Indication	Blood Culture	Sputum Culture	Legionella UAT	Pneumococcal UAT	Other
ICU admission	X	X	X	X	x[a]
Failure of outpatient antibiotic therapy	—	x	x	X	—
Cavitary infiltrates	X	X	—	—	x[b]
Leukopenia	x	—	—	x	—
Alcohol abuse (current)	x	X	x	x	—
Liver disease	x	—	—	x	—
Lung disease	—	x	—	—	—
Asplenia	x	—	—	x	—
Travel within past 2 wk	—	—	x	—	x[c]
Positive Legionella UAT results	—	x	NA	—	—
Positive pneumococcal UAT result	x	x	—	NA	—
Pleural effusion	x	x	x	x	x[d]

Abbreviations: NA, not applicable; UAT, urinary antigen test.
[a] Endotracheal aspirate if intubated, bronchoscopic alveolar lavage, as needed.
[b] Fungal and tuberculosis cultures.
[c] See **Table 1**.
[d] Thoracentesis and pleural fluid cultures.
Adapted from Mandell L, Wunderink R, Anzueto A, et al. Infectious Diseases Society of America/American Thoracic Society consensus guidelines on the management of community-acquired pneumonia in adults. Clin Infect Dis 2007;44(Supplement_2), S40; with permission.

immigration from an endemic country, residing in a homeless shelter, intravenous drug use, or human immunodeficiency virus (HIV) infection. Persons who work with people at high risk for TB infection are also considered high risk.[12,14]

TREATMENT

Most cases of pneumonia can be managed in the outpatient setting. Several severity assessment tools have been developed to help determine appropriate treatment settings. The Pneumonia Severity Index (PSI) considers 20 variables to stratify patients into 1 of 5 risk categories (I–V) based on risk of death within 30 days.[15] Given the number of parameters required, it is not frequently used in general practice. The CURB65 assessment tool was introduced in 2003 by the British Thoracic Society.[16] Similar to the PSI, it calculates risk of 30-day mortality, but instead only uses 5 variables (confusion, urea, respiratory rate, blood pressure, and age >65), with one point awarded for each if present, allowing for greater ease of use.[15,16] The CRB65 can be calculated without blood urea and thus is useful in the outpatient setting. A recent systematic review and meta-analysis found no significant difference in test performance when comparing the 3 severity tools.[15] It was noted that the PSI negative likelihood ratio suggests it may be superior in identifying low-risk patients, and the CURB65 and CRB65 may be superior in identifying high-risk patients.[15] A CURB65 or CRB65 score of 0 or 1 demonstrates low risk of mortality and suggests a patient can be managed in the outpatient setting. A score of 3 or higher should warrant hospital admission. It is always appropriate to consider a patient's social circumstances and treatment wishes when making treatment decisions[12,16] (**Fig. 1**; CURB65 score[12]).

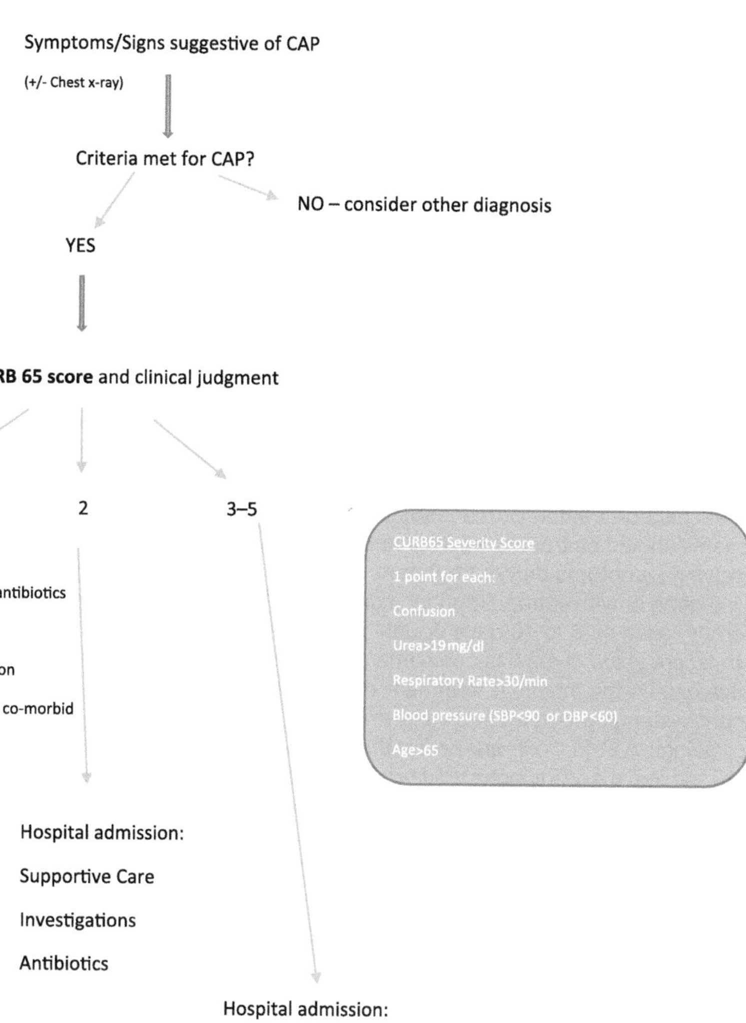

Fig. 1. CURB65 score. (*Adapted from* Lim WS, Baudouin SV, George RC, et al. BTS guidelines for the management of community acquired pneumonia in adults: update 2009. Thorax 2009;64(suppl 3):iii29; with permission.)

When available, treatment of CAP should be guided by local resistance patterns. In previously healthy patients who are appropriate for outpatient treatment, recommended first-line treatment is with a macrolide antibiotic such as azithromycin targeting the most common causal pathogen *S. pneumoniae*. Doxycycline is an alternative option. Patients with comorbidities such as diabetes; chronic heart, lung, renal, or liver disease; alcoholism; asplenia; impaired immune system; or recent antibiotic use within the last 3 months have an increased risk for drug-resistant *S pneumoniae*. As such, a respiratory fluoroquinolone or β-lactam plus a macrolide is recommended (**Table 4**).[11]

Table 4
Outpatient treatment of community-acquired pneumonia

Presence of Comorbidities	Antibiotic Choice
NO	Macrolide or doxycycline
YES	Fluoroquinolone or beta-lactam + macrolide (doxycycline is an alternative for macrolide)

Comorbidities: chronic heart; lung, liver, kidney disease; diabetes; cancer; impaired immune system; alcoholism; asplenia; recent use of antibiotics in previous 3 mo; and risk for multidrug-resistant *S. pneumoniae*.

Adapted from Mandell L, Wunderink R, Anzueto A, et al. Infectious Diseases Society of America/American Thoracic Society consensus guidelines on the management of community-acquired pneumonia in adults. Clin Infect Dis 2007;44(Supplement 2):S45.

A 2014 Cochrane review found no significant differences in efficacy between antibiotic regimens, although there were differences in adverse effects when comparing antibiotics within a single class.[17] Patients appropriate for inpatient non-ICU treatment should also be treated with a respiratory fluoroquinolone or macrolide with β-lactam. Patients should be treated for a minimum of 5 days and should be clinically stable with resolving symptoms before treatment is discontinued.[11,18] Patients with high severity of infection or with extrapulmonary manifestations may benefit from longer duration of therapy, such as 7 to 10 days or until improving.[11,12]

In recent years, there has been emerging data supporting the use of adjunctive corticosteroids in the inpatient treatment of CAP. As this is an area of research, multiple recent systematic reviews and meta-analyses have been published, some with conflicting findings. A 2011 Cochrane review that included relevant CAP studies through the year 2010 showed that corticosteroid use accelerates time to symptom resolution and clinical stability, with infrequent adverse effects.[19] Similarly, a 2015 systematic review by Siemieniuk and colleagues[20] included studies from 2011 through mid-2015. Their analysis of 13 randomized controlled trials found significantly decreased mortality in severe pneumonia, decreased need for mechanical ventilation, decreased occurrence of acute respiratory distress syndrome, decreased time to clinical stability, and shorter duration of hospitalization.[20] Hyperglycemia requiring treatment occurred more frequently in patients treated with corticosteroids.[20,21] The most recent IDSA and BTS guidelines do not make recommendations regarding the routine use of adjunctive corticosteroid for CAP.[11,12] Given the variations in dose and route of administration, an optimal agent and dose is unknown. Further research is needed to determine steroid dosing and duration, as well as what patient populations are most likely to benefit from its use.[20,21]

There are a large number of studies assessing the role of the infection biomarker procalcitonin in diagnosis and monitoring of patients with bacterial infections.[22] A Cochrane 2017 meta-analysis in the primary care setting concluded that the use of procalcitonin to guide initiation and duration of antibiotic treatment results in lower risks of mortality, lower antibiotic consumption, and lower risk for antibiotic-related side effects.[23] Procalcitonin values too low or too high usually exclude bacterial infection, but not always.[24]

Per practitioner discretion and, depending on patient complexity and other comorbidities, a follow-up appointment after successful management in the primary care setting may be arranged. At this appointment, repeat X-ray imaging to confirm resolution of pneumonia is not indicated if the patient seems clinically well. In patients with persistence of symptoms or who have a high risk of lung cancer (age > 50, >30 pack year smoking history), repeat X-ray imaging or low-dose computerized tomography (CT) scan to screen for lung cancer can be considered.[12]

PREVENTION

In the United States, the pneumococcal conjugate vaccine (PCV13 or Prevnar-13) is recommended for all babies and children younger than 2 years, all adults aged 65 years or older, as well as children and adults aged 2 years through 64 years who are at increased risk for pneumococcal disease due to certain medical conditions.[24] The pneumococcal conjugate vaccine has been shown to have an observed 46% reduction in vaccine-type pneumococcal CAP, persisting for at least 4 years after receiving the vaccine.[25,26] The pneumococcal polysaccharide vaccine (PPSV23 or Pneumovax 23) is recommended for all adults aged 65 years or older, all cigarette smokers aged 19 to 64 years, as well as children and adults aged 2 to 64 years with certain medical conditions.[27] A 2013 Cochrane review found that the polysaccharide vaccine is effective in preventing invasive pneumococcal disease in healthy adults. Vaccine efficacy was, however, poorer in adults with chronic illnesses.[28]

NONRESOLVING PNEUMONIA

Pneumonia is considered "nonresolving" if there is an inadequate clinical response despite antibiotic treatment.[11] The incidence of treatment failure is 6% to 15% and is associated with a 5-fold increase in mortality.[29] IDSA broadly classifies nonresponse into 2 different groups: (1) progressive pneumonia characterized by clinical deterioration and (2) persistent pneumonia with absence or delay of clinical stability.[11] Progressive pneumonia with deterioration is characterized by respiratory failure and/or septic shock and typically occurs within 72 hours. Persistent pneumonia with absent or delayed response is typically considered after a time period of 72 hours, because this is often regarded as the median time required for clinical stability.[11,29]

Concern for nonresponse in a patient with pneumonia should initiate a systematic evaluation of possible causes. Host factors that may explain poor response should be considered, including high initial severity score, risk factors for infection with unusual organisms, underlying comorbidities, or risk factors for multi–drug-resistant pathogens (**Table 5**).[24] In areas with high prevalence of HIV or TB, testing is

Table 5
BAD OMEN (nonresolving pneumonia)

Disease/Risk Factor Mnemonic	Listing of Diseases/Conditions/Risk Factors
B	Bronchiolitis obliterans/Bronchiectasis/Influenza B
A	Age >60/Aspiration/Anaerobic infection/Abscess/Influenza A/Atypical pathogens (eg, Legionella, Mycoplasma, hMPV, chlamydia)
D	Drug-resistant pneumonia from *S. Pneumoniae*, gram-negative bacteria, MRSA, ESBL/Drug-induced pneumonitis (eg, amiodarone, MTX, nitrofurantoin, cancer biologics)/Delayed resolution from corticosteroids
O	Opportunistic pathogens (eg, Fungi, mold, *Pneumocystis Jiroveci*); anaerobic bacteria. Consider HIV testing.
M	Misdiagnosis (fungal infections, sarcoidosis, TB)
E	Embolism/Empyema/Eosinophilic pneumonia
N	Neoplasm/Nosocomial bacterial pneumonia

Abbreviations: ESBL, extended-spectrum beta-lactamase organisms; hMPV, human metapneumovirus; MTX, methotrexate.

Adapted from Tan L, Louie S. Unresolved acute pneumonia: a "BAD OMEN". Consultant 2017;57(8):502; with permission.

recommended.[30] Results of initial microbiological tests such as blood or sputum cultures should be reviewed, including any sensitivity data. Repeat blood cultures should be obtained in the setting of clinical deterioration. Additional laboratory testing for *S. pneumonia* and *Legionella pneumophila* via urine antigen testing may be performed, because they may remain positive for days after initiating antibiotic treatment. Additional imaging such as chest CT may be beneficial for assessing interval progression or improvement or identifying pleural effusions, lung abscesses, or pulmonary embolism. If pleural effusions are identified in a patient with treatment failure, thoracentesis should be performed to evaluate for empyema. In select patients, bronchoscopy with protected bronchial sampling or bronchoalveolar lavage (BAL) may be beneficial to provide diagnostic information for infectious causes and noninfectious mimics, such as pulmonary eosinophilia, drug-induced pneumonitis, sarcoidosis, or pulmonary fibrosis.[11,29] Primary or metastatic neoplastic lesions obstructing the bronchus may cause accumulation of secretions distal to the obstruction, predisposing to infection. Both Hodgkin and non-Hodgkin lymphoma can present with lung involvement, with typical radiographic findings of hilar or mediastinal adenopathy, but may also have a presenting pattern that suggests infection.[31]

PNEUMONIA IN THE ELDERLY

Elderly patients with pneumonia may not exhibit typical symptoms or physical examination findings seen in younger adults, such as pleuritic chest pain, cough, fever, and leukocytosis.[32] Signs and symptoms more frequently seen in older adults include falls, decreased appetite, or functional impairment.[32] A change in mental status should prompt evaluation for an infectious cause.[9,11] As with any adult, risk factors for atypical or drug-resistant pathogens should guide treatment. Elderly patients with history of stroke or known dysphagia are at an increased risk for aspiration pneumonia. Residents of nursing homes or long-term care facilities are at an increased risk for methicillin-resistant *Staphylococcus aureus* (MRSA) or multidrug-resistant (MDR) pathogens.[32]

TRAVEL

Evaluation of a returned traveler should include the following: appropriate history covering the travel itinerary (location and activities), onset of illness related to travel, vaccines or prophylaxis received, diet, sexual history, and exposure to animals.[30,33] Respiratory tract infections are among the most common health care complaints affecting returned travelers and are diagnosed in up to 24% of returned patients with fever.[30,34] Although upper respiratory tract infections are more common, the severity and possible mortality associated with lower respiratory tract infections such as pneumonia make it a must-not-miss diagnosis in the returned traveler. As in the United States, *S pneumoniae*, *H. influenzae*, and *S. aureus* are the dominant pneumonia isolates in developing countries. It must be considered that bacterial resistance patterns from different countries may differ in these otherwise commonplace bacteria.[34]

Respiratory symptoms occur in up to half of patients with malaria, and the presentation may seem similar to that of pneumonia. Thus, in a patient returning from a malaria-endemic area, blood smear testing for malaria should be performed.[35] Increased time spent at hotels or on cruise ships in a patient presenting with symptoms of pneumonia should increase suspicion for *Legionella*.[30] Travelers returning from East and Southeast Asia, as well as Australia, with a severe pneumonia may have been exposed to *Burkholderia pseudomallei*—the causative agent of melioidosis, which can cause severe necrotizing pneumonia and has 14% to 40% mortality despite appropriate antibiotic therapy.[30] Severe pneumonia may also be because of viruses such as influenza, Middle

Eastern respiratory syndrome, or hantavirus. A returned traveler with pneumonia with eosinophilia should raise suspicion for helminth infection.[30,34]

Histoplasma capsulatum is a dimorphic fungus that is relatively common in North, Central, and South America and given its growth in bird and bat droppings is associated with activities such as cave exploration. *Coccidioides immitis* is endemic in the southwest United States and northern Mexico, as well as smaller areas in Central America. It is spread through inhalation of spores found in the soil. Fungal infection with *H. capsulatum* and *C immitis* are often asymptomatic but may also present as a flulike illness with fever, malaise, and dry cough 1 to 3 weeks after exposure.[34,36]

Ventilator-Associated Pneumonia

Ventilator-associated pneumonia (VAP) is a type of pneumonia that occurs in patients who have been intubated or mechanically ventilated by means of a tracheostomy for at least 48 hours.[37,38] Mechanical ventilation modifies the oropharyngeal and tracheal environment, allowing oral and gastric secretions to enter the lower airways.[37] It is this change in lower respiratory tract bacterial flora that precipitates the beginning of pneumonia.

VAP is common. Approximately 30% of patients who receive mechanical ventilation will develop VAP.[39]

DIAGNOSTIC CRITERIA

VAP should be suspected when signs of pulmonary infection (fever, purulent secretions, leukocytosis) and radiologic evidence (air bronchograms, infiltrates) are present; bacteriologic confirmation usually follows.[40] Sensitivity and specificity of the diagnostic criteria discussed earlier are 69% and 75%, respectively.[40] Other useful diagnostic criteria have been developed, incorporating additional symptoms and similar signs and laboratory/radiologic criteria.[41] Once VAP is clinically suspected, early empirical treatment is favored. Delaying treatment and/or not appropriately covering for the likely microbial culprit are both associated with higher morbidity and mortality.[42–45]

MICROBIOLOGY

Microbial organisms associated with VAP have been identified (**Table 6**). Early versus late-onset VAP organisms have also been documented.[46,47] Acinetobacter, citrobacter, pseudomonas, and klebsiella are the most predominant late-onset organisms, warranting more aggressive antibacterial intervention.[47]

DIAGNOSTIC TESTING

Bacterial confirmation usually requires secretion sampling, either via bronchoscopic or via nonbronchoscopic methods. Obtaining pleural fluid, when present, under ultrasound guidance, is recommended.[37] Endotracheal aspirates are easily retrieved but have a high false-positive rate in ICU patients due to airway colonization.[37] Bronchoscopic retrieval of distal airway specimens via BAL or protected-specimen brush techniques is the best, but requires a trained bronchoscopist.[37]

ANTIBIOTIC TREATMENT

Selection of antibiotics is typically done empirically and based on whether the patient has any risk factors for MDR pathogens (**Table 7**) and whether onset of VAP is early (defined as within first 4 days of being in the ICU) or late (5 days or later).[37,38,48]

Table 6
Bacterial distribution in ventilator-associated pneumonia

Bacterial Organism	Percentage
Citrobacter freundii	53
Klebsiella pneumoniae	13
Staphylococcus aureus	9.5
Acinetobacter baumannii	7.5
Pseudomonas aeruginosa	3.8
P. aeruginosa + C. freundii	3.8
Coagulase-negative Staphylococci	1.9
Escherichia coli	1.9
Morganella morganii	1.9
Proteus vulgaris	1.9
P. aeruginosa + K. pneumoniae	1.9

Adapted from Thakuria B, Singh P, Agrawal S, et al. Profile of infective microorganisms causing ventilator-associated pneumonia: a clinical study from resource limited intensive care unit. J Anaesthesiol Clin Pharmacol 2013;29(3):363; with permission.

Empirical treatment should also be determined as a result of knowledge of local distribution of pathogens and their antimicrobial susceptibility patterns.[49] Early-onset VAP without MDR risk factors typically should be prescribed one of the following antibiotic options[37]:

- Ceftriaxone
- Fluoroquinolone
- Ampicillin-sulbactam
- Ertapenem

For late-onset and/or MDR factor patients, appropriate antibiotic options would include one or more of the following[37]:

Table 7
Risk factors for multidrug-resistant ventilator-associated pneumonia

Risk Factors for MDR Pathogens	Risk Factors for MDR Pseudomonas and Other Gram-Negative Bacilli	Risk Factors for MRSA
IV antibiotic use within previous 3 mo Sepsis accompanying VAP Adult respiratory distress syndrome before VAP Late-onset VAP (5 d or more in ICU/hospital) Dialysis just before VAP	Treatment in an ICU setting with the following: 1. >10% of gram-negative isolates are resistant to one or more antibiotics indicated for VAP 2. Local antimicrobial susceptibilities are unknown	Treatment in a medical ward/ICU in which: 1. >10%–20% of *Staphylococcus aureus* isolates are MRSA 2. Prevalence of MRSA is unknown

Abbreviations: IV, intravenous; MDR, multidrug-resistant; MRSA, methicillin-resistant *S. aureus*; VAP, ventilator-associated pneumonia.

Adapted from Kalil AC, Metersky ML, Klompas M, et al. Management of adults with hospital-acquired and ventilator-associated pneumonia: 2016 clinical practice guidelines by the Infectious Diseases Society of America and the American Thoracic Society. Clin Infect Dis 2016;63:e61; with permission.

- Antipseudomonal cephalosporins (eg, Cefepime, ceftazidime)
- Antipseudomonal carbapenems (imipenem or meropenem)
- Beta-lactam/beta-lactamase inhibitors (piperacillin-tazobactam) with an antipseudomonal fluoroquinolone (ciprofloxacin) or aminoglycoside plus linezolid or vancomycin (if MRSA risk factors are present)
- Telavancin is indicated for VAP for susceptible isolates of *S. aureus* when other therapies are not suitable.

Dose and frequency of administration of the antibiotic choices discussed earlier are documented extensively elsewhere.[38] Atypical antibiotic choices, such as colistin, polymyxin B, telavancin, inter alia, are rarely indicated but can be used when antimicrobial resistance warrants these agents.[48] Typically, consultation with an infectious disease physician or clinical pharmacist with expertise and familiarity when using these drugs is a sine qua non.[48]

Pediatric Pneumonia

Epidemiology

Pneumonia is a very common affliction of childhood. Pneumonia accounts for 13% of infectious illnesses in infants and toddlers younger than 2 years.[50] Worldwide, approximately 150 million new cases of pneumonia occur annually among children younger than 5 years.[50] Pneumonia is the leading cause of death in children younger than 5 years in developing countries, accounting for 16% of all deaths of children younger than 5 years and killing 920,136 children in 2015.[51,52]

Most childhood pneumonia (CP) can be treated in the outpatient setting. The rate of hospitalization for CP through age 18 years varies per year, but in 2006 it was 201.1 per 100 000.[53] Infants younger than 1 year had the highest rate of hospitalization (912.9 per 100 000), whereas children aged 13 to 18 years had the lowest rate (62.8 per 100 000).[53]

Diagnosis

Signs and symptoms of CP are often nonspecific and depend on several factors including age, microbial organism, and underlying health of the patient. Clinical acumen is key to successfully diagnosing CP. The universal symptom of CP is cough. Other symptoms may include chest pain, headache, arthralgia, nausea, and abdominal pain.[54] Most common signs to look for include fever, tachypnea, labored breathing, rhonchi, crackles, and wheezing.[54] Other physical signs to identify include grunting, nasal flaring, and chest retractions because these increase the likelihood of CP.[55] Diagnostic testing is usually performed, when available, and would include assessment of oxygen saturation by pulse oximetry, chest radiograph, complete blood cell count, respiratory microbial panel by PCR, ultrasound of the chest (when medically indicated), and cultures. Disagreement about whether blood cultures are warranted exists in the literature. As per a recent study, blood cultures have not been shown to assist with clinical management in children hospitalized with pneumonia.[56] The Infectious Diseases Society of America, however, recommends blood cultures for all hospitalized children with pneumonia.[57]

Etiology of pneumonia

Etiologic microbial organisms differ, depending on age of the child. In infants, toddlers, and preschoolers, viruses predominate (**Table 8**). Less common bacterial organisms may infect newborns (see **Table 8**). In older children, bacteria are the more common culprit (**Table 9**). Atypical organisms may be involved when children are immunocompromised or have other underlying comorbidities (see **Table 9**).

Table 8
Etiology of childhood pneumonia (age 0–5 years)

Viruses	Bacteria
RSV	*Streptococcus pneumoniae*
Parainfluenza types 1, 2, 3	Hemophilus influenzae type B
Influenza A and B	Streptococcus pyogenes
Adenovirus	*Staphylococcus aureus*
Rhinovirus	Mycoplasma pneumoniae
Coronavirus	Chlamydia pneumoniae/Chlamydia trachomatis
hMPV	Bordetella pertussis
HSV	***Escherichia coli***
VZV	***Klebsiella pneumoniae***
CMV	***Listeria monocytogenes***
Enterovirus	***Group B Streptococcus***

Abbreviations: CMV, cytomegalovirus; hMPV, human metapneumovirus; HSV, herpes simplex virus; RSV, respiratory syncytial virus; VZV, varicella zoster virus.

Italicized/bolded are more common in newborns (age 0–30 days).

Data from Bennett NJ, Domachowske J, Steele R. Pediatric pneumonia. Medscape. 2017; and Stuckey-Schrock K, Hayes BL, George CM. Community-acquired pneumonia in children. Am Fam Physician 2012;86(7):661–7.

Outpatient versus inpatient

In order to provide optimal care to a child with pneumonia, it is important to determine the severity of the pneumonia and the child's clinical status. Most children will not require inpatient admission; criteria exist to help stratify severity of pneumonia and necessity of hospitalization (**Box 1** and **2**).

Antibiotics

Choosing an antibiotic for CP is initially always an empirical process and based on local and regional microbial susceptibility and resistance patterns, along with the child's age, immunization status, and any underlying, preexisting health

Table 9
Causes of childhood pneumonia (>5 years old)

Bacteria	Viruses	Atypical Organisms
Mycoplasma pneumoniae	CMV	Aspergillus
Streptococcus pneumoniae	Influenza A and B	*Pneumocystis jirovecii*
Staphylococcus aureus	Rhinovirus	*Pseudomonas aeruginosa*
Streptococcus pyogenes	Adenovirus	*Burkholderia cepacia*
Chlamydia pneumoniae	RSV	*Histoplasma capsulatum*
Hemophilus influenzae type B	Parainfluenza	*Cryptococcus neoformans*
	hMPV	*Blastomyces dermatitidis*
	Enterovirus	*Mycobacterium tuberculosis*
		Legionella pneumophila
		Oral anaerobes (aspiration)

Abbreviations: CMV, cytomegalovirus; hMPV, human metapneumovirus; RSV, respiratory syncytial virus.

Data from Refs.[1,5,9]

Box 1
Criteria for childhood pneumonia hospitalization

Infants younger than 3 to 6 months with suspected bacterial CAP

Suspected or documented CAP caused by a pathogen with increased virulence, such as community-associated methicillin-resistant *Staphylococcus aureus*

Temperature greater or equal to 38.5 C (101.3 F)

Children and infants for whom there is concern about careful observation at home or who are unable to comply with therapy or unable to be followed-up

Children and infants who have respiratory distress and hypoxemia (oxygen saturation <92%) (see **Table 2**)

Children and infants with comorbidities (eg, asthma, cystic fibrosis, congenital heart disease, diabetes mellitus, neuromuscular disease)

Poor feeding and/or signs of dehydration

Abbreviation: CAP, community-acquired pneumonia.

Modified from Bradley JS, Byington CL, Shah SS, et al. The management of community-acquired pneumonia in infants and children older than 3 months of age: clinical practice guidelines by the Pediatric Infectious Diseases Society and the Infectious Diseases Society of America. Clin Infect Dis 2011;53(7):e29; with permission.

conditions.[50,54,58,59] Most children can be treated with oral antibiotics in the outpatient setting. First-line and preferred agent is still amoxicillin.[50,54,57,59] Alternative agents are cephalosporins and macrolide antibiotics; however, increasing resistance to penicillin derivatives and macrolides should be noted[60] (**Table 10**). Quinolones can be considered in cases where there are no reasonable alternatives due to MDR pathogens or when an oral antibiotic is deemed optimal.[61] Quinolones

Box 2
Signs of respiratory distress

Tachypnea: RR

Age 0 to 2 months: greater than 60; age 2 to 12 months: greater than 50; age 1 to 5 years: greater than 40; age greater than 5 years: greater than 20

Dyspnea

Retractions: suprasternal, intercostal, or subcostal

Grunting

Nasal flaring

Apnea

Altered mental status

Pulse oximetry measurement less than 90% on room air

Abbreviation: RR, respiratory rate.

Adapted from Bradley JS, Byington CL, Shah SS, et al. The management of community-acquired pneumonia in infants and children older than 3 months of age: clinical practice guidelines by the Pediatric Infectious Diseases Society and the Infectious Diseases Society of America. Clin Infect Dis 2011;53(7):e28; with permission.

Table 10
Outpatient childhood pneumonia antibiotic treatment guidelines

Age	Preferred/First-Line	Alternative/Second-Line
0–5 y		
Viral	No treatment	Antiviral against influenza
Bacterial	Amoxicillin	Amoxicillin-clavulanate/ third-generation cephalosporin
Atypical bacterial	Macrolide	Consult infectious disease
Allergy to any of the above	Third-generation cephalosporin/clindamycin	Quinolone
5–16 y		
Viral	No treatment	Antiviral against influenza
Bacterial	Amoxicillin	Amoxicillin-clavulanate/ third-generation cephalosporin
Atypical bacterial	Macrolide or doxycycline	Quinolone if older than 8 years and suspect MDR organism
Allergy to any of the above	Third-generation cephalosporin/clindamycin	Quinolone

Adapted from Cincinnati Children's Hospital Medical Center. Evidence-based care guideline. Community acquired pneumonia in children 60 days through 17 years of age. Available at: https://www.idsociety.org/uploadedFiles/IDSA/Guidelines-Patient_Care/PDF_Library/2011%20CAP%20in%20Children.pdf Accessed February 20, 2018; with permission.

have been linked to development of childhood tendonitis/tendinopathy, yet recent literature indicates these disabling side effects are rare.[61,62] Inpatient treatment guidelines have also been established (**Table 11**). Isolation of the particular microbial organism is ideal, but not required, in order to determine duration of therapy. Uncomplicated pneumonia treatment in the outpatient setting usually should last 5 to 10 days.[54] Inpatient admission for pneumonia warrants longer duration of antibiotic therapy, typically 7 to 10 days of combined parenteral and oral therapy or at least 1 week after becoming afebrile.[58] Complicated cases of pneumonia will require a minimum of 2 weeks of therapy once lack of fever is confirmed and may be extended for up to 4 weeks.[58] The switch from parenteral to oral therapy may occur after 24 to 48 hours of documented lack of fever but is not always practical in complicated and/or ICU-admitted patients.[63]

SUMMARY

Pneumonia is a common, well-recognized respiratory infection seen in primary care settings. Triage of the usual presenting symptoms will generally set into motion a typical course of action, including physical examination and possibly imaging to confirm clinical suspicion. Further testing depends on treatment venue (outpatient vs inpatient) and other specific criteria (see **Table 3**). Empirical antibiotic therapy is the cornerstone of treatment, and knowledge of local and regional microbial susceptibility and resistance will bolster the success rate of outpatient management of pneumonia, regardless of demographic and/or accompanying morbidities. Special circumstances and scenarios that may occur, including nonresolving pneumonias, pediatric or geriatric populations, travel-related infections, among others, will necessitate a more careful attention to history, physical examination, and antibiotic selection.

Table 11
Inpatient childhood pneumonia antibiotic treatment guidelines

Age/Category	Preferred/First-Line	Alternative/Second-Line
0–6 mo		
Bacterial	IV penicillin derivative and third-generation cephalosporin	Aminoglycoside with PCN derivative; macrolide if suspect atypical organism
6 mo–5 y		
Bacterial	IV penicillin derivative (PCN or ampicillin)	Third-generation cephalosporin
MRSA	Vancomycin or clindamycin (in addition to beta-lactam antibiotic)	Vancomycin or clindamycin (in addition to beta-lactam antibiotic)
Atypical bacterial infection	Macrolide	Macrolide (in addition to beta-lactam antibiotic)
Allergy to any of the above	Third-generation cephalosporin/ clindamycin	Quinolone
5–16 y		
Bacterial	IV penicillin derivative (PCN or ampicillin)	Third-generation cephalosporin
MRSA	Vancomycin or clindamycin (in addition to beta-lactam antibiotic)	Vancomycin or clindamycin (in addition to beta-lactam antibiotic); linezolid in children aged 12 y or older
Atypical bacterial infection	Macrolide	Macrolide (in addition to beta-lactam antibiotic)
Allergy to any of the above	Third-generation cephalosporin/ clindamycin	Quinolone
Severe pneumonia/ ICU admission	Third-generation cephalosporin and macrolide/vancomycin + third-gen ceph + macrolide	Third-generation cephalosporin and doxycycline/vancomycin + third-gen ceph + macrolide + (optional) Nafcillin + antiviral

Abbreviations: Ceph, cephalosporin; IV, intravenous; PCN, penicillin.

Adapted from Cincinnati Children's Hospital Medical Center. Evidence-based care guideline. Community acquired pneumonia in children 60 days through 17 years of age. Available at: file:///C:/Users/sgrief/Downloads/Community%20Acquired%20Pneumona%20Great%20001.pdf. Accessed February 20, 2018; with permission.

REFERENCES

1. McDermott KW, Elixhauser A, Sun R. Trends in hospital inpatient stays in the United States, 2005-2014. HCUP statistical brief #225. Rockville (MD): Agency for Healthcare Research and Quality; 2017. Available at: https://www.hcup-us.ahrq.gov/reports/statbriefs/sb225-Inpatient-US-Stays-Trends.pdf.
2. Rui P, Kang K. National Hospital Ambulatory Medical Care Survey: 2014 emergency department summary tables. Available at: http://www.cdc.gov/nchs/data/ahcd/nhamcs_emergency/2014_ed_web_tables.pdf. Accessed January 16, 2018.
3. Torio C, Moore B. National inpatient hospital costs: the most expensive conditions by payer, 2013. HCUP statistical brief #204. Rockville (MD): Agency for Healthcare Research and Quality; 2016. Available at: http://www.hcup-us.ahrq.gov/reports/statbriefs/sb204-Most-Expensive-Hospital-Conditions.pdf.

4. Jain S, Self WH, Wunderink RG, et al. Community-acquired pneumonia requiring hospitalization among U.S. adults. N Engl J Med 2015;373(5):415–27.
5. Cisneros ED, Lazarte SM. General infectious diseases. In: De Fer T, Sateia H, editors. The Washington manual of outpatient internal medicine. Philadelphia: Lippincott Williams & Wilkins; 2015. p. 523–6.
6. Kaysin A, Viera AJ. Community- acquired pneumonia in adults: diagnosis and management. Am Fam Physician 2016;94(9):698–706.
7. Diehr P, Wood RW, Bushyhead J, et al. Prediction of pneumonia in outpatients with acute cough: a statistical approach. J Chronic Dis 1984;37(3):215–25.
8. Simel DL, Metlay JP. Pneumonia, adult, community-acquired. In: Simel DL, Rennie D, editors. The rational clinical examination: evidence-based clinical diagnosis. New York: McGraw-Hill; 2009. Available at: http://jamaevidence.mhmedical.com.proxy.cc.uic.edu/content.aspx?bookid=845§ionid=61357585. Accessed December 17, 2017.
9. Casey C, Fullerton M, Somerville N. Common questions about pneumonia in nursing home residents. Am Fam Physician 2015;92(7):612–20.
10. Ebell MH. Predicting pneumonia in adults with respiratory illness. Am Fam Physician 2007;76(4):560–2.
11. Mandell L, Wunderink R, Anzueto A, et al. Infectious Diseases Society of America/American Thoracic Society consensus guidelines on the management of community-acquired pneumonia in adults. Clin Infect Dis 2007;44(Supplement 2):S27–72.
12. Lim W, Baudouin S, George R, et al. BTS guidelines for the management of community acquired pneumonia in adults: update 2009. Thorax 2009;64(Suppl 3):iii1–55.
13. Gupta D, Agarwal R, Aggarwal AN, et al. Guidelines for diagnosis and management of community- and hospital-acquired pneumonia in adults: joint ICS/NCCP(I) recommendations. Lung India 2012;29(Suppl 2):S27–62.
14. Tuberculosis (TB) | CDC. Cdcgov. 2018. Available at: https://www.cdc.gov/tb/default.htm. Accessed February 24, 2018.
15. Chalmers J, Singanayagam A, Akram A, et al. Severity assessment tools for predicting mortality in hospitalised patients with community-acquired pneumonia. Systematic review and meta-analysis. Thorax 2010;65(10):878–83.
16. Lim WS, van der Eerden MM, Laing R, et al. Defining community acquired pneumonia severity on presentation to hospital: an international derivation and validation study. Thorax 2003;58(5):377–82.
17. Pakhale S, Mulpuru S, Verheij TJM, et al. Antibiotics for community-acquired pneumonia in adult outpatients. Cochrane Database Syst Rev 2014;2014(10):CD002109.
18. Uranga A, España P, Bilbao A, et al. Duration of antibiotic treatment in community-acquired pneumonia. JAMA Intern Med 2016;176(9):1257.
19. Chen Y, Li K, Pu H, et al. Corticosteroids for pneumonia. Cochrane Database Syst Rev 2011;(3):CD007720.
20. Siemieniuk R, Alonso-Coello P, Guyatt G. Corticosteroid therapy for patients hospitalized with community-acquired pneumonia. Ann Intern Med 2016;164(9):636.
21. Feldman C, Anderson R. Corticosteroids in the adjunctive therapy of community-acquired pneumonia: an appraisal of recent meta-analyses of clinical trials. J Thorac Dis 2016;8(3):E162–71.
22. Sager R, Kutz A, Mueller B, et al. Procalcitonin-guided diagnosis and antibiotic stewardship revisited. BMC Med 2017;15(1):15.

23. Schuetz P, Wirz Y, Sager R, et al. Procalcitonin to initiate or discontinue antibiotics in acute respiratory tract infections. Cochrane Database Syst Rev 2017;(10):CD007498.
24. Tan L, Louie S. Unresolved Acute Pneumonia: a "BAD OMEN". Consultant 2017;500–3.
25. Cdc.gov. Pneumococcal vaccination | what you should know | CDC. [online]. 2017. Available at: https://www.cdc.gov/vaccines/vpd/pneumo/public/index.html. Accessed December 14, 2017.
26. Bonten M, Huijts SM, Bolkenbaas M, et al. Polysaccharide conjugate vaccine against pneumococcal pneumonia in adults. N Engl J Med 2015;372(12):1114–25.
27. Centers for Disease Control and Prevention. Updated recommendations for prevention of invasive pneumococcal disease among adults using the 23-valent pneumococcal polysaccharide vaccine (PPSV23). MMWR Morb Mortal Wkly Rep 2010;59:1102–5.
28. Moberley S, Holden J, Tatham DP, et al. Vaccines for preventing pneumococcal infection in adults. Cochrane Database Syst Rev 2013;(1):CD000422.
29. Sialer S, Liapikou A, Torres A. What is the best approach to the nonresponding patient with community-acquired pneumonia? Infect Dis Clin North Am 2013;27(1):189–203.
30. Trimble A, Moffat V, Collins A. Pulmonary infections in the returned traveler. Pneumonia (Nathan) 2017;9:1.
31. Black A. Non-infectious mimics of community-acquired pneumonia. Pneumonia 2016;8:2.
32. Faverio P, Aliberti S, Bellelli G, et al. The management of community-acquired pneumonia in the elderly. Eur J Intern Med 2014;25(4):312–9.
33. Centers for Disease Control and Prevention. CDC yellow book 2018: health information for international travel. New York: Oxford University Press; 2017.
34. Meltzer E, Schwartz E. Travel-related respiratory infections. In: Schwartz E, editor. Tropical diseases in travelers. Hoboken (NJ): Wiley-Blackwell; 2009. p. 413–26.
35. Fairley JK. General approach to the returned traveler. In: Chapter 5: post-travel evaluation. Centers for disease control and prevention. Available at: https://wwwnc.cdc.gov/travel/yellowbook/2018/post-travel-evaluation/general-approach-to-the-returned-traveler. Accessed February 26, 2018.
36. Segel MJ, Schwartz E. Histoplasmosis and other endemic fungal infections. In: Schwartz E, editor. Tropical diseases in travelers. Hoboken (NJ): Wiley-Blackwell; 2009. p. 282–93.
37. Amanullah S, Mosenifar Z. Ventilator-associated pneumonia overview of nosocomial pneumonias. Medscape 2015.
38. File TM. Treatment of hospital-acquired and ventilator-associated pneumonia in adults. UpToDate 2018.
39. Cook DJ, Walter SD, Cook RJ, et al. Incidence of and risk factors for ventilator-associated pneumonia in critically ill patients. Ann Intern Med 1998;129(6):433–40.
40. Fabregas N, Ewig S, Torres A, et al. Clinical diagnosis of ventilator-associated pneumonia revisited: comparative validation using immediate post-mortem lung biopsies. Thorax 1999;54(10):867–73.
41. Horan T, Gaynes R. Survillence of nosocomial infection. In: Mayhall C, editor. Hospital epidemiology and infection control. 3rd edition. Philadelphia: Lippincott Williams and Wilkins; 2004. p. 1659–702.

42. El Kuti, Patel AA, Coleman CI. Impact of inappropriate antibiotic therapy on mortality in patients with ventilator-associate pneumonia and blood stream infection: a meta-analysis. J Crit Care 2008;23:91.
43. Muscedere JG, Shorr AF, Jiang X, et al. The adequacy of timely empiric antibiotic therapy for ventilator-associate pneumonia: an important determinant of outcome. J Crit Care 2012;27:322.e7.
44. Paul M, Shani V, Muchtar E, et al. Systematic review and meta-analysis of the efficacy of appropriate empiric antibiotic therapy for sepsis. Antimicrob Agents Chemother 2010;54:4851.
45. Swanson JM, Wells DL. Empirical antibiotic therapy for ventilator-associated pneumonia. Antibiotics (Basel) 2013;2:339.
46. Thakuria B, Singh P, Agrawal S, et al. Profile of infective microorganisms causing ventilator-associated pneumonia: A clinical study from resource limited intensive care unit. J Anaesthesiol Clin Pharmacol 2013;29(3):361–6.
47. Rello J, Torres A. Microbial causes of ventilator-associated pneumonia. Semin Respir Infect 1996;11(1):24–31.
48. Kalil AC, Metersky ML, Klompas M, et al. Management of adults with hospital-acquired and ventilator-associated pneumonia: 2016 clinical practice guidelines by the Infectious Diseases Society of America and the American Thoracic Society. Clin Infect Dis 2016;63:e61.
49. Beardsley JR, Williamson JC, Johnson JW, et al. Using local microbiologic data to develop institution-specific guidelines for the treatment of hospital-acquired pneumonia. Chest 2006;130:787.
50. Bennett NJ, Domachowske J, Steele R. Pediatric pneumonia. Medscape 2017.
51. Black RE, Cousens S, Johnson HL, et al, Child Health Epidemiology Reference Group of WHO and UNICEF. Global, regional, and national causes of child mortality in 2008: a systematic analysis. Lancet 2010;375(9730):1969–87.
52. World Health Organization Pneumonia. Fact sheet No. 331. 2016. Available at: http://www.who.int/mediacentre/factsheets/fs331/en/index.html. Accessed February 20, 2018.
53. Lee GE, Lorch SA, Sheffler-Collins S, et al. National hospitalization trends for pediatric pneumonia and associated complications. Pediatrics 2010;126:204–13.
54. Stuckey-Schrock K, Hayes BL, George CM. Community-acquired pneumonia in children. Am Fam Physician 2012;86(7):661–7.
55. Margolis P, Gadomski A. The rational clinical examination. Does this infant have pneumonia? JAMA 1998;279(4):308–13.
56. Neuman MI, Hall M, Lipsett SC, et al. Utility of blood culture among children hospitalized with community-acquired pneumonia. Pediatrics 2017;140(3) [pii: e20171013].
57. Bradley JS, Byington CL, Shah SS, et al. The management of community-acquired pneumonia in infants and children older than 3 months of age: clinical practice guidelines by the Pediatric Infectious Diseases Society and the Infectious Diseases Society of America. Clin Infect Dis 2011;53(7):e25–76.
58. Barson WJ. Pneumonia in children: inpatient treatment. 2018. Available at: http://www.uptodate.com/. Accessed January 16, 2018.
59. Cincinnati Children's Hospital Medical Center. Evidence-based care guideline. Community acquired pneumonia in children 60 days through 17years of age. Available at: file:///C:/Users/sgrief/Downloads/Community%20Acquired%20Pneumona%20Great%20001.pdf. Accessed February 20, 2018.

60. Neuman MI, Kelley M, Harper MB, et al. Factors associated with antimicrobial resistance and mortality in pneumococcal bacteremia. J Emerg Med 2007; 32(4):349–57.
61. Available at: http://www.aappublications.org/news/aapnewsmag/2016/10/31/Fluoroquinolones103116.full.pdf. Accessed February 20, 2018.
62. Available at: https://www.canada.ca/en/health-canada/services/drugs-health-products/medeffect-canada/safety-reviews/summary-safety-review-fluoroquinolones-assessing-potential-risk-persistent-disabling-effects.html. Accessed February 20, 2018.
63. Dagan R, Syrogiannopoulos G, Ashkenazi S, et al. Parenteral-oral switch in the management of pediatric pneumonia. Drugs 1994;47(Suppl 3):43.

Central Nervous System Infections

Richard A. Giovane, MD, Paul Drake Lavender, MD*

KEYWORDS

• Meningitis • Encephalitis • Toxoplasmosis • Tuberculosis • Prions • Cryptococcus

KEY POINTS

- Prompt recognition and treatment of a central nervous system (CNS) infection is crucial for patient survival.
- Diagnosis of CNS infections is typically made by identifying clinical symptoms, evaluation of serology and cerebrospinal fluid studies, and neuroimaging. Specifically, cerebrospinal fluid is analyzed to look at the protein content, opening pressure, glucose levels, and cellular types.
- Prompt treatment of any CNS infection is important to prevent the patient from developing long-term sequelae as well as to decrease morbidity and mortality.
- Treatment is aimed at covering most common pathogens. As such, broad-spectrum antibiotics are preferred as well as antiviral medications.
- Immunodeficiency plays an important role in susceptibility in patients with opportunistic infections, such as toxoplasmosis, tuberculosis, and Cryptococcus.

INTRODUCTION

Infections of the nervous system are potentially life-threatening and are caused by pathogens, such as bacteria, viruses, and fungi. Prompt recognition and treatment of a central nervous system (CNS) infection is crucial for patient survival, as these infections have a high morbidity and mortality. CNS infections include meningitis, encephalitis, and brain abscesses. The CNS comprises the brain and spinal cord. The meninges along with cerebral spinal fluid surround the spinal cord and protect it. The meninges are subdivided into 3 layers from the outside to the inside: the dura, arachnoid, and pia matter.[1] The pia matter is a delicate structure that encases itself around the spinal cord. The arachnoid layer sits above the pia matter between the subarachnoid space that contains spinal fluid. Last, the dura matter is a tougher tissue that is attached to the skull and to the arachnoid layer. Infections occur when

Disclosure Statement: The authors have nothing to disclose.
Department of Family, Internal and Rural Medicine, The University of Alabama, 850 Peter Bryce Boulevard, Box 870377, Tuscaloosa, AL 35401, USA
* Corresponding author.
E-mail address: drake@ua.edu

Prim Care Clin Office Pract 45 (2018) 505–518
https://doi.org/10.1016/j.pop.2018.05.007

primarycare.theclinics.com

pathogens such as bacteria and viruses penetrate the subarachnoid space, eliciting an immune response. This is known as meningitis.[1] This immune response can lead to a release of inflammatory factors, such as cytokines, which leads to localized tissue damage, increased tissue permeability, and disruption of the blood brain barrier. Encephalitis occurs in a similar fashion; however, the inflammation is localized to the brain parenchyma. If not treated, both meningitis and encephalitis can lead to long-term sequalae, such as epilepsy, hydrocephalus, cognitive deficit, and death. Patients with meningitis and encephalitis typically present with the onset of symptoms from hours to days and have nausea, vomiting, headache, photophobia, confusion, fever, and, in some cases, loss of consciousness.

BACTERIAL

The pathogenesis of bacterial meningitis relies on the bacteria possessing pili or fimbriae, which assist on attaching on mucosal walls. Once the bacteria attaches to the epithelium, the bacteria expresses an immunoglobulin (Ig)A protease that cleaves host IgA, which facilitates bacterial colonization onto the epithelium.[2] Once this has occurred, the bacteria will eventually move into the bloodstream and directly infect the meninges and elicit an inflammatory response by the host immune system. This leads to localized inflammation and disruption of the blood brain barrier.

Bacterial meningitis can affect any age group, and the organisms that affect the patient vary by age, as summarized in **Table 1**.

Group B Streptococcus

Group B *Streptococcus* or GBS, is a bacterial infection common in neonates caused by *Streptococcus agalactiae*. Neonates are infected by this bacteria during their descent down the birth canal.[2,3] Risk factors for neonates developing GBS meningitis are infants born to GBS-positive (GBS+) mothers, prolonged rupture of membranes for more than 18 hours, or maternal fever.[3] Patients with suspected GBS meningitis are treated with ampicillin and cefoxtaxime. Of note, cefoxtaxime is favored over ceftriaxone due to ceftriaxone displacing bilirubin and increasing risk of jaundice in the neonate. To prevent GBS meningitis, all mothers are screened at 35 to 37 weeks while pregnant.[4] If the mother is known to be GBS+, she is given penicillin G or ampicillin as an alternative. If the mother has a mild penicillin allergy, then cefazolin can be used; however, an allergic reaction can still occur or clindamycin if the allergy is severe.[4]

Table 1
Common pathogens and treatment for meningitis

Age Group	Pathogen	Treatment
Neonates, infants	*Group B Streptococcus* *Listeria monocytogenes* *Escherichia coli*	Cefoxtaxime Vancomycin Ampicillin
Children (2–18)	*Streptococcus pneumoniae* *Neisseria meningitis* *Haemophilus influenzae*	Ceftriaxone Vancomycin
Adults	*Streptococcus pneumoniae* *Neisseria meningitis* *Listeria monocytogenes*	Ceftriaxone Vancomycin Ampicillin

Listeria monocytogenes

L monocytogenes is common in neonates and in the elderly with compromised immune systems. It is commonly transmitted from unpasteurized milk and dairy products.[2] Symptoms of this infection are consistent with typical bacterial meningitis. Lumbar puncture will show gram-positive rods. Ampicillin and a third-generation cephalosporin are used for treatment.[5]

Escherichia coli

E coli is a common cause of meningitis in neonates and always should be suspected in a neonate with a fever of unknown origin, seizure, failure to thrive, or vomiting.[2,6] A diagnostic lumbar puncture will show gram-negative rods. Ampicillin and a third-generation cephalosporin are used for treatment.[5]

Streptococcus pneumoniae

S pneumoniae is the most common cause of meningitis in adults, accounting for 61% of all bacterial meningitis cases. Patients infected with *S pneumoniae* will exhibit classic meningitis signs; however, a lumbar puncture will reveal gram-positive diplococci.[2,6] Vancomycin, a third-generation cephalosporin, and dexamethasone are used for treatment.

Haemophilus influenzae

H influenzae serotype B is an uncommon cause of meningitis due to vaccination against these bacteria. Infection of this bacteria occurs via direct spread via the sinuses, respiratory tract, and the ear.[2,6] Although uncommon, long-term sequalae of this infection include deafness and intellectual disability. Lumbar puncture will reveal a gram-negative rod. A third-generation cephalosporin is the treatment of choice.

Neisseria meningitis

N meningitis is a common cause of meningitis and it is commonly referred to meningococcal meningitis. The subtypes responsible for meningitis are A, B, C, Y, and W-135.[2,7] Patients at risk are those who are not vaccinated and those living in close quarters, such as military personnel or college students in dormitories. Patients infected with *N meningitis* will have a rapid onset of symptoms, so prompt diagnosis is needed via lumbar puncture, which will show gram-negative diplococci. Patients with *N meningitis* also can go on to develop bilateral adrenal failure, also known as Waterhouse-Friderichsen syndrome. Waterhouse-Friderichsen syndrome occurs due to bleeding within the adrenal glands because of septicemia.[8] This syndrome is characterized by a widespread petechial rash, hypotension, hyperkalemia, hyponatremia, hypoglycemia, and disseminated intravascular coagulation.[8] Treatment of *N meningitis* includes a third-generation cephalosporin and vancomycin. Chemoprophylaxis is given to individuals who had direct contact with the patient in the form of 8 hours or more of close contact (<3 feet) or individuals who had direct contact with the patient's oral secretions. Chemoprophylaxis includes rifampin and ciprofloxacin.[5]

Signs and symptoms of bacterial meningitis vary; however, most patients will complain of headache, neck stiffness, photophobia, malaise, and some may present with altered mental status. Physical examination can be positive for the Kerning sign and Brudzinski sign.[9] The Kerning sign is elicited by having the patient flex his or her hip while supine and then extending their knee. A positive sign is pain while the knee extends. The Brudzinski sign is elicited by flexing the patient's neck and watching for forced flexion of the hip. These tests have a low sensitivity, but high specificity.

Diagnosis of meningitis is done through blood tests, blood cultures, and most importantly a lumbar puncture. A lumbar puncture is done to analyze the cerebrospinal fluid (CSF). Of note, if the patient is suspected to have elevated intracranial pressure from a tumor, abscess, or infection, a lumbar puncture is contraindicated. In bacterial meningitis, the CSF will have low glucose, high protein, and increased neutrophils. **Table 2** summarizes CSF findings for meningitis.[2]

Treatment of bacterial meningitis is dependent on the likely pathogen based off of the patient's age. Generally, the antibiotics used are third-generation cephalosporins in combination with either ampicillin and vancomycin.[6]

VIRAL INFECTIONS

Viral infections in the CNS take 2 primary forms: meningitis and encephalitis.[2,10] Patients with meningitis retain normal cerebral function, whereas a hallmark of encephalitis is altered mental status, motor or sensory deficits, behavior or personality changes, and speech or movement disorders.[11] Although many times definitive etiology of these viral infections of the CNS are not confirmed, viral encephalitis and meningitis do occur frequently and should be recognized.

Encephalitis

Viral encephalitis can be categorized as either primary or postinfectious. Primary encephalitis involves viral infection of the CNS.[2] Biopsy can produce positive viral culture, inclusion bodies on light microscopy, or viral particles on electron microscopy. In postinfectious encephalitis, perivascular inflammation and demyelination occur without the presence of a virus or involvement of neurons and is thought to be an immune-mediated disease.

Most viruses that infect the CNS are capable of causing either meningitis or encephalitis, but typically a particular virus will show a tendency to cause one syndrome more than the other (**Table 3**).[12] Many clues can be used to determine the causative agent of encephalitis, including geographic location, exposure history such as from an insect or animal, and unique clinical syndromes.

Diagnosis of encephalitis is achieved via a combination of clinical findings, neuroimaging, and studies of CSF.[2,13] General findings of altered mental status, seizures, and focal neurologic abnormalities are common regardless of causative agent. Certain viruses have unique findings on physical examination that allow for higher clinical suspicion. Flaccid paralysis progressing into encephalitis is suggestive of West Nile virus.[2,14] Tremors of eyelids, tongue, lips, and extremities are suggestive of either Saint Louis encephalitis or West Nile.[14] Examination of the CSF is not diagnostic but shows an inflammatory picture. Typical CSF findings in viral infections show an elevated white blood cell count with lymphocytosis, elevated protein, and normal glucose.[2,10] Culture of the CSF has limited value and has been replaced by

Table 2
Types of meningitis and cerebrospinal fluid findings

Types of Meningitis	Cell Type	Protein	Glucose	Opening Pressure
Bacterial	Neutrophils	Normal/High	Normal/High	Elevated
Viral	Lymphocytes	High	Normal	Normal
Fungal	Lymphocytes	Elevated	Low	Variable
Tuberculosis	Lymphocytes	Elevated	Low	Variable

Table 3
Viruses and associated syndromes

Virus	Syndrome
Enterovirus	Mild meningitis > Severe meningitis
Mumps/lymphocytic choriomeningitis	Severe meningitis > Mild meningitis > Mild encephalitis
Arbovirus	Mild encephalitis > Fatal encephalitis
Herpes simplex	Fatal encephalitis > Mild encephalitis

polymerase chain reaction testing in most facilities.[10] Antibody testing of serum and CSF has proven reliable in West Nile infections.[14]

Treatment of viral encephalitis focuses on supportive therapy and empiric treatment for herpes simplex virus (HSV) encephalitis. Rapid treatment with acyclovir is recommended while awaiting confirmation of HSV as the causative agent due to the high mortality rate when treatment is delayed.[15]

Meningitis

Viral meningitis, also known as aseptic meningitis, has clinical presentation similar to bacterial meningitis with common symptoms of fever, stiff neck, headache, photophobia, and altered mental status.[10] Most commonly caused by enteroviruses, viral meningitis can also be caused by HSV, human immunodeficiency virus (HIV), West Nile virus, varicella zoster, mumps, and lymphocytic choriomeningitis virus (LCMV).[2] Meningitis caused by enterovirus is most common in summer and fall seasons, but it continues to be a major causative agent throughout the year. HSV can be a cause of viral meningitis, but in contrast to HSV encephalitis, most cases of HSV meningitis are caused by HSV type 2. LCMV is suspected when the patient has exposure to rodents.

Diagnosis of viral meningitis is done after ruling out other infectious causes, particularly bacterial meningitis. The examiner should pay special attention to information in the history and findings on physical examination that can help differentiate between likely infectious sources. Physical examination findings as noted in **Table 4** can help differentiate between causative agents.[2]

Management of possible viral meningitis should include strong consideration of bacterial causes and possible need for empiric antibiotics. Fungal and mycobacterial infections also should be considered. Supportive care is indicated for all viral meningitis, and despite utilization of empiric antiviral medication for HSV encephalitis, there is no clear role for use of acyclovir in HSV meningitis.

Table 4
Physical examination findings and possible infectious agents

Physical Examination Finding	Possible Infectious Agent
Diffuse maculopapular rash	Enterovirus, human immunodeficiency virus
Oropharyngeal thrush	Human immunodeficiency virus
Genital lesions	Herpes simplex type 2
Parotitis	Mumps
Asymmetric flaccid paralysis	West Nile virus

FUNGAL INFECTION

Cryptococcus

Cryptococcus is an opportunistic fungal infection that typically affects immunocompromised patients, especially those with HIV and a CD4 count of less than 100.[2,16] The 2 main species of *Cryptococcus* that cause CNS infections are *Cryptococcus neoformans* and *Cryptococcus gatti*. Of note, *C neoformans* is an acquired immunodeficiency syndrome (AIDS)-defining illness, although patients in other immunocompromised states, such as those receiving chemotherapy, also can develop this infection. *C gatti*, however, can occur in immunocompetent patients.[17]

An initial *Cryptococcus* infection usually occurs in the lungs, then spreads to the CNS, which then affects the surrounding nervous tissue.[18] Patients infected exhibit classic signs of meningitis, such as neck stiffness, fever, malaise, photophobia, and vomiting.[2,18]

The diagnosis of *Cryptococcus* is usually reserved for patients who have a high suspicion for it, such as patients with HIV and a CD4 count of less than 100.[16] A lumbar puncture should be done to test for *Cryptococcus* antigen in the spinal fluid, which is the definitive test. Patients with *Cryptococcus* typically have a low white blood cell count, low glucose, an elevated protein in their spinal fluid, and an increased opening pressure.[19] The spinal fluid can be stained with India ink to visualize *Cryptococcus*.[19] The *Cryptococcus* antigen also can be present in urine and sputum, but these tests have poor sensitivity. Other modalities of testing include polymerase chain reaction, enzyme immunoassay, and latex agglutination.[20] It is important to remember that for patients with suspected elevated intracranial pressure or a mass lesion, a computed tomography (CT) scan of the head should be done before doing a lumbar puncture.

Treatment for *Cryptococcus* involves starting the patient on amphotericin B and flucytosine for 2 weeks.[21] After this time, a repeat lumbar puncture is done to confirm sterility of the spinal fluid. If the spinal fluid is sterile, then the patient is switched to oral fluconazole for 8 weeks.[21] The patient will then take oral fluconazole daily for 1 year for suppression therapy. During initial therapy, it is important to monitor for signs of increased intracranial pressure. If the patient has elevated intracranial pressure, then serial lumbar punctures are recommended with a goal of intracranial pressure less than 20 mm Hg.[21] Patients who are HIV positive and are being treated for *Cryptococcus* should be monitored for immune reconstitution inflammatory syndrome (IRIS). This occurs in patients who are immunocompromised and are being treated for opportunistic infections. As their immune status improves, the immune system overcompensates and produces an inflammatory state.[22] Patients can develop acute respiratory distress syndrome or worsening neurologic deficits. Treatment is supportive and corticosteroids have been shown to have some benefit in treating IRIS.[22]

Candida

Candidiasis refers to the range of infections caused by a species of the fungal genus *Candida*. *Candida* species are considered normal flora in the gastrointestinal and genitourinary tracts, but can become invasive in the setting of immunologic imbalance in the host.[2] Infections with *Candida* are most commonly benign and localized to mucous membranes. More invasive focal infections may occur either from hematogenous spread or due to the presence of devices such as CNS shunts[2,23]

Candidal meningitis is the most common neurologic fungal infection. Candidal meningitis is seen primarily in immunocompromised hosts, particularly premature neonates, patients with HIV, and in patients who have had neurosurgical procedures.[23]

Meningitis is most often seen as a result of Candidemia from disseminated infections, but can also enter the CNS via a ventricular shunt or at the time of craniotomy.[23,24]

The symptoms typically seen with candidal meningitis include fever, stiff neck, altered mental status, and headache, and are often indistinguishable from symptoms of bacterial meningitis.[24] Generalized encephalopathy may be the presenting symptoms of multiple cerebral microabscesses.

Diagnosis of CNS *Candida* infection should be suspected if there is treatment failure for meningitis of bacterial or mycobacterial source, if *Candida* species are isolated from CSF obtained with a lumbar puncture, or if fungemia is discovered in a patient with an elevated white blood cell count in the CSF.[1,6] Culture results from the CSF have been found to be inconsistent, with only approximately 80% of patients with candidal infections testing positive.[24] It should be noted that *Candida* isolated from the CSF should not be viewed as contaminant, even in the presence of other pathogens. The beta-D-glucan assay, which detects a cell wall component of fungi in the CSF, can be a useful adjunct study to CSF culture.[25] Neuroimaging may be used to help identify microabscesses and response to treatment, and MRI has proven to be the study of choice for this purpose.[26]

Initial treatment of candidal meningitis is typically with a combination of amphotericin B and flucytosine.[27,28] Different formulations exist for amphotericin B; however, the most potent form is liposomal amphotericin B, which readily penetrates into the CNS. It is fungicidal against almost all species of *Candida*, whereas flucytosine has excellent penetration into the CNS as well as anti-candidal activity.[27] Fluconazole is often used as step-down therapy after initial treatment with amphotericin.[27] Other antifungals, including Posaconazole, Isavuconazole, and Caspofungin do not achieve adequate CNS concentrations and should not be used for candidal CNS infections.[29]

Duration of treatment depends on several factors. For patients with acute meningitis, lumbar puncture should be repeated weekly for the first few weeks to be sure CSF changes are normalizing.[27] If abscesses are seen on presentation, therapy should continue until resolution is seen on MRI, CSF studies have returned to normal, and the patient's symptoms have resolved.[27] MRI should be repeated at 2 weeks, then monthly until findings have resolved. For patients with chronic meningitis, lumbar puncture should be performed as with acute meningitis, with particular attention paid to white blood cell counts, and protein and glucose concentrations, because culture outcomes are not reliable in these cases.[27] Implanted CNS devices should be removed, if possible, from infected patients. If it is not possible to remove a ventricular device, administration of amphotericin may be performed through the device, but this is often limited by toxicity symptoms of headache, nausea, and vomiting.

Toxoplasmosis

Toxoplasmosis is caused by the intracellular protozoan parasite, *Toxoplasma gondii*, and is typically acquired via ingestion of infectious oocytes from soil or cat litter contaminated with feline feces, or from ingestion of undercooked meat.[2] Toxoplasmosis is the most common CNS infection in patients with AIDS, caused by a reactivation of latent infection in patients when CD4 cell counts fall below 100 cells/μL.[30]

Patients with toxoplasmic encephalitis typically present with headache, altered mental status, or other neurologic symptoms, such as hemiparesis, memory loss, and seizures.[30] Fever is often present, but is not a reliable finding. Focal neurologic symptoms or seizures are also common. A wide range of mental status changes can be present, from confusion to coma.

Definitive diagnosis requires a matching clinical syndrome, identification of one or more mass lesions on neuroimaging, and positive identification of the organism via biopsy.[31,32] To avoid brain biopsy and its extensive associated sequela, presumptive diagnosis is considered adequate for treatment initiation. Presumptive diagnosis can be made if patient has a CD4 cell count less than 100 cells/μL, has not been receiving prophylactic treatment for toxoplasmosis, has a positive serology for antibody to *T gondii*, encephalitis symptoms, and brain lesions identified on neuroimaging.[32] MRI is considered the imaging study of choice, as it is more sensitive in identifying lesions associated with toxoplasmic encephalitis than CT.

Treatment of toxoplasmic encephalitis is divided into initial treatment and maintenance treatment. A combination of sulfadiazine, pyrimethamine, and leucovorin is commonly used for initial therapy, with clindamycin substituted for sulfadiazine if a sensitivity to this medication arises.[33,34] Corticosteroids may be used as an adjunct therapy for patients with mass effect arising from brain lesions or edema.[34] Maintenance therapy usually consists of the same medications and can be stopped if the CD4 cell count is more than 200 cells/μL for at least 6 months.[35]

For patients with HIV, the risk of developing toxoplasmic encephalitis can be reduced by testing for IgG serology. If the patient's anti-toxoplasma IgG is positive, and the patient has CD4 cell counts less than 100 cells/μL, trimethoprim-sulfamethoxazole can be given as prophylaxis.

Tuberculosis

Mycobacterium tuberculosis is the second most common infectious cause of death in adults worldwide.[2] CNS infections caused by tuberculosis fall into 3 categories: tuberculous meningitis, intracranial tuberculoma, and spinal tuberculous arachnoiditis.[2,36] In areas of the world in which the prevalence of tuberculosis is high, dissemination of disease is commonly seen in children and young adults. In areas in which the prevalence is low (North America and Western Europe), tuberculosis outside the pulmonary system is seen primarily as reactivation disease in adults with immune deficiency, and in these areas the primary CNS form of disease is tuberculous meningitis.

Tuberculous meningitis is most commonly caused by generalized infection. In infants and children, this is typically due to disseminated primary infection, whereas in adults with immune deficiency this is usually due to reactivation disease.[37] Tuberculous meningitis manifests in 3 phases: a prodromal phase, a meningitic phase, and a paralytic phase.[37] The prodromal phase lasts 2 to 3 weeks and presents with low-grade fever, malaise, and mental status changes. The meningitic phase exhibits classic meningitis symptoms of meningismus, headache, neurologic changes, and a progression of mental status changes. The paralytic phase is the final phase, exhibiting coma, seizures, and hemiparesis.[37]

CNS tuberculosis presents a diagnostic challenge, and a high level of clinical suspicion is needed. CSF assays are of premium value for diagnostic purposes, typically revealing a lymphocytic pleocytosis, increased protein, and low glucose levels.[38] Neuroimaging is recommended in the form of contrast-enhanced MRI instead of CT.

CNS tuberculosis is treated with 4-drug therapy (isoniazid, rifampin, pyrazinamide, and ethambutol) for 2 months, followed by a prolonged continuation phase with isoniazid and rifampin for an additional 7 to 10 months.[39] Isoniazid resistance is known to be quite common, and several alternative antibiotic agents have been recommended, including fluoroquinolones, ethionamide, streptomycin, and amikacin.[39] Surgical treatment is not indicated unless patients have hydrocephalus or mass lesions that are ineffectively managed by medical therapy.

Lyme Disease

Lyme disease is a zoonotic infection that is spread from a genus of ticks called *Ixodes*. These ticks transmit a harmful bacterium to humans via a tick bite.[2] The bacteria that causes Lyme disease is a spirochete called *Borrelia burgdorferi*, which is transmitted to humans, usually from younger ticks, called nymphs.[40,41] Nymphs have a higher success rate at transmitting the bacteria, as they are smaller and therefore less likely to be noticed on the host. The natural reservoir of the *Ixodes* tick are deer and the white-footed mouse, with the latter having an increased chance of transmitting Lyme disease via tick feedings.[41,42] Once the tick latches onto a human, it takes 36 to 48 hours of feeding to transmit the *B burgdorferi* from the tick's midgut to the salivary glands. *B burgdorferi* will migrate to the dermis and illicit a host immune response in the form of a rash called erythema migrans, which has a characteristic "bullseye target" appearance (**Fig. 1**).[2]

During this initial infection period, neutrophils are not recruited to the site of infection; this allows for faster dissemination of the bacteria.[43]

Lyme disease can be distinguished into 3 separate phases: early localized, early disseminated, and late disease.[40,42] Early localized Lyme disease is characterized erythema migrans; an erythematous rash with a central clearing that mimics a bullseye. This rash usually occurs 1 to 2 weeks after the initial infection. It should be noted that every patient infected with *B burgdorferi* will not always go on to develop this rash.

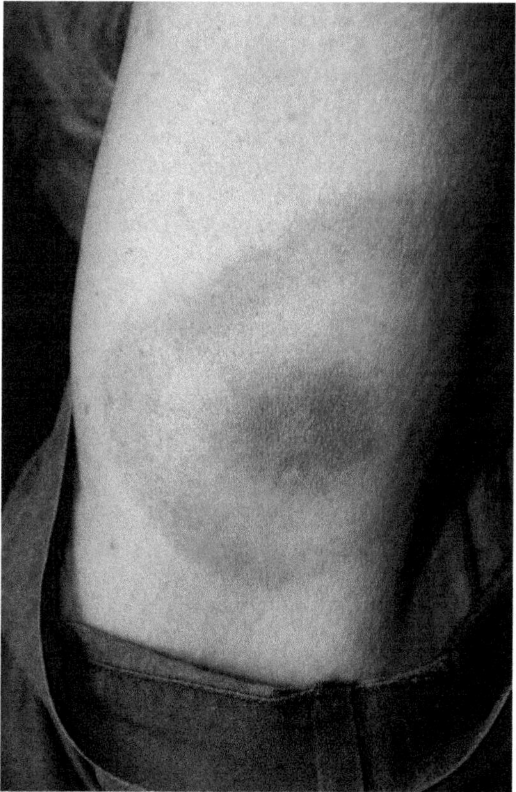

Fig. 1. Erythema migrans. (*Courtesy of* Centers for Disease Control and Prevention Public Health Image Library/James Gathany.)

Other symptoms include headache and fever. Early disseminated Lyme disease is characterized by the spread of *B burgdorferi* to the heart and CNS. The usual time period for this to occur is in days to months. Lyme disease can cause atrioventricular blocks of the heart, as well as myocarditis.[2] Lyme disease can affect the nervous system by causing facial nerve palsy, radiculopathy, meningitis, and encephalitis. Patients with Lyme meningitis have classic bacterial meningitis symptoms, such as head stiffness, photophobia, and confusion.[40] Patients may also go on to develop encephalitis, which is characterized by memory loss, insomnia, and altered mental status. Late Lyme disease occurs after months to years without treatment. Arthritis of larger joints is common during this stage of illness, with most patients experiencing joint swelling and tenderness of their knees and hips.[2] Lyme encephalopathy occurs during the late stage and is characterized by migraines, psychosis, somatoform delusions, and vertigo.

Lyme disease is a clinical diagnosis; however, not all patients will present with erythema migrans or symptoms consistent with Lyme disease.[44] If Lyme is suspected, a 2-step approach to diagnose is recommended. The first step is an enzyme immunoassay. If this step is negative, then no further testing is needed. If positive or inconclusive, then a Western blot is done.[41]

Treatment for Lyme disease depends on the patient's age. For patients who are 8 years and older, doxycycline, amoxicillin, or cefuroxime are recommended.[45] In patients who are younger than 8 or who are pregnant, amoxicillin or cefuroxime are recommended. Most symptoms caused by Lyme disease respond well to antibiotic therapy.[45] As Lyme disease is a spirochete, patients may experience Jarisch-Herxheimer reaction characterized by fever, chills, tachycardia, and hypotension that is self-limited and unavoidable. Patients can be given ibuprofen or aspirin to help with symptoms.[2]

Prophylaxis is also recommended with doxycycline in patients who meet all of the following criteria: (1) the tick is identified as an *Ixodes* tick, (2) the tick has been attached for more than 36 hours, (3) prophylaxis can be started within 72 hours of exposure, (4) local rate of tick infections is greater than 20%, and (5) doxycycline is not contraindicated.[46] If the patient cannot take doxycycline, then no prophylaxis is recommended.

PRIONS

Prions are groups of misfolded proteins that induce disease in the CNS. In a healthy person, prions form proteins called PRP^{C} that are susceptible to proteases; enzymes that break down abnormal proteins.[2,46] In the disease state, prion proteins undergo a misfolded state from alpha helixes to beta sheets, which form PRP^{SC} that are resistant to proteases and induce a collective form of disease called transmissible spongiform encephalopathies (TSEs).[47] TSEs can be further classified as Kuru, Creutzfeldt-Jakob disease (CJD), Gerstmann-Sträussler-Scheinker syndrome, and fatal familial insomnia (FFI).

The mechanism by which prions cause disease is due to the aggregation of these prion proteins in the extracellular space, which causes amyloid deposition that subsequently leads to plaque accumulation and the formation of vacuoles that destroy neurons.[6] The mechanism by which healthy prions PRP^{C} gets converted to PRP^{SC} is unknown; however, the main way in which a human gets infected by a prion is by ingestion.[47]

CJD is the most common form of TSE.[48] A patient develops CJD 3 specific ways: sporadic, which is due to misfolded proteins; familial, which is due to gene mutations; and acquired, which is from being exposed to tissue from an affected patient.[48] Like other prion diseases, CJD is due to misfolded prion proteins that accumulate and cause cellular disruption. Diagnosis of CJD can be challenging; however, it is routinely done via electroencephalogram (EEG), MRI, and CSF analysis. EEG will show a sharp wave pattern that is triphasic or biphasic. CSF analysis will show an elevated amount of 14-3-3 protein.[49] MRI shows increased signal intensity of the putamen and caudate nucleus.

Kuru was one of the first prion disease identified, as it was prominent in cannibal tribes of Southeast Asia during rituals.[50] Unlike other TSEs, Kuru has a predictable progression of illness, with the first signs of tremors and postural ataxia. As the disease progresses, the patient becomes unable to ambulate, has worsening tremors, and ataxia.[2] In later stages, severe dementia develops. Diagnosis of Kuru is difficult to establish, as laboratory work usually comes back unremarkable. EEG, however, does show sharp wave complex, but this is seen with other prion diseases. Like all prion diseases, treatment is supportive, as no medications exist to slow the progression of the disease or to cure it.

Gerstmann-Sträussler-Scheinker syndrome is an autosomal dominant form of TSE in which a codon is changed from proline to leucine for the gene that codes for PRP on chromosome 20.[51] A characteristic feature of this syndrome is the development of cerebellar ataxia and dysarthria with dementia occurring later. Patients will also have nystagmus as well.[51] As with other prion diseases, diagnosis can be challenging. In Gerstmann-Sträussler-Scheinker syndrome, CSF is normal, imaging is unremarkable, and EEG may show slowing. A definitive diagnosis can be done via genetic testing, which will show PRNP gene mutations.[51]

FFI is another autosomal dominant TSE in which a mutation occurs on the protein PRP C due to a missense mutation.[52] Mean age onset of this disease is 50 years old with patients dying within 1 year of onset of symptoms.[52] Symptoms can be divided into 4 stages. In the first stage, the patient develops insomnia with paranoia and phobias.[53,54] In the second stage, the patient begins hallucinating. During the third stage, the patient is unable to sleep at all and begins having rapid weight loss. The final stage occurs when the patient develops dementia. Of note, patients will not respond to sedatives to initiate sleep and in FFI, it will hasten the disease.[53]

REFERENCES

1. Scheld WM, Koedel U, Nathan B, et al. Pathophysiology of bacterial meningitis: mechanism(s) of neuronal injury. J Infect Dis 2002;186(Suppl 2):S225–33.
2. Parikh V, Tucci V, Galwankar S. Infections of the nervous system. Int J Crit Illn Inj Sci 2012;2(2):82–97.
3. Eichenwald EC. Perinatally transmitted neonatal bacterial infections. Infect Dis Clin North Am 1997;11(1):223–39.
4. Centers for Disease Control and Prevention. Active bacterial core surveillance (ABCs) report, emerging infections program network, group B Streptococcus, 2003. 2004. Available at: https://www.cdc.gov/groupbstrep/about/prevention.html. Accessed March 1, 2018.
5. Centers for Disease Control and Prevention. Meningitis treatment. Available at: https://www.cdc.gov/meningitis/bacterial.html. Accessed March 1, 2018.
6. Durand ML, Calderwood SB, Weber DJ, et al. Acute bacterial meningitis in adults. A review of 493 episodes. N Engl J Med 1993;328(1):21–8.
7. Sun YH, Bakshi S, Chalmers R, et al. Functional genomics of *Neisseria meningitidis* pathogenesis. Nat Med 2000;6(11):1269–73.

8. Migeon CJ, Kenny FM, Hung W, et al. Study of adrenal function in children with meningitis. Pediatrics 1967;40(2):163–83.
9. Heckenberg SG, De gans J, Brouwer MC, et al. Clinical features, outcome, and meningococcal genotype in 258 adults with meningococcal meningitis: a prospective cohort study. Medicine (Baltimore) 2008;87(4):185–92.
10. Logan SA, Macmahon E. Viral meningitis. BMJ 2008;336(7634):36–40.
11. Rotbart HA. Viral meningitis. Semin Neurol 2000;20(3):277–92.
12. Ziai WC, Lewin JJ. Update in the diagnosis and management of central nervous system infections. Neurol Clin 2008;26(2):427–68, viii.
13. Kupila L, Vuorinen T, Vainionpää R, et al. Etiology of aseptic meningitis and encephalitis in an adult population. Neurology 2006;66(1):75–80.
14. Mazurek JM, Winpisinger K, Mattson BJ, et al. The epidemiology and early clinical features of West Nile virus infection. Am J Emerg Med 2005;23(4):536–43.
15. Gordon B, Selnes OA, Hart J, et al. Long-term cognitive sequelae of acyclovir-treated herpes simplex encephalitis. Arch Neurol 1990;47(6):646–7.
16. Chayakulkeeree M, Perfect JR. Cryptococcosis. Infect Dis Clin North Am 2006; 20:507–44 (v–vi).
17. Park BJ, Wannemuehler KA, Marston BJ, et al. Estimation of the current global burden of cryptococcal meningitis among persons living with HIV/AIDS. AIDS 2009;23(4):525–30.
18. Cox GM, Perfect JR. *Cryptococcus neoformans* var *neoformans* and *gattii* and *Trichosporon* species. In: Edward LA, editor. Topley and Wilson's microbiology and microbial infections. 9th edition. London: Arnold Press; 1997.
19. Zerpa R, Huicho L, Guillén A. Modified India ink preparation for *Cryptococcus neoformans* in cerebrospinal fluid specimens. J Clin Microbiol 1996;34(9): 2290–1.
20. Leber AL, Everhart K, Balada-llasat JM, et al. Multicenter evaluation of the biofire filmarray meningitis encephalitis panel for the detection of bacteria, viruses and yeast in cerebrospinal fluid specimens. J Clin Microbiol 2016;54(9):2251–61.
21. Perfect JR, Dismukes WE, Dromer F, et al. Clinical practice guidelines for the management of cryptococcal disease: 2010 update by the Infectious Diseases Society of America. Clin Infect Dis 2010;50(3):291–322.
22. Haddow LJ, Colebunders R, Meintjes G, et al. Cryptococcal immune reconstitution inflammatory syndrome in HIV-1–infected individuals: literature review and proposed clinical case definitions. Lancet Infect Dis 2010;10(11):791–802.
23. Nguyen MH, Yu VL. Meningitis caused by *Candida* species: an emerging problem in neurosurgical patients. Clin Infect Dis 1995;21(2):323–7.
24. Sánchez-portocarrero J, Pérez-cecilia E, Corral O, et al. The central nervous system and infection by *Candida* species. Diagn Microbiol Infect Dis 2000;37(3): 169–79.
25. Lyons JL, Erkkinen MG, Vodopivec I. Cerebrospinal fluid (1,3)-β-D-glucan in isolated *Candida* meningitis. Clin Infect Dis 2015;60(1):161–2.
26. Lai PH, Lin SM, Pan HB, et al. Disseminated miliary cerebral candidiasis. AJNR Am J Neuroradiol 1997;18(7):1303–6.
27. Pappas PG, Kauffman CA, Andes DR, et al. Clinical practice guideline for the management of candidiasis: 2016 update by the Infectious Diseases Society of America. Clin Infect Dis 2016;62(4):e1–50.
28. Slavoski LA, Tunkel AR. Therapy of fungal meningitis. Clin Neuropharmacol 1995; 18(2):95–112.
29. Deresinski SC, Stevens DA. Caspofungin. Clin Infect Dis 2003;36(11):1445–57.

30. Porter SB, Sande MA. Toxoplasmosis of the central nervous system in the acquired immunodeficiency syndrome. N Engl J Med 1992;327(23):1643–8.
31. Luft BJ, Remington JS. Toxoplasmic encephalitis in AIDS. Clin Infect Dis 1992; 15(2):211–22.
32. Cohn JA, Mcmeeking A, Cohen W, et al. Evaluation of the policy of empiric treatment of suspected *Toxoplasma encephalitis* in patients with the acquired immunodeficiency syndrome. Am J Med 1989;86(5):521–7.
33. Dannemann B, Mccutchan JA, Israelski D, et al. Treatment of toxoplasmic encephalitis in patients with AIDS. A randomized trial comparing pyrimethamine plus clindamycin to pyrimethamine plus sulfadiazine. The California Collaborative Treatment Group. Ann Intern Med 1992;116(1):33–43.
34. Nath A, Sinai AP. Cerebral toxoplasmosis. Curr Treat Options Neurol 2003;5(1): 3–12.
35. Panel on Opportunistic Infections in HIV-Infected Adults and Adolescents. Guidelines for the prevention and treatment of opportunistic infections in HIV-infected adults and adolescents: recommendations from the Centers for Disease Control and Prevention, the National Institutes of Health, and the HIV Medicine Association of the Infectious Diseases Society of America. Available at: http://aidsinfo.nih.gov/contentfiles/lvguidelines/adult_oi.pdf. Accessed March 3, 2018.
36. Al-deeb SM, Yaqub BA, Sharif HS, et al. Neurotuberculosis: a review. Clin Neurol Neurosurg 1992;94(Suppl):S30–3.
37. Kennedy DH, Fallon RJ. Tuberculous meningitis. JAMA 1979;241(3):264–8.
38. Lewinsohn DM, Leonard MK, Lobue PA, et al. Official American Thoracic Society/Infectious Diseases Society of America/Centers for Disease Control and Prevention clinical practice guidelines: diagnosis of tuberculosis in adults and children. Clin Infect Dis 2017;64(2):e1–33.
39. Thwaites G, Fisher M, Hemingway C, et al. British Infection Society guidelines for the diagnosis and treatment of tuberculosis of the central nervous system in adults and children. J Infect 2009;59(3):167–87.
40. Pachner AR. Early disseminated Lyme disease: Lyme meningitis. Am J Med 1995;98(4A):30S–7S.
41. Centers for Disease Control and Prevention. 2010. Lyme disease.
42. Steere AC. Lyme disease. N Engl J Med 1989;321(9):586–96.
43. Sanchez E, Vannier E, Wormser GP, et al. Diagnosis, treatment, and prevention of Lyme disease, human granulocytic anaplasmosis, and babesiosis: a review. JAMA 2016;315(16):1767–77.
44. Case definitions for infectious conditions under public health surveillance. Centers for Disease Control and Prevention. MMWR Recomm Rep 1997;46(RR-10): 1–55.
45. Halperin JJ, Shapiro ED, Logigian E, et al. Practice parameter: treatment of nervous system Lyme disease (an evidence-based review): report of the quality standards subcommittee of the American Academy of Neurology. Neurology 2007;69(1):91–102.
46. Wormser GP, Dattwyler RJ, Shapiro ED, et al. The clinical assessment, treatment, and prevention of Lyme disease, human granulocytic anaplasmosis, and babesiosis: clinical practice guidelines by the Infectious Diseases Society of America. Clin Infect Dis 2006;43(9):1089–134.
47. Haywood AM. Transmissible spongiform encephalopathies. N Engl J Med 1997; 337(25):1821–8.
48. Prusiner SB. Molecular biology of prion diseases. Science 1991;252(5012): 1515–22.

49. Puoti G, Bizzi A, Forloni G, et al. Sporadic human prion diseases: molecular insights and diagnosis. Lancet Neurol 2012;11(7):618–28.
50. Kretzschmar HA, Ironside JW, Dearmond SJ, et al. Diagnostic criteria for sporadic Creutzfeldt-Jakob disease. Arch Neurol 1996;53(9):913–20.
51. Gajdusek DC, Zigas V. Degenerative disease of the central nervous system in New Guinea; the endemic occurrence of kuru in the native population. N Engl J Med 1957;257(20):974–8.
52. Johnson RT, Gibbs CJ. Creutzfeldt-Jakob disease and related transmissible spongiform encephalopathies. N Engl J Med 1998;339(27):1994–2004.
53. Mastrianni JA, Nixon R, Layzer R, et al. Prion protein conformation in a patient with sporadic fatal insomnia. N Engl J Med 1999;340(21):1630–8.
54. Plazzi G, Schutz Y, Cortelli P, et al. Motor overactivity and loss of motor circadian rhythm in fatal familial insomnia: an actigraphic study. Sleep 1997;20(9):739–42.

Common Gastrointestinal Infections

Jarrett Sell, MD, AAHIVS[a,*], Bevin Dolan, MD[b]

KEYWORDS

• Gastrointestinal infections • Diarrhea • Food-borne illness • Traveler's diarrhea

KEY POINTS

- Viral infections, with norovirus being the most common, account for most cases of acute diarrhea in the United States.
- Nontyphoidal *Salmonella* species are the leading cause in the United States of hospitalization and death from gastrointestinal infections.
- The immunocompromised, children under the age of 5, and adults over 65 years of age are the most severely affected.
- For most patients in the United States presenting with diarrhea, no testing is necessary if the presentation is consistent with a viral cause and of mild to moderate severity.

INTRODUCTION

Gastrointestinal infections account for a large burden of acute and chronic disease worldwide. Diarrhea is defined as 3 or more stools in 24 hours and is the most common manifestation. It is defined as acute if lasting less than 7 days, prolonged if lasting 7 to 13 days, persistent if lasting 14 to 29 days, and chronic if lasting 30 days or longer.[1] Common bacterial, viral, and parasitic pathogens are spread via food, via contaminated water, or from person to person. According to the World Health Organization, diarrhea is the cause of 4% of deaths globally and kills approximately 2.2 million people each year.[2] Those in developing countries, and particularly children, are most affected. In the United States, not all cases are actively reported, but it is approximated that 179 million cases of acute diarrhea in adults occur each year, resulting in 500,000 hospitalizations and more than 5000 deaths.[3] Nationally, children less than 5 years old account for the largest portion of infections, but those older than 65 years old account for greatest number of hospitalizations and deaths.[4]

Despite modern advances in food preparation and delivery, gastrointestinal infections in the United States are commonly caused by food-borne pathogens. In

Disclosure Statement: The authors have nothing to disclose.
[a] Department of Family and Community Medicine, Penn State Health Hershey Medical Center, 500 University Drive, Hershey, PA 17033, USA; [b] Delaware Valley Infectious Disease Associates, 100 East Lancaster Avenue, MOB East Suite 556, Wynnewood, PA 19096, USA
* Corresponding author.
E-mail address: jsell@pennstatehealth.psu.edu

Prim Care Clin Office Pract 45 (2018) 519–532
https://doi.org/10.1016/j.pop.2018.05.008

2011, it was found that norovirus (58%) caused the most food-borne infections followed by nontyphoidal *Salmonella* spp (11%), *Clostridium perfringens* (10%), and *Campylobacter* spp (9%). Nontyphoidal *Salmonella* spp (35%) was the leading cause of hospitalization followed by norovirus (26%), *Campylobacter* spp (15%), and *Toxoplasma gondii* (8%). Nontyphoidal *Salmonella* spp (28%) also caused the most deaths followed by *T gondii* (24%), *Listeria monocytogenes* (19%), and norovirus (11%).[3]

Diarrhea also accounts for the largest number of travel-related illness in the United States, with acute diarrhea accounting for 22% of travel-related diagnoses in US residents.[5] Areas with the highest risk of acquiring traveler's diarrhea include Africa, South Asia, Latin America, and the Middle East. Risk is increased for those taking medications that lower gastric acid.[6] Traveler's diarrhea (**Table 1**) is more likely bacterial in contrast to infectious diarrhea acquired in the United States, which is most commonly viral. Protozoa are less common causes of traveler's diarrhea but may result in longer duration or persistence of symptoms upon return to the United States.

CLINICAL MANIFESTATIONS

History

A comprehensive history is important to determine potential infectious causes of gastrointestinal diseases with a focus on sick contacts, food exposures, and travel history (**Table 2**). The onset, duration, severity, and frequency of diarrhea should be determined with attention to the stool volume and character. It is important to note if the stool has been watery or contains blood or mucus. Fever, tenesmus, and the presence of blood in stool may be more suggestive of invasive bacterial pathogens. Additional systemic symptoms, such as decreased urine output, weakness, dizziness, and confusion, may be signs of dehydration. Pathogens that primarily affect the small bowel are more likely to cause watery larger volume diarrhea with bloating, gas, and cramping. Those that affect the large bowel may cause more frequent, small volume, or painful bowel movements.

Environmental exposure or a history of immunocompromise may help identify specific pathogens. History of prior abdominal surgeries, radiation exposure, or recent antibiotic use should be obtained. A detailed sexual history may also be relevant because anal receptive sex, sharing of toys, or oral-anal contact may increase the risk of transmission of fecal pathogens, particularly *Shigella*, *Salmonella*, *Campylobacter*, *Escherichia coli*, *Entamoeba histolytica*, and *Giardia*.[7]

Physical Examination

A comprehensive physical examination in patients with suspected gastrointestinal infections should focus on a thorough abdominal examination with consideration

Table 1
Common causes of traveler's diarrhea

Bacterial	Viral	Parasitic
Shiga-toxin producing *E coli*	Rotavirus	*Giardia lamblia*
Other *E coli* types	Norovirus	*Cryptosporidium*
Salmonella		*Cyclospora*
Campylobacter		*E histolytica*
Shigella		
Aeromonas		
Vibrio		

Table 2
Common sources of water or food-borne illnesses

Source	Pathogen
Camping, untreated river water	*Giardia*
Fried rice	*Bacillus cereus*
Raw milk	*Salmonella, Campylobacter, Listeria,* Shiga toxin-producing *E coli*
Seafood	*Vibrio cholerae, Vibrio parahaemolyticus*
Undercooked meat	*Bacillus cereus, Campylobacter, C perfringens, Listeria, Salmonella,* STEC, *Staphylococcus aureus, Yersinia*

of a rectal examination to identify blood or stool quality. The examiner should also look for signs of dehydration, such as orthostatic vital signs, dry mucous membranes, skin tenting, or delayed capillary refill. After the acute phase of diarrhea, examination may be helpful to identify postinfectious complications of enteric pathogens, as listed in **Table 3**.

DIAGNOSIS/MANAGEMENT

Differential Diagnosis

A thorough history and physical examination may point to a clear infectious cause, whereas the differential may also include other noninfectious causes, such as medication adverse effects, other intrinsic gastrointestinal diseases, or endocrine disorders that affect the gastrointestinal system (**Table 4**).

General Diagnostic Approach

For most patients in the United States presenting with diarrhea, no testing is necessary if the presentation is consistent with a viral cause and of mild to moderate severity.[1] The Infectious Disease Society of America (IDSA), based on low quality of evidence, recommends that those with fever, bloody, or severe diarrhea should be evaluated for treatable enteropathogens, such as *Salmonella*, *Shigella*, and *Campylobacter*.[1] Recent travel to an endemic area or known exposure would be other reasons to consider specific testing. Stool testing is recommended for those with diarrhea and fever, bloody stools, mucoid stools, severe abdominal pain or cramping, diarrhea lasting longer than 14 days, or signs of sepsis.[1] Stool testing is most commonly obtained to specifically assess for *Salmonella*, *Shigella*, *Campylobacter*, *Yersinia*, *C difficile*, and

Table 3
Postinfectious complications of enteric pathogens

Postinfectious Complication	Commonly Associated Organisms
Hemolytic uremic syndrome	*Shigella dysenteriae* serotype 1, STEC
Reactive arthritis	*Campylobacter, Salmonella, Shigella*
Erythema nodosum	*Campylobacter, Salmonella, Shigella, Yersinia*
Guillain-Barre syndrome	*Campylobacter*
Hemolytic anemia	*Campylobacter, Yersinia*
Irritable bowel syndrome (IBS)	*Campylobacter, Salmonella, Shigella,* STEC, *Giardia*

Data from Shane AL, Mody RK, Crump JA, et al. 2017 Infectious Diseases Society of America clinical practice guidelines for the diagnosis and management of infectious diarrhea. Clin Infect Dis 2017;65(12):1963–73.

Table 4
Noninfectious causes of diarrhea

Cause	Examples
Medication adverse effects	Antibiotics Metformin Orlistat Acarbose Nonsteroidal anti-inflammatory drugs Metoclopramide Iron Fibrates Proton pump inhibitors Lithium Aminosalycilates (5-ASA) ACE inhibitors Laxatives Colchicine Calcitonin Chemotherapy Antacids Protease inhibitors Magnesium Weight loss supplements
Gastroenterologic diseases	Inflammatory bowel disease Irritable bowel syndrome Ischemic colitis Mesenteric ischemia Diverticulitis Malabsorption Colorectal cancer Celiac disease Lactose intolerance Short bowel syndrome Constipation with overflow
Endocrine diseases	Hyperthyroidism Adrenal insufficiency Carcinoid tumors

Data from Chassany O, Michaux A, Bergmann JF. Drug-induced diarrhoea. Drug Saf 2000;22(1):53–72; and Schiller LR, Pardi DS, Sellin JH. Chronic diarrhea: diagnosis and management. Clin Gastroenterol Hepatol 2017;15(2):182–93.e3.

Shiga toxin-producing *E coli* (STEC). Blood cultures should be collected for those with signs of sepsis, the immunosuppressed, infants <3 months of age, or those with a febrile illness of unclear cause. Stool nonmicrobiologic diagnostic tests have historically been considered in evaluating persons with suspected gastrointestinal infections, but the IDSA in their 2017 guideline recommends against testing for fecal leukocytes and lactoferrin, based on moderate evidence of lack of benefit.[1] Additional testing may be necessary to diagnose postinfectious complications of enteric pathogens (see **Table 3**).

Abdominal imaging with ultrasound, computed tomography (CT), or MRI may be considered in those with peritoneal signs or to evaluate for other noninfectious causes, such as those listed in **Table 4**. More invasive endoscopic examination may be considered in those with persistent diarrhea of unclear cause, particularly in those with AIDS or a suspected noninfectious cause.

PATHOGEN-SPECIFIC DIAGNOSIS, MANAGEMENT, AND PREVENTION

Bacteria

Campylobacter

Campylobacter are gram-negative spiral, rod-shaped, or curved bacteria and are a common bacterial cause of gastrointestinal infections in the United States. *Campylobacter jejuni* causes most human infections and is transmitted via undercooked poultry and unpasteurized milk.[8] Symptoms typically present 1 to 3 days after exposure and last a week. Most cases of infection are self-limited with fever, abdominal pain/cramping, and diarrhea, with blood in a third of cases. Stool culture remains the gold standard for diagnosis with increasing utilization of culture independent diagnostic testing (CIDT).[9] Treatment is supportive. Azithromycin may be considered if symptoms are more severe, because treatment may reduce duration of diarrhea. A 2014 systemic review and meta-analysis showed postinfection rates of reactive arthritis (2.86%), irritable bowel syndrome (4.01%), and Guillain Barré syndrome (0.07%).[10]

Salmonella

Salmonella is a motile, gram-negative anaerobic rod, and nontyphoidal species are a common cause of traveler's diarrhea and gastroenteritis in the United States. Nontyphoidal *Salmonella* causes the most deaths worldwide and is more prevalent in the summer. Exposure commonly is due to food (eg, eggs, unpasteurized dairy, undercooked poultry) or animals (eg, turtles, iguanas, poultry). Symptoms are typically self-limited. Stool culture and/or CIDT should be considered in those with more severe symptoms and those at risk for transmission, such as food handlers or health care workers. Blood culture should also be considered in those with sepsis, the immunocompromised, the hospitalized, or those with prosthetic heart valves or joints. Antibiotics should be reserved for those at greater risk for complications (**Box 1**) because they may not reduce diarrhea nor fever duration and risk increasing fecal carriage. Postinfectious sequelae of nontyphoidal *Salmonella* may include reactive arthritis in 5.8% and irritable bowel syndrome in 3.3%.[11]

Shigella

Shigella are gram-negative, anaerobic nonmotile rod-shaped bacteria closely related to *E coli* and is one of the leading causes of diarrhea worldwide, with milder disease severity in the United States (**Table 5**). *Shigella* and enteroinvasive *E coli* (EIEC) are the primary causative agents of bacillary dysentery (**Table 6**), characterized by bloody

Box 1
Criteria for consideration of antibiotics for treatment of nontyphoidal *Salmonella* infection

- Patients less than 3 months old or greater than 50 year old
- Patients with valvular heart disease
- Patients with severe atherosclerosis
- Patients with malignancy
- Patients with prosthetic joints, heart valves, or vascular grafts
- Patient who are immunocompromised
- Patients with bacteremia

Data from Shane AL, Mody RK, Crump JA, et al. 2017 infectious diseases society of America clinical practice guidelines for the diagnosis and management of infectious diarrhea. Clin Infect Dis 2017;65(12):1963–73.

Table 5
Shigella subtypes

Subtype	Global Prevalence	Severity of Disease
Shigella sonnei	Most common subtype in the United States	Least severe
Shigella dysenteriae	Rare in the United States	Most severe
Shigella flexneri	Primary cause of endemic disease in developing countries	More severe
Shigella boydii	Most commonly found in Indian subcontinent. Rare in the United States	Mild

Data from Centers for Disease Control and Prevention. Questions & Answers | Shigella – Shigellosis | CDC. Available at: https://www.cdc.gov/shigella/general-information.html. Accessed April 9, 2018.

diarrhea. Toxin mediated symptoms occur 1 to 2 days after exposure and include diarrhea, fever, abdominal pains, and tenesmus, lasting an average of 5 to 7 days. Shigellosis has been found to be more common in men who have sex with men (MSM) (odds ratio [OR] 8.24), persons with HIV (OR 8.17), direct oral-anal contact (OR 7.5), and foreign travel (OR 20.0).[12] Diagnosis may be made via stool culture or stool polymerase chain reaction (PCR), although differentiating *Shigella* from EIEC and other *E coli* species may require specialized laboratories. Most cases do not require antibiotic treatment. A Cochrane review found that antibiotics reduce the duration of dysentery in patients with moderately severe illness, but there was insufficient evidence to recommend a specific antibiotic class as superior.[13] Shigella species develop antibiotic resistance through both clonal spread and horizontal gene transfer, and increased fluoroquinolone and azithromycin resistance has been noted in the United States, particularly in MSM.[14]

Escherichia coli

E coli has 6 subtypes that cause gastrointestinal symptoms (**Box 2**), with Shiga toxin-producing E. coli (STEC) being the most common subtype in food-borne outbreaks. Specifically, *E coli* O157:H7 is the STEC type that is found in 36% of STEC infections and can cause more severe symptoms when compared with non-O157 types. Symptoms typically start 3 to 4 days after exposure and can cause diarrhea, abdominal pain,

Table 6
Differential diagnosis of dysentery

	Organisms
Bacterial	*Shigella* Enteroinvasive E. coli (EIEC) Nontyphoidal *Salmonella* *Yersinia enterocolitis* *Campylobacter enterocolitis* Enterohemorrhagic *E coli* *C difficile* *Aeromonas* *Vibrio*
Parasitic	Amebiasis Schistosomiasis
Viral	Cytomegalovirus

Data from Pfeiffer ML, DuPont HL, Ochoa TJ. The patient presenting with acute dysentery–a systematic review. J Infect 2012;64(4):374–86.

and fever, lasting an average of 5 to 7 days' duration.[15] Transmission is typically from unpasteurized milk, unpasteurized apple cider, soft cheeses, infected water, or contact with cattle. Antibiotics are not recommended and may increase the risk of hemolytic uremic syndrome,[16] which occurs in 4% to 17% of cases of STEC[17] and presents typically 7 days after onset of diarrhea with decreased urination, fatigue, and pallor.

Yersinia

Y enterocolitica is a facultative anaerobic gram-negative coccobacillus that is more common in the winter and commonly transmitted by eating raw or undercooked pork, unpasteurized milk, untreated water, or contact with animals. The incubation period is 4 to 6 days and diagnosis can be made by isolation from stool, blood, bile, wound, throat swab, mesenteric lymph nodes, cerebrospinal fluid, or peritoneal fluid.[18] Antibiotic therapy can be considered for more severe cases but has no effect on postinfectious complications, such as reactive arthritis and erythema nodosum.[18]

Listeria

Listeria is more common in older adults, the immunocompromised, and particularly pregnant women. *L monocytogenes* is a gram-positive, anaerobic motile bacillus transmitted via contaminated food (see **Table 2**) and maternal-fetal transmission. Listeriosis can cause bacteremia, meningitis, miscarriage, fetal loss, and death with 15% of cases in the United States occurring in pregnant women, with Hispanic women being at greater risk.[19] In pregnant women, *Listeria* presents with fever (65%), flu-like symptoms (32%), abdominal or back pain (21.5%), vomiting/diarrhea (7%), headache (10.5%), myalgia (4%), or sore throat (4%),[20] requiring a high index of suspicion during pregnancy. The American College of Obstetricians and Gynecologists does not recommend routine testing for asymptomatic women.[21] Invasive listeriosis in nonpregnant individuals is more common in those older than 65 years of age, with 89% of cases resulting in hospitalization and 23% in death in 2014.[19] Diagnosis can be made via culture of blood or cerebrospinal fluid. Empiric antibiotic treatment of pregnant women may be considered during outbreaks or in those that are symptomatic and with fever.[21] Those that are immunocompromised or pregnant should be encouraged to avoid foods commonly associated with *Listeria* (**Box 3**).

Clostridium perfringens

C perfringens is a spore-forming gram-positive bacterium that is a common cause in the United States of food-borne illness, in raw meat and poultry. Its spores can survive high

Box 2
***Escherichia coli* diarrheal subtypes, as classified by the Centers for Disease Control and Prevention**

- Shiga toxin-producing E coli (STEC) also known as Verocytotoxin-producing *E coli* or enterohemorrhagic *E coli*
- Enterotoxigenic *E coli*
- Enteropathogenic *E coli*
- Enteroaggregative *E coli*
- Enteroinvasive E. coli (EIEC)
- Diffusely adherent *E coli*

Data from Questions and Answers | E.coli | CDC. Available at: https://www.cdc.gov/ecoli/general/index.html. Accessed April 9, 2018.

Box 3
Foods commonly associated with *Listeria monocytogenes*

- Mexican-style cheese, such as queso fresco, queso blanco
- Unpasteurized dairy products
- Raw meats, delicatessen meats, hot dogs, cold cuts, pâtés, and meat spreads
- Smoked or raw seafood
- Soft cheeses, such as feta and brie or blue-veined cheeses

Data from Centers for Disease Control and Prevention (CDC). Vital signs: listeria illnesses, deaths, and outbreaks–United States, 2009-2011. MMWR Morb Mortal Wkly Rep 2013;62(22):448–52. Available at: http://www.ncbi.nlm.nih.gov/pubmed/23739339. Accessed January 1, 2018.

temperatures, germinating and reproducing in incorrectly stored or reheated foods. The toxin produced by *C perfringens* causes diarrhea and abdominal cramps within 6 to 24 hours of exposure and typically lasts 24 hours with spontaneous resolution. Fever and vomiting are uncommon with *C perfringens* infections, and the illness is not spread from person to person. Treatment is supportive with no role for antibiotic use.

Clostridium difficile

C difficile is a gram-positive, spore forming, anaerobic bacillus spread via fecal oral transmission that can survive on dry inanimate surfaces for up to 5 months,[22] making infection control particularly important. *C difficile* infection (CDI) has become common in both community and health care environments, causing 12.1% of health care-associated infections.[23] Multiple recurrent CDI is associated with older age, female gender, use of antibiotics, proton pump inhibitors, corticosteroids within 90 days of diagnosis, chronic kidney disease, and nursing homes.[24] A 2014 systemic review found that mortality was associated with older age, comorbidities, hypoalbuminemia, leukocytosis, acute renal failure, and infection with ribotype 027.[25] Community-acquired CDI was found in a 2013 meta-analysis to be greatest with use of the following antibiotics: clindamycin (OR 20.43), fluoroquinolones (OR 5.65), cephalosporins (OR 4.47), penicillins (OR 3.25), macrolides (OR 2.55), and sulphonamides/trimethoprim (OR 1.84).[26]

Fever, cramping, abdominal discomfort, passage of mucus or occult blood in the stool, and peripheral leukocytosis are common. It is important to distinguish CDI from colonization, because asymptomatic *C difficile* colonization prevalence can be as high as 15% in healthy adults and 18% to 90% among healthy newborns and infants.[27] Diagnosis of CDI is made in those that are symptomatic and over 2 years of age by the presence of stool toxin. Stool toxin in children under 2 years of age does not confirm diagnosis because of the high rate of colonization, requiring exclusion of other causes of diarrhea.[28] Less commonly, diagnosis is made by histopathology, endoscopy (eg, pseudomembranous colitis), or CT (eg, severe colitis, megacolon or ileus).

Medical management can be based on disease severity, as is outlined in **Table 7**. Complications of severe *C difficile* colitis include dehydration, electrolyte disturbances, hypoalbuminemia, toxic megacolon, bowel perforation, hypotension, renal failure, systemic inflammatory response syndrome, sepsis, and death. Surgical colectomy may be considered for severely ill patients. A 2017 study showed that despite increased infection rates, *C difficile*-associated fatality decreased from 3.6% in 2004 to 1.6%.[29] Newer treatment methods for recurrent or refractory cases include fidaxomicin therapy, monoclonal antibodies, and fecal microbiota transplantation. There is insufficient evidence to recommend probiotics for treatment of CDI,[30] but a Cochrane review showed moderate evidence of benefit for prevention.[31]

Table 7
Treatment based on severity categorization for *Clostridium difficile* infection

Disease Severity	Criteria	Treatment
Mild-moderate	WBC ≤15,000 cells/μL Cr ≤1.5 times baseline	Metronidazole 500 mg PO tid × 10–14 d
Severe	WBC ≥15,000 cells/μL Cr ≥1.5 times baseline	Vancomycin 125 mg PO qid × 10–14 d
Severe-complicated	Meets criteria for severe disease PLUS hypotension, shock, ileus, megacolon, or perforation	Vancomycin 500 orally or per nasogastric tube qid PLUS metronidazole 500 mg IV q8h (consider rectal vancomycin if complete ileus)

Abbreviations: Cr, creatinine; WBC, white blood cell count.

Adapted from Cohen SH, Gerding DN, Johnson S, et al. Clinical practice guidelines for Clostridium difficile infection in adults: 2010 update by the Society for Healthcare Epidemiology of America (SHEA) and the Infectious Diseases Society of America (IDSA). Infect Control Hosp Epidemiol 2010;31(5):447; with permission.

Viruses

Norovirus

Noroviruses are highly contagious and a significant cause of gastroenteritis worldwide.[32] Prolonged viral shedding, persistence in the environment, and the small inoculum required to cause infection contribute to increased transmission.[33] Norovirus causes approximately 20 million cases of acute gastroenteritis and up to 800 deaths per year in the United States, with most cases presenting during the winter.[34] Outbreaks occur in health care facilities, schools, daycare centers, restaurants, and cruise ships. In countries where the rotavirus vaccine has been implemented, norovirus has surpassed rotavirus as the predominant cause of acute gastroenteritis in children.[35]

The incubation period is between 24 to 48 hours, and treatment is mainly supportive, with correction of dehydration and electrolyte abnormalities as the primary focus.[33] Polymerase chain reaction (PCR) testing which is highly sensitive and specific and allows for viral typing, is considered to be the gold standard for diagnosis, with immunoassays having inferior sensitivity to PCR.[36] Early identification, reporting, and implementation of infection control measures such as contact precautions, hand washing with soap and water, environmental disinfection with bleach solutions, mask use for individuals who may be exposed to vomitus, visitor restrictions, and ward closures may help to reduce transmission.[37]

Rotavirus

Rotavirus is the most common cause of severe diarrhea in infants and children under 5 years of age worldwide and has been responsible for up to 600,000 deaths annually.[38] Disease can occur year-round but typically peaks in the winter and spring. Most unvaccinated children have evidence of rotavirus infection by the age of 5.[38] Rotavirus has an incubation period of 48 hours, causing vomiting, fever, and watery diarrhea lasting 3 to 8 days.[39] Less commonly, development of seizures, necrotizing enterocolitis, intussusception, central nervous system involvement, and death can occur. Stool enzyme immunoassays are most commonly used for diagnosis, although PCR is more sensitive. Alternative diagnostic methods include culture, electron microscopy, and serology to detect antibodies to rotavirus. Treatment is primarily supportive. Although improvements in water quality and sanitation have led to decreased incidence of some enteric pathogens, the incidence of rotavirus infection has been largely unaffected. Vaccination, on the other hand, which was introduced in the Unites States in 2006, is estimated to prevent more than 60,000 hospitalizations each year.[40]

Parasites

Cryptosporidum

Cryptosporidium was more common during the AIDS epidemic and can be transmitted via water, animal exposure, as well as person-to-person contact. A small inoculum (10–100 oocysts) may transmit infection, with spores surviving for months in water or soil and resistant to water purification chemicals, resulting in outbreaks in lakes and swimming pools.[41] Cryptosporidiosis typically causes self-limited watery diarrhea, nausea, vomiting, and abdominal pain, with more severe, protracted symptoms and extraintestinal disease in the immunocompromised or malnourished children, who may exhibit respiratory tract involvement or failure to thrive.[41]

Cryptosporidium is detected by microscopy, requiring special staining for visualization, PCR, or stool antigen assays, which are costlier. Both PCR and immunoassays offer improved sensitivity over microscopy.[42] Nitazoxanide shortens the duration of diarrhea and parasite excretion in immunocompetent hosts.[43] In immunocompromised hosts, nitazoxanide may still be of some benefit, but at higher doses and longer duration. For patients with HIV and low CD4 counts (<50 cells/μL), antiretroviral therapy is the primary treatment because nitazoxanide has been of little benefit.[44]

Giardia

Giardia intestinalis is among the most common causes of human parasitic infections in the United States, with approximately 20,000 cases reported annually.[45] *Giardia* can be transmitted via water, via food, or person to person. Most outbreaks occur in summer months, because of increased recreational exposure to contaminated water. Human infection occurs after ingestion of as few as 10 cysts, causing both acute and chronic infections. Common symptoms include diarrhea, nausea, vomiting, malaise, abdominal cramping, steatorrhea, and weight loss. In patients with chronic infection, significant weight loss can occur. First-line treatment options for *Giardia* include metronidazole 250 mg orally 3 times daily for 5 to 7 days, tinidazole 2 g orally once, or nitazoxanide 500 mg orally twice a day for 3 days. Albendazole, paromomycin, and furazolidone have been used as alternative therapies.

Entamoeba histolytica

Amebic dysentery is caused by the protozoan parasite, *E histolytica*, via fecal-oral transmission of cysts. Risk factors include communal living, oral and anal sex, immunosuppression, and travel to endemic areas.[46] *E histolytica* can cause mild diarrhea or fulminant dysentery. Severe disease can be fatal or cause colonic ulcers, toxic megacolon, perforation, chronic carriage or amebic liver abscesses. Of note, only 10% to 20% of infected patients develop symptoms.[47]

Available methods for detecting *E histolytica* infection include antibody testing, stool microscopy, culture, and enzyme-linked immunosorbent assay (ELISA) or PCR-based stool assays. Antibody testing has limited utility in patients from endemic areas because it can be difficult to distinguish between active infection and prior exposure. Microscopy is poorly sensitive and *E histolytica* is difficult to distinguish from nonpathogenic *Entamoeba* species. Stool assays using PCR and ELISA-based antigen detection are highly sensitive and specific but may not be available in resource-limited settings.[48]

Symptomatic infections are generally treated with 7 to 10 days of metronidazole 500 to 750 mg orally 3 times a day, followed by a luminal agent such as paromomycin, for the treatment of intraluminal cysts.[49,50] Colonization can be treated with solely an intraluminal agent, such as paromomycin 25 to 35 mg/kg/d orally divided 3 times a day for 7 days or diloxanide furoate 500 mg orally 3 times a day for 10 days.[50] Treatment is recommended even in the absence of symptoms due to the risk of developing invasive disease and spread to close contacts.[46]

Special Populations

Persons with HIV are at increased risk of acute and chronic diarrhea because of a combination of immunosuppression, direct HIV viral effects, adverse medication effects and behaviors that may increase exposure. HIV enteropathy can result from direct effects of HIV on gastrointestinal tract cells and gut-associated lymphoid tissue.[51] After the introduction of highly active antiretroviral therapy in 1996, there was a reduction in opportunistic infections as the cause of chronic diarrhea from 53% to 13% in patients with AIDS, whereas the overall incidence of chronic diarrhea did not decrease.[52] Lymphoma and Karposi sarcoma are other noninfectious causes of diarrhea. In those with HIV and bacterial diarrhea, *C difficile* was the most common cause in persons studied from 1992 to 2002.[53] An acid-fast smear or immunofluorescent stain should be requested to look for *Cryptosporidium*, *Isospora*, and *Cyclospora*. In patients with CD4 counts less than 100 cells/μL, the possibility of *Microsporidium* should also be investigated via trichrome staining of a stool specimen. Biopsy may be required to confirm infection with *Mycobacterium avium complex* or cytomegalovirus.[54,55]

REFERENCES

1. Shane AL, Mody RK, Crump JA, et al. 2017 infectious diseases society of America clinical practice guidelines for the diagnosis and management of infectious diarrhea. Clin Infect Dis 2017;65(12):1963–73.
2. WHO. Water-related diseases. Geneva (Switzerland): WHO; 2016. Available at: http://www.who.int/water_sanitation_health/diseases-risks/diseases/diarrhoea/en/. Accessed February 17, 2018.
3. Scallan E, Hoekstra RM, Angulo FJ, et al. Foodborne illness acquired in the United States-major pathogens. Emerg Infect Dis 2011;17(1):7–15.
4. CDC. Foodborne diseases active surveillance network (FoodNet): foodnet surveillance report for 2014 (final report). Atlanta, (GA): 2014. Available at: https://www.cdc.gov/foodnet/pdfs/2014-foodnet-surveillance-report.pdf. Accessed April 10, 2018.
5. Harvey K, Esposito DH, Han P, et al. Surveillance for travel-related disease–GeoSentinel Surveillance System, United States, 1997-2011. MMWR Surveill Summ 2013;62:1–23. Available at: http://www.ncbi.nlm.nih.gov/pubmed/23863769. Accessed January 1, 2018.
6. Wei L, Ratnayake L, Phillips G, et al. Acid-suppression medications and bacterial gastroenteritis: a population-based cohort study. Br J Clin Pharmacol 2017;83(6):1298–308.
7. Mitchell H, Hughes G. Recent epidemiology of sexually transmissible enteric infections in men who have sex with men. Curr Opin Infect Dis 2018;31(1):50–6.
8. Friedman CR, Hoekstra RM, Samuel M, et al. Risk factors for sporadic *Campylobacter* infection in the united states: a case-control study in foodnet sites. Clin Infect Dis 2004;38(s3):S285–96.
9. Information for Health Professionals | Campylobacter | CDC. Available at: https://www.cdc.gov/campylobacter/technical.html. Accessed April 9, 2018.

10. Keithlin J, Sargeant J, Thomas MK, et al. Systematic review and meta-analysis of the proportion of Campylobacter cases that develop chronic sequelae. BMC Public Health 2014;14(1):1203.
11. Keithlin J, Sargeant JM, Thomas MK, et al. Systematic review and meta-analysis of the proportion of non-typhoidal Salmonella cases that develop chronic sequelae. Epidemiol Infect 2015;143(7):1333–51.
12. Aragon TJ, Vugia DJ, Shallow S, et al. Case-control study of shigellosis in San Francisco: the role of sexual transmission and HIV infection. Clin Infect Dis 2007;44(3):327–34.
13. Christopher PR, David KV, John SM, et al. Antibiotic therapy for Shigella dysentery. Cochrane Database Syst Rev 2010;(8):CD006784.
14. Heiman KE, Karlsson M, Grass J, et al. Notes from the field: shigella with decreased susceptibility to azithromycin among men who have sex with men — United States, 2002–2013. MMWR Morb Mortal Wkly Rep 2014; 63(6):121–6.
15. Questions and Answers | E.coli | CDC. Available at: https://www.cdc.gov/ecoli/general/index.html. Accessed April 9, 2018.
16. Freedman SB, Xie J, Neufeld MS, et al. Shiga toxin–producing *Escherichia coli* infection, antibiotics, and risk of developing hemolytic uremic syndrome: a meta-analysis. Clin Infect Dis 2016;62(10):1251–8.
17. Keithlin J, Sargeant J, Thomas MK, et al. Chronic sequelae of *E. coli* O157: systematic review and meta-analysis of the proportion of *E. coli* O157 cases that develop chronic sequelae. Foodborne Pathog Dis 2014;11(2):79–95.
18. Information for Health & Lab Professionals | Yersinia | CDC. Available at: https://www.cdc.gov/yersinia/healthcare.html. Accessed April 10, 2018.
19. Centers for Disease Control and Prevention (CDC). Vital signs: listeria illnesses, deaths, and outbreaks–United States, 2009-2011. MMWR Morb Mortal Wkly Rep 2013;62(22):448–52. Available at: http://www.ncbi.nlm.nih.gov/pubmed/23739339. Accessed January 1, 2018.
20. Mylonakis E, Paliou M, Hohmann EL, et al. Listeriosis during pregnancy: a case series and review of 222 cases. Medicine (Baltimore) 2002;81(4):260–9.
21. Committee on Obstetric Practice. American college of obstetricians and gynecologists. committee opinion no. 614. Obstet Gynecol 2014;124(6):1241–4.
22. Kramer A, Schwebke I, Kampf G. How long do nosocomial pathogens persist on inanimate surfaces? a systematic review. BMC Infect Dis 2006;6(1):130.
23. Magill SS, Edwards JR, Bamberg W, et al. Multistate point-prevalence survey of health care–associated infections. N Engl J Med 2014;370(13):1198–208.
24. Ma GK, Brensinger CM, Wu Q, et al. Increasing incidence of multiply recurrent Clostridium difficile infection in the United States: a cohort study. Ann Intern Med 2017;167(3):152–8.
25. Abou Chakra CN, Pepin J, Sirard S, et al. Risk factors for recurrence, complications and mortality in Clostridium difficile infection: a systematic review. PLoS One 2014;9(6):e98400.
26. Deshpande A, Pasupuleti V, Thota P, et al. Community-associated clostridium difficile infection antibiotics: a meta-analysis. J Antimicrob Chemother 2013; 68(9):1951–61.
27. Furuya-Kanamori L, Marquess J, Yakob L, et al. Asymptomatic Clostridium difficile colonization: epidemiology and clinical implications. BMC Infect Dis 2015; 15(1):1–11.
28. Cohen SH, Gerding DN, Johnson S, et al. Clinical practice guidelines for Clostridium difficile infection in adults: 2010 update by the society for healthcare

epidemiology of america (SHEA) and the infectious diseases society of America (IDSA). Infect Control Hosp Epidemiol 2010;31(5):431–55.
29. Shrestha MP, Bime C, Taleban S. Decreasing Clostridium difficile –associated fatality rates among hospitalized patients in the United States: 2004-2014. Am J Med 2017;131(1):90–6.
30. Pillai A, Nelson R. Probiotics for treatment of Clostridium difficile-associated colitis in adults. Cochrane Database Syst Rev 2008;(1):CD004611.
31. Goldenberg JZ, Ma SS, Saxton JD, et al. Probiotics for the prevention of Clostridium difficile-associated diarrhea in adults and children. Cochrane Database Syst Rev 2013;(12):CD006095.
32. Ahmed SM, Hall AJ, Robinson AE, et al. Global prevalence of norovirus in cases of gastroenteritis: a systematic review and meta-analysis. Lancet Infect Dis 2014; 14(8):725–30.
33. Robilotti E, Deresinski S, Pinsky BA. Norovirus. Clin Microbiol Rev 2015;28(1): 134–64.
34. Norovirus | U.S. Trends and Outbreaks | CDC. Available at: https://www.cdc.gov/norovirus/trends-outbreaks.html. Accessed February 17, 2018.
35. Nguyen GT, Phan K, Teng I, et al. A systematic review and meta-analysis of the prevalence of norovirus in cases of gastroenteritis in developing countries. Medicine (Baltimore) 2017;96(40):e8139.
36. Division of Viral Diseases, National Center for Immunization and Respiratory Diseases, Centers for Disease Control and Prevention. Updated norovirus outbreak management and disease prevention guidelines. MMWR Recomm Rep 2011; 60(RR-3):1–18. Available at: http://www.ncbi.nlm.nih.gov/pubmed/21368741. Accessed April 10, 2018.
37. Barclay L, Park GW, Vega E, et al. Infection control for norovirus. Clin Microbiol Infect 2014;20(8):731–40.
38. Parashar UD, Hummelman EG, Bresee JS, et al. Global illness and deaths caused by rotavirus disease in children. Emerg Infect Dis 2003;9(5):565–72. Available at: http://www.ncbi.nlm.nih.gov/pubmed/12737740. Accessed April 10, 2018.
39. Rotavirus | Clinical Disease Information | CDC. Available at: https://www.cdc.gov/rotavirus/clinical.html. Accessed April 10, 2018.
40. Cortes JE, Curns AT, Tate JE, et al. Rotavirus vaccine and health care utilization for diarrhea in U.S. children. N Engl J Med 2011;365(12):1108–17.
41. Yoder JS, Wallace RM, Collier SA, et al. Centers for Disease Control and Prevention (CDC). Cryptosporidiosis surveillance–United States, 2009-2010. MMWR Surveill Summ 2012;61(5):1–12. Available at: http://www.ncbi.nlm.nih.gov/pubmed/22951493. Accessed April 10, 2018.
42. Cama VA, Mathison BA. Infections by intestinal coccidia and giardia duodenalis. Clin Lab Med 2015;35(2):423–44.
43. Rossignol JF, Ayoub A, Ayers MS. Treatment of diarrhea caused by Cryptosporidium parvum: a prospective randomized, double-blind, placebo-controlled study of nitazoxanide. J Infect Dis 2001;184(1):103–6.
44. Rossignol JF. Nitazoxanide in the treatment of acquired immune deficiency syndrome-related cryptosporidiosis: results of the United States compassionate use program in 365 patients. Aliment Pharmacol Ther 2006;24(5):887–94.
45. Yoder JS, Gargano JW, Wallace RM, et al. Centers for Disease Control and Prevention (CDC). Giardiasis surveillance–United States, 2009-2010. MMWR Surveill Summ 2012;61(5):13–23. Available at: http://www.ncbi.nlm.nih.gov/pubmed/22951494. Accessed April 10, 2018.

46. Petri WA, Singh U. Diagnosis and management of amebiasis. Clin Infect Dis 1999;29:1117–25.
47. Marie C, Petri WA. Amoebic dysentery. BMJ Clin Evid 2013;2013. Available at: http://www.ncbi.nlm.nih.gov/pubmed/23991750. Accessed February 17, 2018.
48. Skappak C, Akierman S, Belga S, et al. Invasive amoebiasis: a review of Entamoeba infections highlighted with case reports. Can J Gastroenterol Hepatol 2014;28(7):355–9.
49. Ximénez C, Morán P, Rojas L, et al. Novelties on amoebiasis: a neglected tropical disease. J Glob Infect Dis 2011;3(2):166.
50. Haque R, Huston CD, Hughes M, et al. Amebiasis. N Engl J Med 2003;348(16): 1565–73.
51. MacArthur RD, DuPont HL. Etiology and pharmacologic management of noninfectious diarrhea in HIV-infected individuals in the highly active antiretroviral therapy era. Clin Infect Dis 2012;55(6):860–7.
52. Call SA, Heudebert G, Saag M, et al. The changing etiology of chronic diarrhea in HIV-infected patients with CD4 cell counts less than 200 cells/mm3. Am J Gastroenterol 2000;95(11):3142–6.
53. Sanchez TH, Brooks JT, Sullivan PS, et al. Bacterial diarrhea in persons with HIV infection, United States, 1992-2002. Clin Infect Dis 2005;41(11):1621–7.
54. CMV | Herpes | Adult and Adolescent Opportunistic Infection | AIDSinfo. Available at: https://aidsinfo.nih.gov/guidelines/html/4/adult-and-adolescent-opportunistic-infection/337/cmv. Accessed April 10, 2018.
55. MAC | Adult and adolescent opportunistic infection | AIDSinfo. Available at: https://aidsinfo.nih.gov/guidelines/html/4/adult-and-adolescent-opportunistic-infection/326/mac. Accessed April 10, 2018.

Role of Complementary and Alternative Therapies in Infectious Disease

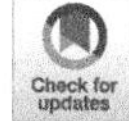

Jeffrey H. Baker, MD[a,*], Juan Qiu, MD, PhD[b], Kristen Grine, DO[a]

KEYWORDS

• Acupuncture • Ayurveda • Complementary and alternative medicine • Homeopathy • Infectious disease • Natural products • Supplements

KEY POINTS

- Complementary and Alternative Medicine (CAM) is increasingly being used in Western countries despite the lack of conclusive research studies.
- Several CAM modalities have only shown variable therapeutic efficacy in infectious disease management.
- Clinicians should be familiar with these therapies in order to advise patients about alternative therapeutic options when treating infections.

INTRODUCTION

Complementary and alternative medicine (CAM) therapies are terms used to signify nonmainstream medical practices. The National Center for Complementary and Integrative Health (NCCIH) uses the term "complementary" therapy when a nonmainstream practice is used with conventional medicine, whereas same the nonmainstream practice, when used in place of conventional medicine, is viewed as an "alternative" therapy.[1] Key data from the 2012 US National Health Interview Survey revealed that approximately 33% of adults and 12% of children had used complementary health approaches, similar numbers from previous survey in 2007.[1] It was estimated that Americans spent 12.8 billion out-of-pocket dollars on "natural products," while spending 14.7 billion dollars on complementary practitioner visits.[2] Given the magnitude of CAM use, it is essential that clinicians are prepared to advise their patients of the benefits and potential hazards of these therapies. The NCCIH then divides the practices of CAM into 3 groups: natural products (dietary supplements as vitamins, minerals, herbs and probiotics), mind-body practices (osteopathic and chiropractic manipulation, acupuncture, massage, yoga and

Disclosure Statement: The authors have nothing to disclose.
[a] Department of Family and Community Medicine, Penn State University College of Medicine, Penn State Hershey Medical Group, 476 Rolling Ridge Drive, #101, State College, PA 16801, USA; [b] Department of Family and Community Medicine, Penn State University College of Medicine, Penn State Hershey Medical Group, 32 Colonnade Way, State College, PA 16803, USA
* Corresponding author.
E-mail address: jbaker3@pennstatehealth.psu.edu

Prim Care Clin Office Pract 45 (2018) 533–539
https://doi.org/10.1016/j.pop.2018.05.009 primarycare.theclinics.com

meditation, relaxation techniques), and other forms of therapies (naturopathy, homeopathy, Ayurvedic medicine, traditional Chinese medicine, and other traditional healings).[1]

Natural Products: Supplements for Infections

There is no one product, no panacea "for what ails you" in integrative infectious disease therapy. There are only scattered randomized controlled trials to make recommendations for individual natural products in identifiable infections. The *Cochrane Database of Systematic Reviews* is a valuable source for these assessments. The data presented in **Table 1** represent and reflect those Cochrane studies and reviews.

Table 1
Natural products

Name	Use	Evidence	Recommendation	Notes
Multivitamins	Infection prevention in elderly	Systematic review[3] RCT[4]	No benefit No benefit	
Vitamin C	Viral URI Prevent/treat pneumonia	Cochrane review[5] Cochrane review[6]	No benefit Possible benefit	May have benefit where vitamin intake is low. ≥1 g/d has better results
Vitamin D	Prevent URI	Review/ meta-analysis[7,8]	Probable benefit	Those at risk for deficiency do better[7]; conflicting findings[8]
Zinc	Viral URI	Meta-analysis[9]	Probable benefit	≥80 mg/d
Garlic	Viral URI	Cochrane review[10]	Insufficient evidence	
Echinacea	Viral URI	Cochrane review[11]	Insufficient evidence	Effect variable among spp of Echinacea
Ginseng	Viral URI	Systematic review[12]	Insufficient evidence	
Cranberry	Prevent/treat UTI	Cochrane review[13,14]	No benefit	
Probiotics	Vulvovaginal candidiasis	Cochrane review[15]	Probable benefit	Adjuvant therapy to ABx
	Bacterial vaginosis	Cochrane review[16]	Insufficient evidence	
	Prevent UTI	Cochrane review[17]	No benefit	
	Viral URI	Cochrane review[18]	Possible benefit	Quality of evidence low to very low
	Acute diarrhea	Cochrane review[19]	Probable benefit	Unsure which probiotic spp are helpful
	Prevent ABx diarrhea in pediatrics	Cochrane review[20]	Beneficial	Lactobacillis, Bifidobacterium, Streptococcus, Saccharomyces helpful alone or in combination
	Prevent *C diff* in adults	Cochrane review[21]	Beneficial	Helpful in groups high at risk for infection
	Treat *C diff*	Cochrane review[22]	No benefit	
	Treat *H pylori*	Systematic review[23]	Possible benefit	In combination with ABx therapy

Respiratory Infections

Upper respiratory infections (URI) or the "common cold" is the disease state most often investigated for the use of supplements for treatment. Cochrane reviews of primary research are recognized as the standard for evidence-based health care resources. They have undertaken reviews of vitamin C,[5,6] garlic,[10] and *Echinacea* species.[11] Other systematic reviews have compiled research on the treatment of URI involving vitamin D,[7,8] zinc,[9] and ginseng.[12] A summary of the findings is in **Table 1**, Natural Products. These systematic reviews voiced concerns over the lack of large study groups and lack of randomized controlled trial structures. Further research using large randomized controlled trials is needed.

Gastrointestinal Infections

With the advent of probiotic use, multiple studies have been done on gastrointestinal illnesses and reviewed with systematic analysis. The significant reviews included acute diarrhea,[19] *Clostridium difficile* treatment and prevention,[21,22] antibiotic-associated diarrhea,[20] and treatment of *Helicobacter pylori*[23] (see **Table 1**). Further research needs to focus on which group or species of probiotics will be useful and beneficial in these treatment strategies.

Vulvovaginal Candidiasis and Bacterial Vaginosis

Probiotics have also been studied in the prevention and treatment of bacterial vaginosis[15] and vulvovaginal candidiasis.[16] The review of candidal vulvovaginosis research noted that there is only low-quality evidence that the use of probiotics as adjuvant therapy to current treatment could increase the rate of short-term cure and relapse, but that furthermore, more comprehensive study is needed. There is not enough research evidence at present to either support or not support the use probiotics for a diagnosis of bacterial vaginosis.[15] Reviewers cited a lack of large, randomized controlled trials to support clinical consideration.

Urinary Tract Infections

Despite common clinical use, 2 separate Cochrane reviews[14,15] did not find support to recommend the use of cranberry in the treatment or prevention of urinary tract infections (UTIs). Because of varied study groups reviewed, this area of research will likely have further study.

Human Immunodeficiency Virus Infections

A quandary for research has been using natural products for human immunodeficiency virus (HIV) infection. A 2017 Cochrane systematic review found no reliable evidence to add supplements to HIV treatment regimens to provide clinical improvements, but that deficient patients might benefit by at least increasing to daily allowances of micronutrients.[24] However, ongoing research is suggesting that promising plant substances are also known to modulate cellular factors, which are also involved in the replication of HIV and hence their role as potential candidates for therapy.[25] This area has the potential for ongoing future research.

Recommendations

For viral respiratory infections, the use of vitamin C, vitamin D, zinc, and probiotics has benefit in treating the infection. Of note, the beneficial effects of vitamin C and D are most associated with vitamin C and D deficiency, that is, the greatest benefit in treatment is felt by those deficient in the vitamin.

There is probable benefit in using probiotics with antifungal agents as adjuvant therapy in treating vulvovaginal candidiasis.

Probiotics hold the greatest promise for treatment of acute diarrheal illness and preventing antibiotic-associated diarrhea, in preventing *C difficile* in at-risk populations, and in treating *H pylori* infections.

Mind-Body Practices: Acupuncture for Infectious Diseases

In traditional chinese medicine (TCM), a disease is thought to originate from an imbalance of Qi or poor flow of Qi. Acupuncture is a component of TCM that works to restore the balance of Qi, thus allows self-healing. Acupuncture is performed by inserting needles and applying heat or electrical stimulation at very precise acupuncture points on the surface of the body.

The study of acupuncture is challenging using the standard randomized, double-blinded, placebo-controlled trials due to the physical nature of the intervention. The randomized controlled trials of acupuncture for infectious diseases are limited. Systematic reviews suggest that acupuncture is effective in preventing recurrent UTI in women,[26] decreasing chronic prostatitis symptoms,[27] and may provide short-term benefits for treating acute hordeolum when compared with conventional treatments.[28] A meta-analysis suggested that acupuncture is effective in the treatment of chronic pelvic inflammatory disease.[29] A systematic review and meta-analysis suggested that acupuncture improves pain and rash of acute herpes zoster.[30] Acupuncture was shown to be effective in preventing and treating common cold symptoms in a randomized controlled trial.[31]

Despite the study limitation, acupuncture may be a reasonable complementary option for interested patients with some chronic or recurrent infectious diseases in decreasing the symptoms and recurrence of the diseases.

Other Alternative Therapies: Ayurveda and Communicable Diseases

Ayurveda emphasizes the promotion of health to optimize the body's response to disease. Ayurveda originates from India based on Hindu healers' teachings. Examples of Ayurvedic medicine include herbal medications, yoga, meditation, self-awareness, and breathing exercises. It encourages interconnectedness through the maintenance of mental and spiritual well-being, which can be achieved through the practice of truth, sympathy, respecting others, altruism, and eating properly. Prevention as well as cure of the disease is goal of Ayurveda medicine.

Ayurveda medicine believes communicable diseases are spread through physical contact, expired air, eating with others, sharing beds, clothes, and cosmetics. Not following one's duty hampers one's immunity, thus indirectly exposing an individual to infection. The goal is to improve immunity and prevent spread of disease.

Ayurvedic medicine has emerged as a way to complement tradition infectious disease management. This partnership has become a necessity with the emergence of antibiotic resistance from both overprescribing and the food industry. Ayurvedic botanicals produce biological active secondary metabolites that have the potential to inhibit infectious activity. The alkaloids have the ability to interrupt cell division. The phenolics and polyphenols (**Table 2**) are compounds found in plants with various mechanisms to disrupt cellular microbe function (**Table 3**).[32,33]

Homeopathy

The research in homeopathy is limited and has methodologic flaws that do not allow conclusions about the efficacy of therapy.[34–36] More rigorous research in this area is needed in order to make future recommendations. Cochrane reviews have discussed

Table 2
Phenolics and polyphenols

Flavonoids	Found in vegetables, seeds, fruits, and nuts; possess the ability to disrupt the permeability of the microbial membrane
Quinones	Found in all plant parts; have the ability to inactivate a cell and cause loss of function
Tannins	Found in all plant parts; affect the cell envelope and adhesion mechanisms
Coumarins	Plants produce to combat bacterial infections functions as well as antifungal
Terpenes	The largest group of secondary metabolites; found in many essential oils. It is thought that this group can disrupt the microbial membrane
Lectin	Larger than polypeptides; disrupt cellular membranes
Polypeptides	Disrupt cellular membranes
Saponins	Have the ability to form soapy lathers when mixed with water

recent popular preparations of Oscillococcinum (Anas barbariae 200CK HPUS, domesticated duck liver and heart preparation) and Umcka (preparation containing extract of the root of *Pelargonium sidoides*), not finding rigorous evidence to make recommendations for their use.

SUMMARY

The recommendations that can be made regarding the use of supplements for infectious disease are in using vitamin C and zinc for treating an acute URI and using vitamin D to prevent pneumonia in susceptible children. Acupuncture has been shown effective in preventing and treating URI symptoms, treating acute hordeolum, and reducing the pain and rash of acute Herpes zoster outbreaks. In women, acupuncture helps prevent recurrent UTI as well as pelvic inflammatory symptoms, decreasing chronic prostatitis symptoms. In men, acupuncture reduces the symptoms of chronic prostatitis. Probiotics are gaining a place in the prevention and treatment of gastrointestinal infections, noted to be helpful in treating acute diarrhea or *H pylori* infection, as well as vulvovaginitis. They also are beneficial in preventing antibiotic-induced diarrhea in children and *C difficile* infections in adults.

There is promise ahead, especially as the research on the microbiome explodes with advancing technology, more specific testing, and rigorous outcomes for the use of probiotics, as current therapies alter an individual's microbiome. CAM research is faced with significant design challenges in trying to apply outcomes to the randomized controlled trials that mark the current academic culture. CAM therapies are often individualized and not fully applicable across a spectrum within a disease.

Table 3
Ayurvedic medicine: botanic mechanisms of antimicrobial activity

Prevention of biofilms	A protective outer layer of microbial groups
Inhibition of efflux pumps	Disrupts the outer membrane of the microbe
Reduced virulence	Less pathogenic microbe
Immunomodulation	Rev up host immune system
Innate immunity	Increase macrocytic activity
Acquired immunity	Improved B- and T-cell activity
Antiviral activity	Combat various viral activities

Mechanisms of actions are poorly understood, and therefore, study results are often inconclusive. As more patients will ask about CAM therapies and divulge their use, it remains imperative that clinicians recognize the difficulties of research providing conclusive evidence as they advise their patients regarding these therapies.

REFERENCES

1. Available at: https://nccih.nih.gov/health/integrative-health. Accessed February 25, 2018.
2. Available at: https://nccih.nih.gov/research/statistics/NHIS/2012. Accessed February 25, 2018.
3. El-Kadiki A, Sutton AJ. Role of multivitamins and mineral supplements in preventing infections in elderly people: systematic review and meta-analysis of randomised controlled trials. BMJ 2005;330(7496):871.
4. Avenell A, Campbell MK, Cook JA, et al. Effect of multivitamin and multimineral supplements on morbidity from infections in older people (MAVIS trial): pragmatic, randomised, double blind, placebo controlled trial. BMJ 2005;331(7512):324–9.
5. Hemila H, Chalker E. Vitamin C for preventing and treating the common cold. Cochrane Database Syst Rev 2013;(1):CD000980.
6. Hemilä H, Louhiala P. Vitamin C for preventing and treating pneumonia. Cochrane Database Syst Rev 2013;(8):CD005532.
7. Martineau AR, Joliffe DA, Hooper RL, et al. Vitamin D Supplementation to prevent acute respiratory tract infections: systematic review and meta-analysis of individual participant data. BMJ 2017;356:i6583.
8. Aglipay M, Birken CS, Parkin PC, et al. Effect of high-dose vs standard-dose wintertime vitamin D supplementation on viral upper respiratory tract infections in young healthy children. JAMA 2017;318(3):245–54.
9. Hemilia H, Chalker E. The effectiveness of high-dose zinc acetate lozenges on various common cold symptoms: a meta-analysis. BMC Fam Pract 2015;16:24.
10. Lissiman E, Bhasale AL, Cohen M. Garlic for the common cold. Cochrane Database Syst Rev 2014;(11):CD006206.
11. Karsch-Völk M, Barrett B, Kiefer D, et al. Echinacea for preventing and treating the common cold. Cochrane Database Syst Rev 2014;(2):CD000530.
12. Seida JK, Durec T, Kuhle S. North American *(Panax quinquefolius)* and Asian Ginseng *(Panax ginseng)* preparations for prevention of the common cold in healthy adults: a systematic review. Evid Based Complement Alternat Med 2011;2011:282151.
13. Jepson RG, Mihaljevic L, Craig JC. Cranberries for treating urinary tract infections. Cochrane Database Syst Rev 1998;(4):CD001322.
14. Jepson RG, Williams G, Craig JC. Cranberries for preventing urinary tract infections. Cochrane Database Syst Rev 2012;(10):CD001321.
15. Xie H, Feng D, Wei D, et al. Probiotics for vulvovaginal candidiasis in non-pregnant women. Cochrane Database Syst Rev 2017;(11):CD010496.
16. Senok AC, Verstraelen H, Temmerman M, et al. Probiotics for the treatment of bacterial vaginosis. Cochrane Database Syst Rev 2009;(4):CD006289.
17. Schwenger EM, Tejani AM, Loewen PS. Probiotics for preventing urinary tract infections in adults and children. Cochrane Database Syst Rev 2015;(12):CD008772.
18. Hao Q, Dong B, Wu T. Probiotics for preventing acute upper respiratory tract infections. Cochrane Database Syst Rev 2015;(2):CD006895.

19. Allen SJ, Martinez EG, Gregorio GV, et al. Probiotics for treating acute infectious diarrhoea. Cochrane Database Syst Rev 2010;(11):CD003048.
20. Goldenberg JZ, Lytvyn L, Steurich J, et al. Probiotics for the prevention of pediatric antibiotic-associated diarrhea. Cochrane Database Syst Rev 2015;(12):CD004827.
21. Goldenberg JZ, Yap C, Lytvyn L, et al. Probiotics for the prevention of Clostridium difficile-associated diarrhea in adults and children. Cochrane Database Syst Rev 2017;(12):CD006095.
22. Pillai A, Nelson RL. Probiotics for treatment of Clostridium difficile-associated colitis in adults. Cochrane Database Syst Rev 2008;(1):CD004611.
23. Kafshdooz T, Akbarzadeh A, Majdi Seghinsara A, et al. Role of probiotics in managing of Helicobacter pylori infection: a review. Drug Res (Stuttg) 2017;67(02): 88–93.
24. Visser ME, Durao S, Sinclair D, et al. Nutritional supplements for people being treated for active tuberculosis. Cochrane Database Syst Rev 2016;(6).
25. Kurapati KRV, Atluri VS, Samikkannu T, et al. Natural products as Anti-HIV agents and role in HIV-Associated Neurocognitive Disorders (HAND): a brief overview. Front Microbiol 2015;6:1444.
26. Eells SJ, Bharadwa K, McKinnell JA, et al. Recurrent urinary tract infections among women: comparative effectiveness of 5 prevention and management strategies using a markov chain monte carlo model. Clin Infect Dis 2014;58(2):147–60.
27. Franco JV, Turk T, Jung JH, et al. Non-pharmacological interventions for treating chronic prostatitis/chronic pelvic pain syndrome. Cochrane Database Syst Rev 2018;26(1):CD012551.
28. Cheng K, Law A, Guo M, et al. Acupuncture for acute hordeolum. Cochrane Database Syst Rev 2017;(2):CD011075.
29. Fan LL, Yu WH, Liu XQ, et al. A meta-analysis on effectiveness of acupuncture and moxibustion for chronic pelvic inflammatory disease. Zhen Ci Yan Jiu 2014;39(2):156–63.
30. Coyle ME, Liang H, Wang K, et al. Acupuncture plus moxibustion for herpes zoster: a systematic review and meta-analysis of randomized controlled trials. Dermatol Ther 2017;30(4):1–8.
31. Kawakita K, Shichidou T, Inoue E, et al. Preventive and curative effects of acupuncture on the common cold: a multicentre randomized controlled trial in Japan. Complement Ther Med 2004;12(4):181–8.
32. Kalamkar GS, Sawai RV, Rampurkar MV. Role of ayurveda in communicable diseases, National Seminar on Empowering and Empanelling Ayurveda System of Medicine. Satara (India), March 26–27, 2015.
33. Gupta PD, Birdi TJ. Development of botanicals to combat antibiotic resistance. J Ayurveda Integr Med 2017;8(4):266–75.
34. Fashner J. Letter: homeopathic remedies for treatment of the common cold. Am Fam Physician 2013;87(1):7.
35. Mathie RT, Frye J, Fisher P. Homeopathic oscillococcinum® for preventing and treating influenza and influenza-like illness. Cochrane Database Syst Rev 2015;(1):CD001957.
36. Timmer A, Günther J, Motschall E, et al. Pelargonium sidoides extract for treating acute respiratory tract infections. Cochrane Database Syst Rev 2013;(10):CD006323.

Health Guidelines for Travel Abroad

Jason Lohr, MD[a,b,*], Norman Benjamin Fredrick, MD[c], Leesha Helm, MD, MPH[d], Jeffrey Cho, MD, MPH[b]

KEYWORDS

• Travel health • Travel abroad • Pretravel Assessment • Posttravel Assessment

KEY POINTS

- Primary care providers manage the majority of travel medical care. The purpose of the pretravel visit are risk assessment and mitigation.
- Encourage travelers to enroll in the Smart Traveler Enrollment Program for travel advisories.
- The Centers for Disease Control and Prevention travel website offers destination-specific, point-of-care resources for clinicians and travelers.
- Travelers who are visiting friends and relatives are a high-risk group.
- The most common syndromes in returning travelers are gastrointestinal, febrile, and dermatologic.

INTRODUCTION

Most travel medical care is provided by patients' primary care physicians; only 10% of international travelers visit a travel clinic. The main purposes for travel include vacationing, visiting friends and family, business, and for educational purposes.

PRETRAVEL CONSULTATION

The purposes of the pretravel consultation are to estimate risk and provide recommendations to mitigate risk.

Disclosure Statement: The authors have nothing to disclose.
[a] CMO, SAC Health System, 250 South G Street, San Bernardino, CA 92410, USA; [b] Family Medicine Residency Program, Loma Linda University, 1200 California Street, Suite 240 Redlands, CA 92374, USA; [c] Family and Community Medicine and Public Health Sciences, Global Health Center, Pennsylvania State University College of Medicine, 500 University Drive, Hershey, PA 17033, USA; [d] Department of Family Medicine, Pennsylvania State University College of Medicine, Penn State Health, PGY-3, 500 University Drive, Hershey, PA 17033, USA
* Corresponding author. 250 South G Street, San Bernardino, CA 92410.
E-mail address: JLLohr@sachealthsystem.org

Prim Care Clin Office Pract 45 (2018) 541–554
https://doi.org/10.1016/j.pop.2018.05.012
0095-4543/18/
primarycare.theclinics.com

TRAVELER BACKGROUND

The initial pretravel assessment should focus on specific aspects regarding the health background of the traveler (**Box 1**). A full history and physical examination, including a review of immunizations, allergies, medications, and chronic medical conditions should be explored. Special attention and tailored recommendations should be given to those with chronic disease states, including congestive heart failure, diabetes, mental health issues, and immunocompromised states. It is important to note recent hospitalizations and surgeries and to assess the risk associated with traveling after these events. Prior travel history may provide clues regarding intolerance to certain antimalarials or other medications.

TRIP SPECIFICS

Review the itinerary of the traveler, including types of travel, the reason for travel, and accommodations. Country-specific risks and travel advisories should be discussed in detail with the traveler by reviewing resources like the Smart Traveler Enrollment Program (https://step.state.gov/). By assessing these specific aspects, the provider can obtain a wealth of knowledge that can be synthesized to help the traveler manage possible risks.

Box 1
Risk assessment

Medical history

- Medications
- Allergies
- Immunizations
- Chronic disease states
- Mental health
- Hospitalizations
- Surgeries
- Pregnancy or breastfeeding
- Previous travel
- Previous use of antimalarials, antibiotics
- Plans for repeat travel in next 1 to 2 years

Trip itinerary

- Location
- Dates and season
- Activities, mass gatherings
- Reasons for travel
- Accommodations
- Travel insurance

Data from Centers for Disease Control and Prevention. CDC yellow book 2018: health information for international travel. New York: Oxford University Press; 2017.

TRAVEL RECOMMENDATIONS TO REDUCE RISK

Preparedness for Exacerbations of Chronic Disease States

Travel can be stressful and demanding for individuals with chronic disease states. Before travel, clinicians should direct travelers to recommendations provided by national associations related to their chronic medical states for travel guidelines. In addition, travelers should be directed to check in with the US embassy or consulate in their area of travel to clarify any restrictions on medications with which they may need to travel.

Travel Insurance and International Health Care

Many health insurances do not provide adequate coverage for international travel, including repatriation and medical evacuation.[1] The following resources can be used to help travelers make a decision regarding the need for travel insurance, travel health insurance, and medical evacuation insurance.

- Department of State (www.travel.state.gov)
- International Association for Medical Assistance to Travelers (www.iamat.org)

Accessing Local Reputable Medical Facilities

The International Association of Medical Assistance to Travelers maintains a list of clinics available to members: www.iamat.org/doctors_clinics.cfm. In addition, the Joint Commission International maintains a list of accredited, certified health care facilities: www.jointcommissioninternational.org.

Health Kit

Medications for chronic conditions and prevention of disease states specific to regions of travel should be procured before initiation of travel. Individuals with preexisting conditions or allergies should consider wearing a medical alert bracelet or card in their wallet. See **Table 1** for a list of suggested travel health kit items.

Table 1
Health kit item checklist

Prescription Medications	Over-the-Counter Medications	Injury/Illness Prevention
Regular medications	Tylenol	Insect repellant for skin and clothing[a]
Diarrheal antibiotics	Aspirin	Bed net[a]
Antimalarial[a]	Ibuprofen	Alcohol-based sanitizer, hand wipes
Medication for altitude sickness[a]	Antacid	Latex condoms
Contact lenses/glasses[a]	Laxative	Ear plugs
Epinephrine pen[a]	Oral rehydration	Safety equipment (helmet, child safety seat)
Diabetes testing supplies and insulin[a]	Loperamide	Sunscreen
Needles or syringes[a]	Antihistamine	Water purification tablets
Medical bracelet or necklace[a]	Decongestant	
Preexposure or postexposure HIV medications[a]	Cough suppressant or drops	
	Sleep aid	
	Saline eye or nose drops	

Abbreviation: HIV, human immunodeficiency virus.
[a] If indicated.
Data from Centers for Disease Control and Prevention. CDC yellow book 2018: health information for international travel. New York: Oxford University Press; 2017.

Providers should recommend travelers carry documentation of the following:

- Health insurance, supplemental insurance,
- Proof of vaccinations,
- List of medications and preexisting conditions, and
- Contact card with emergency contact, location of travel, hospitals and clinics, US embassy or consulate number, health care provider contact information.

Important Travel Risks

The World Health Organization has cited that, among deaths in travelers, 18% to 24% are caused by injuries, whereas only 2% are caused by infectious disease.[1]

Motor vehicle safety

Among US travelers in foreign countries, motor vehicle accidents are the leading cause of death, making up approximately 27% of all nonnatural deaths in 1 study.[1] Contributing factors include lack of familiarity with infrastructure in the area of traveled, lack of seat belt use, alcohol use, travel fatigue, poor visibility, and increased risk for road-related accidents.[1] Prevention strategies include using seatbelts and child safety seats, avoiding night-time driving, increasing awareness of driving hazards, using helmets when driving motorcycles or motorbikes, avoiding alcohol or cellphone use before or during driving, using marked taxis for travel, avoiding travel in overcrowded buses, and remaining alert while crossing streets.[1]

Swimming

Drowning is the fourth leading cause of death of international US travelers.[1] Avoidance of swimming alone and the use of a life jacket with water-related activities should be encouraged. Swimming should be avoided when local water conditions or currents are unknown and if a traveler has recently used alcohol.

Crime and violence

Of nonnatural death causes in foreign travelers, 21% can be attributed to crime and violence.[1] Clinicians should encourage travelers to familiarize themselves with crime trends in the areas they are traveling to. Information can be accessed from the Overseas Security Advisory Council website (www.osac.gov). Travelers can also familiarize themselves with security updates by accessing the Department of State's Bureau of Consult Affairs recommendations for travel safety at http://travel.state.gov. Special precaution should be taken to protect against pickpocketing and individuals should attempt to keep money worn under clothing secured to the neck or waist. Travelers should limit traveling alone or at night time, keep all valuables secure, keep all doors and windows locked, use recommended safe modes of transportation, and avoid resistance if confronted in a robbery. The nearest US embassy should be contacted if concerns related to crime, violence, accidents, medical concerns, or specific travel questions arise.

Counterfeit, adulterated, or expired medications

Travelers should be educated about the risks of procuring medications while traveling including but not limited to medication side effects secondary to use of inappropriately compounded medications, counterfeit medications, and use of uncommon medication additives.[1] Clinicians should recommend obtaining all medications before travel to ensure that individuals are using authentic medications with known side effects and appropriate dosing.

Infections While Abroad

Immunizations

Maintenance of an accurate immunization history is necessary to provide adequate protection for the traveler. Immunization records should be obtained and reviewed and, if unreliable, titers for measles, mumps, rubella, and hepatitis A should be obtained. Sufficient time should be taken before travel to ensure travel-specific vaccines can be administered and appropriate immunity achieved (**Table 2**). The risks and benefits of immunizations should be discussed. In addition, vaccines with waning immunity should be addressed as well, especially in the case of immunocompromised travelers. Assessing return travel to similar areas with the next 1 to 2 years from the initial trip will help clinicians to assess the need for specific immunizations. Travelers should be given an updated immunization record to travel with. Country-specific recommendations for vaccines can be accessed by clinicians at the Centers for Disease Control and Prevention (CDC) travel website (https://wwwnc.cdc.gov/travel).

Malaria

Several important diseases are transmitted by mosquitos, of which malaria is among the most important. Most of the 1700 cases of malaria diagnosed in the United States annually are among returned travelers.[1] **Box 2** outlines strategies for malaria prevention.

From dawn to dusk, mosquitoes that transmit Dengue, Yellow Fever, Zika, and Chikungunya are active and bite whereas, from dusk to dawn, mosquitoes that carry malaria, West Nile, and Japanese encephalitis are active. Providers should review the CDC's Malaria Maps, and Malaria Information by Country Table and take note of the special considerations mentioned on the drug selection guide: https://www.cdc.gov/malaria/travelers/drugs.html.

Antimalarials should always be purchased before travel, because in some countries drugs that are sold may be counterfeit.[1] Clinicians should also warn travelers that if symptoms of malaria occur, including flulike illness while traveling or after returning home, immediate medical attention should be sought. Antimalarials alone do not prevent transmission and should be used in conjunction with preventive measures, including repellants for skin and clothing in addition to appropriate clothing and mosquito netting.[1,6]

Traveler's diarrhea

Traveler's diarrhea often occurs suddenly with loose, frequent stools in about 30% to 70% of travelers.[7] Poor food handling practices are thought to put travelers at highest risk for traveler's diarrhea. Preventative measures include specific food and beverage selection, frequent handwashing, frequent use of alcohol-based hand sanitizers with greater than 60% alcohol content, and consideration of vaccination against typhoid and hepatitis A.[8] **Table 3** contains recommendations for traveler's diarrhea treatment based on severity.

Respiratory illness

Respiratory illness occurs in 20% of returning travels, with upper respiratory infections being the most common respiratory illness. Risks include exposures in hotels, cruise ships, aircrafts and tour group. Individuals with comorbidities including asthma and chronic obstructive pulmonary disease are at higher risk for respiratory illnesses.[1] Prevention tips include minimizing contact with individuals with cough or congestive symptoms, frequent handwashing, and vaccination before travel. Viral etiologies such as rhinovirus, are more common causal

Table 2
Travel vaccines, including routine vaccines of high priority in travelers

Vaccine	Indication	Administration
Hepatitis A	All travelers ≥1 y of age	2 doses
Hepatitis B	All travelers	• 3 doses • Administer ≥6 mo before travel
Influenza	All travelers ≥6 mo of age	• 1 dose • Booster: annual
Tetanus, diphtheria, pertussis (Td, Tdap)	All travelers	• Td every 5 y for adult travelers • Tdap: Adolescents age 11–18 y, or age ≥19 if no Tdap administered prior • Pregnancy between 27 and 36 wk gestation
Cholera	• Age 18–64 • Individuals at high risk (health care workers)	• 1 dose • Booster: undetermined
Japanese encephalitis	• Travelers to high-risk areas (Asia, Western Pacific) • >1 mo travel • Travel to rural areas	• 2 doses on days 0 and 28 • Booster: 1 y
Meningococcal meningitis	• Travelers to specific areas of Africa associated with meningitis • Travelers to crowded spaces (dormitories)	• Age 2–55, 1 dose MenACWY • Age ≥56 who have never received the vaccine, 1 dose MPSV4 • Booster: 5 y after last dose if individual received dose at age ≥7
Polio	• Travelers to countries with increased prevalence of polio (eg, Pakistan, Afghanistan, Nigeria)	• 4 dose childhood series (2, 4, 6–18 mo, and 4–6 y of age) Plus • Single dose inactivated virus for all adults ○ Booster: not indicated ○ Administer 4 wk to 12 mo before travel
Rabies	• Travelers to remote, rural areas • Long-term travelers • Wildlife workers, spelunkers	• 3 doses on days 0, 7, 21 or 28 • Booster: If at high risk, check serology every 2 y, and administer booster if low antibodies • If low risk: No booster indicated
Typhoid fever	• All travelers to low-income nations, rural travel, or high-risk areas • Duration of travel >1 mo	• Oral: 1 tab taken every other day for 7 d for 5-y protection • IM: 1 dose for 2 y of protection • Booster: repeat oral or IM at appropriate interval
Yellow fever	• Travelers to tropical Africa and South America • Not indicated for travelers <9 mo of age	• Single dose • Contraindicated in immunosuppressed individuals • Increased risk of adverse events for first time recipients age >60 y

Abbreviations: IM, intramuscularly; MPSV4, meningococcal polysaccharide vaccine.
Data from Refs.[1–5]

agents, although coronaviruses (Middle East respiratory syndrome in the Arabian Peninsula) and avian influenza (Asia) should also be included in a clinician's differential.[1] Viral causes can also put individuals at risk for superimposed bacterial infections.

Box 2
Strategies to prevent malaria

Long-sleeved pants, shirts, and socks

Permethrin-treated clothing

Permethrin-treated bed nets

Mosquito repellants ($\geq$20% DEET)

Chemoprophylaxis

Data from Alpern JD, Dunlop SJ, Dolan BJ, et al. Personal protection measures against mosquitoes, ticks, and other arthropods. Med Clin North Am 2016;100(2):303–16.

Bloodborne illness

Travelers should be cautioned against obtaining tattoos and piercings in low-income areas of the world, because the risk of human immunodeficiency virus and hepatitis C transmission secondary to use of unclean needles is high in these areas.[1]

Exposure to human immunodeficiency virus

Travelers should be cautioned about the risk of human immunodeficiency virus specifically associated with certain practices, including needle sharing, risky sexual behaviors, or exposure in a health care setting. In the case of health care workers or individuals who plan to be involved with high-risk behaviors, the physician should discuss having postexposure prophylaxis available to them in case of exposure. Preexposure prophylaxis can reduce the risk of human immunodeficiency virus infection by up to 70%.[1] Immediate attention by a physician should be sought out if concern for exposure arises to ensure appropriate counseling and the possible need for postexposure prophylaxis.

Sexual health

Travelers should be cautioned against high-risk sexual activities that may lead to the transmission of sexually transmitted infections, unwanted pregnancy, or bloodborne infections. Consistent contraceptive methods should be used in a traveler who does

Table 3
Treatment of traveler's diarrhea based on severity

Mild: tolerable diarrhea, does not interfere for activity, often resolves within 2–5 d	Moderate: distressing diarrhea, interferes with activity	Severe: incapacitating diarrhea, prevent activity
Loperamide or bismuth subsalicylate; hydration	Hydration Antibiotics may be used including 1. Fluoroquinolones 2. Azithromycin 3. Rifaximin Loperamide can be used in conjunction with antibiotics or as a monotherapy.	Emergency care Antibiotics should be used including 1. Azithromycin (preferred) 2. Fluoroquinolones or rifaximin (can be used for nondysenteric, severe traveler's diarrhea).

Data from de Saussure PPH. Management of the returning traveler with diarrhea. Therap Adv Gastroenterol 2009;2(6):367–75.

decide to be sexually active. Health care resources overseas should be provided for travelers, including reputable clinics to seek out if concerns for sexually transmitted infections and/or pregnancy arise.

Venous Thrombosis and Embolism

Travelers at increased risk for development of deep venous thrombosis who are traveling long distances should be advised to walk as often as possible, use appropriately fitted compression stockings that provide 15 to 30 mm Hg at the ankle, hydration, and to perform calf exercises as often as possible. The use of aspirin for deep venous thrombosis prevention is not recommended.[1]

Jet lag

When traveling between time zones, travelers can often develop a mismatch between their natural 24-hour circadian rhythm and the time of day. When traveling through more than 3 time zones, sleep-related difficulty, mood changes, mental clarity, and gastrointestinal disturbance can occur with jet lag. During the pretravel assessment, the clinician can discuss this in detail with the traveler and set expectations. Changes to diet and physical activity, sunlight exposure, the use of melatonin and melatonin-receptor analogs, consideration of hypnotic medications with discussion of risks and benefits, and a combination of these therapies can be discussed with the traveler before initiation of travel. Avoidance of alcohol as a sleep aid should be discussed with travelers as well as encouraging hydration during the trip.

SPECIAL POPULATIONS

Immunocompromised Travelers

According to the 2018 CDC Yellow Book, immunocompromised travelers make up 1% to 2% of travelers seen in US travel clinics.[1] The immunocompromised status may be due to a medical condition, medication, or treatment. Common examples are noted in **Box 3**.

Special points to remember for immunocompromised travelers:

- Response to vaccines may be limited.
- Live vaccines are contraindicated in severely immunosuppressed individuals.

Box 3
Examples of immunocompromised travelers

Chronic oral steroids greater than or equal to 20 mg per day of prednisone or equivalent

Posttransplant on medication

Renal failure on dialysis

Current or recent (<3 months) chemotherapy

Asplenia

Chronic liver disease

Human immunodeficiency virus infection with a CD4 count of less than 200

Autoimmune diagnosis on biologics

Data from Centers for Disease Control and Prevention. CDC yellow book 2018: health information for international travel. New York: Oxford University Press; 2017.

- Increased risk of foodborne and waterborne infections (*Salmonella*, *Shigella*, *Campylobacter*, *Giardia*, *Listeria*, and *Cryptosporidium*).
- Avoid swallowing water during water-based activities.
- Avoid eating raw seafood.

Traveling while pregnant

Key points for pregnant travelers[1]:

- Obstetric emergencies are sudden and can be life threatening. Having an emergency plan and access to appropriate obstetric care is recommended.
- Before booking, check with the airline or cruise ship regarding any limitations on travel. Some limit travel based on gestational age.
- During air travel the cabin is pressurized to 6000 to 8000 feet. This will not affect a fetus in a normal pregnancy, but could cause fetal problems in women with cardiovascular conditions, sickle cell disease, or severe anemia (hemoglobin <8 g/dL).
- During air travel, frequent stretching, walking, and isometric exercises are recommended to decrease risk of deep venous thrombosis, which is increased in pregnancy.
- Treatment of choice for traveler's diarrhea is hydration and, if indicated, azithromycin.
- Owing to the risk of birth defects, the CDC recommends that pregnant women do not travel to areas where Zika is present. If travel cannot be avoided, avoidance of mosquito bites is extremely important. More information can be found at the CDC Zika website (http://www.cdc.gov/zika/pregnancy/index.html).
- Most live virus vaccines are contraindicated during pregnancy except for yellow fever, for which pregnancy is considered a precaution by the Advisory Committee on Immunization Practices.
- Malaria is more serious in pregnant than in nonpregnant women and puts both the mother and the fetus at risk. Malaria chemoprophylaxis is highly encouraged. Chloroquine and mefloquine (depending on the region) are the drugs of choice. Doxycycline and primaquine are contraindicated due to possible effects on the fetus, whereas atovaquone-proguanil lacks available safety data.

Traveling with Children

According to the CDC, an estimated 1.9 million American children travel internationally each year.[1] Typically, children are exposed to the same risks as adults, but the consequences can be more severe and children are less likely to receive travel advice than adults.

The most common health problems among child travelers were[1]:

- Diarrheal illnesses,
- Dermatologic diagnosis (animal/insect bites, cutaneous larva migrans, sunburn),
- Febrile illnesses (malaria), and
- Respiratory disorders.

Key points when traveling with children[1]:

- Diarrheal diseases are more common and can be more likely to cause dehydration. Treatment should focus on oral rehydration solution and if indicated antibiotics for traveler's diarrhea. Children should be given a nonfluoroquinolone such as azithromycin, which can be given as a single daily dose (10 mg/kg) for 3 days.

- Car crashes and drowning are the leading 2 causes of death in children while traveling. Car seats are often not available so parents should bring their own. Life vests should always be used around water.
- Avoidance of mosquito and other bug bites is critical, especially in malaria endemic areas. Repellents with DEET should not be used on infants less than 2 months and after 2 months, only repellents with 30% or less DEET should be used.
- Malaria prophylaxis is also recommended for children in malaria endemic areas. Dosing will need to be adjusted based on weight. Doxycycline should not be given to children less than 8 years old because of the risk of teeth staining, and atovaquone-proguanil should not be used in children weighing less than 5 kg.
- Rabies is more common in children owing to less fear in approaching animals. If there is exposure to any animal bite, seek medical care immediately. Consider rabies vaccine if planning to spend more than 3 months in endemic area.

Visiting Friends and Relatives

A traveler who is returning home to visit friends or relatives is considered a visiting friends and relatives traveler. Today, visiting friends and relatives travelers make up more than one-half of all international travelers.[1] They are least likely to seek pretravel advice and more likely to develop problems while traveling because they typically stay longer at a destination, eat local food in people's homes, and often do not take the same precautions as other travelers.

Key points for visiting friends and relatives travelers[1]:

- Malaria risk is 8 to 10 times higher than for a non-visiting friends and relatives traveler. Malaria immunity weans after living outside of a malaria endemic region, so when returning to the endemic region, malaria prophylaxis and mosquito bite avoidance is recommended. Malaria prevention medication should be started several weeks before international travel.
- Foodborne illnesses are more common and any immunity to local bacteria can also wean with time after living outside the community. Avoidance of food at room temperature, raw fruits and vegetables, tap water, and ice from tap water is recommended.
- These travelers are also at increased risk of tuberculosis and sexually transmitted diseases.

POSTTRAVEL ASSESSMENT

General Approach

Worldwide, 8% of travelers develop illnesses severe enough to seek a health care provider.[1] The majority of travelers present to primary care for posttravel illnesses. Data gathered from a directed history can elucidate the cause of a traveler's symptoms. Knowledge of the travel itinerary and incubation periods is essential to narrowing down a differential diagnosis based on geography and timing after travel.

Common Syndromes

According to a large-scale study by GeoSentinal, a global surveillance network, the most common syndromes in returned travelers are gastrointestinal (34.0%), febrile (23.3%), and dermatologic (19.5%).[9]

Table 4
Top infectious causes of persistent traveler's diarrhea listed in decreasing order of frequency in each column

Protozoa	Bacteria
1. *Giardia lamblia* (most common overall)	1. *Clostridium difficile*
2. *Entamoeba histolytica*	2. *Campylobacter jejuni*
3. *Cryptosporidium parvum*	3. *Salmonella* spp.
4. *Cyclospora cayatanensis*	4. *Shigella* spp.

Data from de Saussure PPH. Management of the returning traveler with diarrhea. Therap Adv Gastroenterol 2009;2(6):367–75.

Gastrointestinal Illness

Many cases of traveler's diarrhea can be treated empirically, and 80% to 90% of cases are bacterial. See **Table 4** for top infectious causes of persistent traveler's diarrhea. Azithromycin should be preferentially used in travelers returning from South and Southeast Asia owing to the increasing resistance to fluoroquinolones.[7] Severe symptoms, including fever, tenesmus, and gross blood, should prompt further testing, including stool culture. If stool is tested for ova and parasites, 3 or more stool specimens should be collected to increase sensitivity.[7] Some organisms, such as *Cryptosporidium* and *Cyclospora*, require specific testing. Testing for *Clostridium difficile* should be performed if the traveler recently used antibiotics or malaria chemoprophylaxis. A minority of travelers have persistent diarrhea lasting more than 2 weeks, which can be from (1) persistent infection or an untreated coinfection, (2) postinfectious processes like postinfectious irritable bowel syndrome, which can be diagnosed using the Rome criteria, or (3) unmasking of a previously undiagnosed gastrointestinal disease.[7]

Febrile Illness

Fever in a returned traveler needs to be evaluated immediately owing to the potential for a rapidly progressing, life-threatening illness like malaria. Those who arrive from areas where malaria is endemic should be evaluated with thick and thin blood films and malarial antigen tests, if available. Blood smears should be repeated if suspicion is high and initial smears are negative. Other important causes to consider include dengue fever, enteric fever (typhoid, paratyphoid), and rickettsial diseases (eg, African tick bite fever), among others. It is also important to keep in mind other common causes of fever including influenza, which occurs year round in tropical climates. See **Table 5** for the top febrile illnesses to consider in returned travelers based on location. Those with fever accompanied by alarming symptoms should be thoroughly

Table 5
Top febrile illnesses to consider in returned travelers based on location

Febrile Illness	Location
Malaria (21%)	Sub-Saharan Africa, Oceania (especially Papua New Guinea)
Dengue fever (6%)	Southeast Asia, Central and South America, Caribbean
Enteric fever (2%)	South Central Asia (ie, Indian subcontinent)
Rickettsioses (2%)	Southern Africa (especially African tick bite fever in South Africa)

Data from Leder K, Torresi J, Libman MD, et al. GeoSentinel surveillance of illness in returned travelers, 2007–2011. Ann Intern Med 2013;158(6):456–68.

Box 4
Top 10 tropical[a] dermatologic conditions to consider in returned travelers

1. Cutaneous larva migrans
2. Arthropod bite
3. Myiasis (bot fly, tumbu fly)
4. Injuries including animal bites
5. Scabies
6. Cutaneous leishmaniasis
7. Tungiasis
8. Swimmer's itch
9. Rickettsial infection
10. Dengue fever

[a] Many cosmopolitan causes (eg, cellulitis) excluded from this list.

Data from Lederman ER, Weld LH, Elyazar IR, et al. Dermatologic conditions of the ill returned traveler: an analysis from the GeoSentinel Surveillance Network. Int J Infect Dis 2008;12(6):593–602; and O'Brien BM. A practical approach to common skin problems in returning travellers. Travel Med Infect Dis 2009;7(3):125–46.

evaluated as soon as possible, which may be best conducted in the emergency department. In 25% to 40% of patients with fever, no specific cause was identified.[9,10]

Dermatologic Conditions

Rashes are common in returned travelers. One of the most common skin findings is the classic pruritic migratory serpiginous rash of cutaneous larva migrans.[11] Exposure occurs when skin (eg, bare feet) comes in contact with contaminated sand or soil. Animal bites and scratches, most commonly received from dogs and monkeys, are also common in returned travelers and may require rabies postexposure prophylaxis in up to 12% of cases.[9] See **Box 4** for the top tropical dermatologic conditions to consider in returned travelers.

Screening Asymptomatic Returned Travelers

Currently, there are no CDC guidelines for asymptomatic returned travelers.

Table 6
Common medications for altitude illness

Drug	Indication	Dose
Acetazolamide	AMS, HACE prevention	125 mg PO BID starting 12 h prior
	AMS treatment	250 mg PO BID
Dexamethasone	AMS, HACE prevention	4 mg PO every 12 h
	AMS, HACE treatment	8 mg PO once, then 4 mg PO every 6 h
Nifedipine	HAPE prevention/treatment	30 mg SR PO every 12 h

Abbreviations: AMS, acute mountain sickness; BID, twice per day; HACE, high altitude cerebral edema; HAPE, high altitude pulmonary edema; PO, by mouth.

Data from Centers for Disease Control and Prevention. CDC yellow book 2018: health information for international travel. New York: Oxford University Press; 2017.

Box 5
Recommendations to prevent motion sickness

Air	Sit at window seat over wing and look out window
Motor vehicle	Sit in front seat, semireclining position, avoid head motion, view horizon
Sea	Chose cabin in middle of ship near the waterline

Data from Centers for Disease Control and Prevention. CDC yellow book 2018: health information for international travel. New York: Oxford University Press; 2017.

SPECIAL CIRCUMSTANCES SECTION

Altitude Illness

Altitude illness is most common at altitudes of 8200 feet (2500 m) or more, although it can occur at lower elevations.[1] The main issue in altitude sickness is hypoxemia, which is exacerbated during sleep. Respiratory depressants such as alcohol and sleep medications should be avoided; acetazolamide and stimulants may speed acclimatization. Moderate-to-vigorous physical activity can exacerbate hypoxemia and should be avoided for the first 48 hours. Physical conditioning does not predict acclimatization. Contraindications to traveling to altitude include severe heart or lung disease, sickle cell anemia, high-risk pregnancy, and cerebral pathology.

There are 3 altitude syndromes: acute mountain sickness, high altitude cerebral edema, and high altitude pulmonary edema. Treatment involves immediate descent, medications (**Table 6**), oxygen supplementation, and pressurization bags if rapid descent is not feasible.

SCUBA Diving

SCUBA-related illnesses can be divided into 2 categories: barotrauma and decompression illness. The primary risk factors are dive depth, bottom time, and speed of ascent.[1] Decompression illness can occur even when all precautions are taken. The Divers Alert Network is a resource that can be accessed by both divers and health care providers at http://www.diversalertnetwork.org/ or at their 24-hour emergency hotline (919-684-9111).

Motion Sickness

Motion sickness is not a true pathology, but a normal response to the external stimulation that is created by the vestibular system. The most common forms are sea sickness, motor vehicle sickness, and air sickness. It has been noted to be more common in women and less common in frequent travelers either owing to habituation or self-selection. See **Box 5** and **Table 7** for recommendations for motion sickness prevention and management.

Table 7
Common preventive medications for motion sickness

Drug	Dose	Side Effects
Dimenhydrinate (Dramamine)	50 mg PO every 4–6 h	Sedation
Meclizine (Antivert)	25–50mg 1 hour before travel, every 24 h	Mild sedation
Scopolamine patch (Transderm Scop)	1 patch applied every 72 h	Dry mouth, blurry vision

Abbreviation: PO, by mouth.

Data from Centers for Disease Control and Prevention. CDC yellow book 2018: health information for international travel. New York: Oxford University Press; 2017.

Box 6
Mass gathering examples

Measles exposure at amusement parks in the United States.

Meningitis (meningococcal vaccine is required for the Hajj) and respiratory infections (Coronavirus) among Hajj pilgrims.

Concern for Zika at Rio, Brazil Olympics.

Exposure to flu during sports events, concerts, conventions.

Mass Gatherings

Defined as at least 1000, but can be more than 25,000, people gathered at a specific location for a specific purpose.[1] Often these gatherings can strain the local resources and increase the risk of disease transmission among the attendees. Common challenges among attendees are hypothermia, heat exhaustion, dehydration, sunburn, but worsening of underlying chronic diseases (eg, heart failure, diabetes) also occurs. And at times there can be other dangers such as unsafe transportation, stampedes, collapse of structures, fire, terrorism and other forms of violence. See **Box 6** for examples of mass gatherings.

REFERENCES

1. Centers for Disease Control and Prevention. CDC yellow book 2018: health information for international travel. New York: Oxford University Press; 2017.
2. Centers for Disease Control and Prevention. Vaccines & immunizations. 2017. Available at: https://www.cdc.gov/vaccines/terms/usvaccines.html. Accessed February 1, 2018.
3. Amicizia D, Domnich A, Panatto D, et al. Epidemiology of tick-borne encephalitis (TBE) in Europe and its prevention by available vaccines. Hum Vaccin Immunother 2013;9(5):1163–71.
4. Centers for Disease Control and Prevention (CDC). Tick-borne encephalitis among US travelers to Europe and Asia—2000-2009. MMWR Morb Mortal Wkly Rep 2010;59(11):335–8.
5. Lo Re V 3rd, Gluckman SJ. Travel immunizations. Am Fam Physician 2004;70(1): 89–99.
6. Alpern JD, Dunlop SJ, Dolan BJ, et al. Personal protection measures against mosquitoes, ticks, and other arthropods. Med Clin North Am 2016;100(2):303–16.
7. de Saussure PP. Management of the returning traveler with diarrhea. Therap Adv Gastroenterol 2009;2(6):367–75.
8. Innis BL, Snitbhan R, Kunasol P, et al. Protection against hepatitis A by an inactivated vaccine. JAMA 1994;271(17):1328–34.
9. Leder K, Torresi J, Libman MD, et al. GeoSentinel surveillance of illness in returned travelers, 2007–2011. Ann Intern Med 2013;158(6):456–68.
10. Thwaites GE, Day NP. Approach to fever in the returning traveler. N Engl J Med 2017;376(6):548–60.
11. Lederman ER, Weld LH, Elyazar IR, et al. Dermatologic conditions of the ill returned traveler: an analysis from the GeoSentinel Surveillance Network. Int J Infect Dis 2008;12(6):593–602.

Approach to Aquatic Skin Infections

Brintha Vasagar, MD, MPH[a,*], Vasudha Jain, MD[b], Anthony Germinario, MD[b], Heber J. Watson, DO[b], Michael Ouzts, DO[b], Richard John Presutti, DO[c], Salvador Alvarez, MD[d]

KEYWORDS

- Aquatic infection • Skin infection • *Vibrio* • *Aeromonas* • *Edwardsiella* • *Erysipelothrix* • *Mycobacterium*

KEY POINTS

- Although *Staphylococcus* and *Streptococcus* are the most common causative agents of skin infection, consider other species in aquatic infections.
- Skin and soft tissue infections from an aquatic source can rapidly progress to necrotizing fasciitis.
- Mortality is decreased by starting empiric antibiotics without waiting for culture results and considering early surgical evaluation if indicated.

INTRODUCTION

Aquatic-based infections can present a treatment challenge for primary care physicians because of the likely polymicrobial nature of the infection and the possibility of uncommon pathogenic organisms.[1–3] Skin and soft tissue infections (SSTIs) acquired in aquatic environment are usually the result of wound exposure to the multitude of organisms present. Microbiologic cultures in this setting most commonly yield polymicrobial gram-negative organisms.[1] All aquatic wounds should receive routine wound care, including irrigation, removal of foreign bodies, tetanus prophylaxis, and wound culture if possible. Although *Staphylococcus* and *Streptococcus* species that colonize the skin are the most common etiologic agents associated with salt water and freshwater infections, other significant pathogens can include *Vibrio*, *Aeromonas*, *Edwardsiella*, *Erysipelothrix*, and *Mycobacterium* as seen in **Table 1**.[4,5] Early detection and

Disclosure: The authors have nothing to disclose.

[a] Department of Family Medicine, Medical University of South Carolina, 5 Charleston Center, Charleston, SC 29425, USA; [b] Department of Family Medicine, Tidelands Health MUSC Family Medicine Residency Program, 4320 Holmestown Road, Myrtle Beach, SC 29578, USA; [c] Department of Family Medicine, Mayo School of Medicine, 4500 San Pablo Road, Jacksonville, FL 32224, USA; [d] Department of Internal Medicine, Mayo School of Medicine, 4500 San Pablo Road, Jacksonville, FL 32224, USA

* Corresponding author. 4320 Holmestown Road, Myrtle Beach, SC 29588.
E-mail address: vasagar@musc.edu

Prim Care Clin Office Pract 45 (2018) 555–566
https://doi.org/10.1016/j.pop.2018.05.010
0095-4543/18/

Table 1
Most common uniquely marine organisms

Bacteria	Type	Location	Characteristic Presentation
Vibrio spp (*Vulnificus*, *Parahaemolyticus*, *Alginolyticus*, and *Damsela*)	Facultative anaerobic gram-negative rod	Oceans, coastal waterways, but may survive in freshwater	"Salt loving"; virulent infection associated with severe cellulitis, osteomyelitis, necrotizing fasciitis, and septicemia.
Aeromonas hydrophila	Facultative gram-negative rod	Freshwater and aquariums	Onset similar to standard cellulitis but within 24 h bullae with purulent discharge may develop. If improperly treated, may develop gas within the soft tissue, necrotizing fasciitis, or osteomyelitis. May be coinfected with *Pseudomonas* spp.
Edwardsiella tarda	Facultative, anaerobic, gram-negative rod	Fresh and brackish water	Associated with wounds caused by fish or suffered in infected waters; causes abscess formation and invasive infections in the immunocompromised.
Erysipelothrix rhusiopathiae	Gram-positive bacillus	Saltwater and fish handling	"Fish-handler's disease"; causes erysipeloid (ring-shaped lesion with a sharply demarcated purplish/red border, associated with intense pain); may mimic septic arthritis or result in disseminated endocarditis.
Mycobacterium marinum	Atypical nontuberculous mycobacterium	Marine and freshwater	"Swimming pool granulomas"; may take weeks or months to manifest clinically; begins with a focal area or erythema followed by an ulceration and may progress to cellulitis, myelitis, tenosynovitis, septic arthritis, osteomyelitis, or a disseminated infection; most likely requires surgical debridement.

Data from Crosby SN, Snoddy MC, Atkinson CT, et al. Upper extremity myonecrosis caused by *Edwardsiella tarda* resulting in transhumeral amputation: case report. J Hand Surg Am 2013;38(1):129–32; and Noonburg GE. Management of extremity trauma and related infections occurring in the aquatic environment. J Am Acad Orthop Surg 2005;13(4):243–53.

appropriate management of aquatic infections can significantly decrease morbidity and mortality. This article reviews the pathophysiology, presentation, and management for the most common water-borne pathogens causing SSTI.

VIBRIO SPECIES

Vibrio spp are halophilic, gram-negative bacilli found worldwide in salt and brackish water.[6,7] *Vibrio* thrives at water temperatures of 9°C to 31°C, and has typically been associated with tropical and subtropical waters but, with global warming leading to increased water temperatures, outbreaks have been seen as far north as Denmark.[8] Although more than 100 species of Vibrionaceae exist, only 12 have been known to be pathogenic in humans and most are associated with gastroenteritis following ingestion of contaminated shellfish.[7,9,10] SSTIs are usually seen when open wounds or broken skin are exposed to contaminated water, although the species may survive on the skin as reported in a case of infection resulting from acupuncture needle insertion after exposure to brackish water.[11] Of the Vibrio spp, *Vibrio vulnificus* and *Vibrio parahaemolyticus* are the most commonly isolated in SSTIs.

V vulnificus is the best studied of the *Vibrio* spp causing SSTI, likely because of the associated risk of high mortality.[12] Of the three *V vulificus* biotypes associated with SSTI, biotype 1 is the most common and can cause sepsis with a high mortality rate of up to 50%; biotype 2 is mostly seen in eels but can on rare occasion cause human wound infection; and biotype 3 can cause severe infection, but mortality is much improved at only 8%.[7] There are about 100 nonfoodborne *V vulnificus* infections annually in the United States, with patients significantly more likely to be male, older, and white, than those who acquired foodborne illness.[13] At highest risk for sepsis from nonfoodborne exposure are patients with liver disease (adjusted odds ratio, 4.1), hematologic disease (adjusted odds ratio, 3.2), malignancy (adjusted odds ratio, 3.2), immunodeficiency, end-stage renal disease, or iron storage diseases.[7,13,14]

V vulnificus possesses several toxins that aid in its virulence, including hemolysin, which stimulates the release of iron from hemoglobin and has cytotoxic effects. The organism thrives with elevated iron levels, which may explain why liver disease and iron storage diseases are risk factors for infection.[7] VvpE, an extracellular metalloprotease, may be specifically relevant to SSTI, because it leads to edema and bullous lesions that are seen in severe infection. Although the roles of these toxins in the cytotoxicity of *V vulnificus* remains unclear, studies of mutant strains show that RtxA1, which stimulates necrotic cell death and apoptosis, may be the critical toxin in disease severity.[7] Interestingly, estrogens may provide some protective benefits because males are much more likely to experience illness.

SSTIs caused by *V vulnificus* have three clinical stages: initially inflammatory, followed by bullous, and finally gangrenous.[15] The most common site infection can vary geographically, with the right upper limb most common in Taiwan versus the lower limbs most common in Japan.[16] Symptoms usually present within 7 to 12 days of exposure and can rapidly progress to more serious infection, including bullae and cellulitis with pain and swelling. More serious infections are seen as necrotizing fasciitis or gangrene, with increased mortality and risk of sepsis.[7] The necrotizing fasciitis caused by *Vibrio* spp (type III) progresses rapidly, which makes the urgent identification and treatment of the infection paramount.[17]

Although less commonly seen, other strains of *Vibrio* also cause SSTI. *V parahaemolyticus* typically causes a milder infection, although it can also progress to necrotizing fasciitis. Typically, symptoms develop within 1 day of exposure as pain, swelling, and ecchymosis.[17] *Vibrio cholera non-O1, non-0139* infections typically present as cellulitis, and may include bullae or hemorrhagic lesions, with the possibility of progression to necrotizing fasciitis. SSTI with *V cholera non-O1, non-0139* is more commonly seen in males and people with underlying liver disease, hematologic disease, or diabetes.[9] Although much less common with only 20 cases published worldwide, *Vibrio demselae* may be more severe than other *Vibrio* spp because it typically presents with necrotizing fasciitis. It is distinguished microbiologically by its impressive B-hemolysis.[10] Finally, *Vibrio alginolyticus* usually causes a benign SSTI requiring only local treatment, although it can progress to ulcer or abscess, cellulitis, or, rarely, necrotizing fasciitis.[8]

Diagnosis of Vibrio

Diagnosis is based on clinical history and confirmed with culture. Culture results for *Vibrio* spp can take 1 to 3 days and antibiotics should not be delayed.

Treatment of Vibrio

The Centers for Disease Control and Prevention has recommended ceftazidime, 1 to 2 g intravenously (IV)/intramuscularly every 8 hours, plus doxycycline, 100 mg IV/by mouth twice a day for 7 to 14 days, as initial empiric treatment of suspected *Vibrio* infection based on history and presentation, although cefotaxime plus minocycline or tetracycline may also be used.[6,7,15] These infections are not commonly seen in children, but in such cases trimethoprim-sulfamethoxazole (TMP-SMX) and an aminoglycoside may be used.[6,7] In more severe SSTI, such as necrotizing fasciitis, early debridement and fasciotomy are critical in improving mortality.[7,15] Prognosis improves with early surgical evaluation, and worsens with unclear history, older age, more extensive skin lesions, progression to sepsis, leukocytes less than 10,000 cells/mm^3, platelets less than 100,000/mm^3, serum creatinine greater than 1.3 mg/dL, and serum albumin less than 2.5 mg/dL.[12,15,16]

Prevention

Those with significant risk factors, such as liver disease, should avoid exposure to bodies of warm salt water when they have open wounds or broken skin.

AEROMONAS HYDROPHILA

The *Aeromonas* spp are gram-negative bacilli that are divided into two groups: the first group contains motile, mesophilic species that can cause disease in humans; and the second group contains nonmotile, psychrophilic species causing disease in only fish. The *Aeromonas* spp are found in freshwater marine systems and can tolerate polluted environments. They can grow to large numbers in warmer temperatures and are also found in surface water, drinking water, and waste water.[18] A virulent subtype of *Aeromonas hydrophilia* was isolated from a wound infection and showed genes for toxin production, toxin secretion, and bacterial motility. The *Aeromonas* spp are oxidase positive, ferment glucose, and grow in temperatures ranging from 0°C to 42°C. A potent virulence factor of *A hydrophila* is cytotoxic enterotoxin and it has shown to contribute in the pathogenesis of deep wound infections.[19,20] The first published outbreak of *A hydrophila* was reported in 2004 in mud football players in Western Australia who were predisposed to infection from *A hydrophila* because of cuts and skin abrasions.[18] In addition to freshwater, there have been multiple cases of *A hydrophila* SSTI and sepsis 2 to 11 days after leech therapy. Results showed aquariums filled with tap water further aided in the colonization of leeches with *A hydrophila* and recommendations to use noncarbonated bottled water and regular cleaning of the aquarium was made to lower the risk of infections following leech therapy.[21]

A hydrophila infections most commonly present as mild SSTIs of body parts immersed in contaminated freshwater during warmer months. Some forms of *A hydrophila* can present as self-limited mild diarrhea with no evidence of SSTIs.[18,20] The most typical presentation is cellulitis and affects men three times more than women. A prospective study done in France showed that 74% of the SSTIs related to *A hydrophila* presented as purulent lesions and 26% of them as abscesses.[6] Within 24 hours of exposure, the wound starts to show erythema, edema, and purulent drainage. If such wounds are left untreated or improperly treated they can progress to fever, chills, and invasive infections including necrotizing fasciitis, myositis, and osteomyelitis, especially in immunocompromised patients.[6] Infections related to *A hydrophila* tend to mimic streptococcal soft tissue infections, which can delay treatment with the appropriate antibiotic therapies.[22]

Diagnosis

Diagnosis is made based on Gram stain and culture of the wound. *A hydrophila* are seen as oxidase positive gram-negative rods. On Gram stain, *Aeromonas* spp can often be confused with other oxidase-positive organisms, such as *Vibrio*, but are further distinguished by resistance to O/129. Final diagnosis is made from wound culture, but identification may require clinical suspicion because analysis for *Aeromonas* is not part of standard protocol.[18]

Treatment

Treatment of *A hydrophila* that only presents with mild diarrhea is usually self-limited and does not typically require any antibiotic therapy.[18,20] Treatment of SSTI related to *A hydrophila* includes wound drainage and debridement in conjunction with TMP-SMX, carbapenems, tetracyclines, chloramphenicol, aminoglycosides, fluoroquinolones, or third-generation cephalosporins. *Aeromonas* spp are resistant to penicillins and first-generation cephalosporins, and strains associated with leech therapy have been found to be fluoroquinolone-resistant.[23–25] Most *Aeromonas* spp infections are treatable with monotherapy and studies with combination therapy do not show better outcomes.[23] Antibiotic selection can also be further broken down by region; for example, infection with *A hydrophila* after traveling to Taiwan or Spain should not be treated with TMP-SMX because the prevalence of TMP-SMX-resistant strains is high. Antibiotic therapy should be continued for 7 to 10 days for SSTIs.[18] According to guidelines from Infectious Diseases Society of America, patients with necrotizing infections of the skin, muscle, and fascia should be treated with doxycycline 100 mg IV every 12 hours, plus ciprofloxacin, 500 mg IV every 12 hours, or ceftriaxone, 1 to 2 g IV every 24 hours.[23]

EDWARDSIELLA TARDA

Edwardsiella tarda is a gram-negative, facultative anaerobic, motile bacillus that is a member of the Enterobacteriacae family. It is found in a variety of aquatic fish and reptile species worldwide, and has been associated with gastrointestinal and SSTI in humans.[26] Less commonly, bacteremia and other extraintestinal infections have occurred with a high mortality rate in *E tarda* bacteremia.[27,28] Reported cases are highest in Japan, the United States, and China and have been most commonly associated with brackish and freshwater exposure, and ingestion of raw fish and eel.[28] It has been cultured from the stool of many animals that inhabit these waters, such as fish, crustaceans, amphibians, and lizards, and being cultured directly from waters.[29–31] Most infections present during warmer weather months of May to November. In multiple case reports and literature reviews, independent risk factors for extraintestinal infection and complication have been identified as immunocompromised state, hepatobiliary disease, diabetes mellitus, and malignancy, and high iron state (hemoglobinopathy and neonatal stage).[28,32–36]

Although most cases are classified as gastroenteritis, there is significant risk of SSTI, which can present as abscess formation or necrotizing fasciitis, with significant morbidity and mortality. One literature review study showed 23.4% of *E tarda* infections were SSTI.[28] Wounds sustained in fresh and brackish water, wounds associated with fish, reptile, and crustacean exposure, and open wounds exposed to an infected source have highest risk of *E tarda* infection. Presentation of SSTI is consistent with typical wound infection, with erythema, warmth, pus and drainage, and tenderness. Abscess formation is common in *E tarda* infection with one small single-hospital study finding five out of five cases of skin infection requiring surgical drainage of abscess, and one case of myonecrosis and one case of bacteremia.[29] Multiple studies have showed greater than 50% of *E tarda* cellulitis infections progress to abscess.[37]

Because of its relative rarity, there have been limited studies specifically related to pathogenicity in *Edwardsiella* sp. *E tarda* has a similar virulence profile and is similar biochemically and clinically to *Salmonella* species.[26,36] It is an organism that is capable of chemotactic mobility, allowing for rapid spread. Janda and colleagues[36] also found HEp-2 cell invasive capabilities, cell-associated hemolysins, heat-stable enterotoxinlike activity, siderophore production, and plasmid production. This organism thrives in an iron-rich environment and stains positive for Congo red absorption, likely indicative of increased iron acquisition. There is significant risk for bacteremia and atypical infection in hyperferremic hosts, as demonstrated by increased severity of illness in the neonatal stage and in those with sickle cell hemoglobinopathy. In high-iron states, these bacteria are upregulated and have been shown to express iron-cofactor superoxide dismutase, an enzyme that inhibits the human immune response mediated by macrophages.[27] *E tarda* is capable of hemolysis via cell-associated hemolysins activity in iron-deficient environments, which may lead to further complications. Furthermore, *E tarda* has demonstrated mannose-resistant hemagglutination and enteroinvasive and epithelial-invasive mechanisms, which likely play a role in infectious skin changes, with epithelial cell destruction and inflammation.[36]

Diagnosis

Diagnosis is made by wound culture. Blood culture may be positive in disseminated infection. Empiric antibiotic treatment should not be delayed while awaiting culture results. Because gastrointestinal disease is typically self-limiting, stool culture is usually not needed.

Treatment

Uncomplicated SSTIs typically respond well to empiric antibiotic therapy. Complicated infections, especially extraintestinal infections, have poorer outcomes. There is an approximate 50% mortality rate in *E tarda* bacteremia, even when treated appropriately. Like most Enterobactericeae species, *E tarda* is resistant to macrolides, streptogramins, glycopeptides, and lincosamides because of its outer membrane. There is natural sensitivity to most β-lactam antibiotics including cephalosporins, tetracyclines, aminoglycosides, nitrofurantoin, fosfomycin, quinolones, chloramphenicol, and antifolates.[37] If *E tarda* infection is confirmed by wound culture, typical treatment consists of second-, third-, or fourth-generation cephalosporins, although penicillins and carbapenems also have been used effectively.[37] Because this infection is rare, and there have been limited studies regarding appropriate therapy, treatment should be tailored to individual sensitivities. No study has evaluated sufficient numbers of treatment courses to provide appropriate dosage recommendations. Dose and course, therefore, should reflect typical antibiotic regimens for SSTI. Given risk for complication, threshold for further investigation should be low in a patient with suspected or confirmed *E tarda* skin infection. Surgical intervention may be necessary, and should clinical evaluation cause any concern of complicated infection, imaging and surgical consultation should be obtained.

ERYSIPELOTHRIX RHUSIOPATHIAE

Erysipelothrix rhusiopathiae is a facultative, non-spore-forming, gram-positive bacillus. Because it is a rare organism, it often proves difficult to isolate and may be mistaken for other more common organisms unless clinical suspicion is raised.[38] *E rhusiopathiae* exists ubiquitously in the environment and is found in swine and other domestic animals, birds, and fish. It has been shown to exist specifically on the mucoid exterior slime of fish.[39] Infection with this organism typically occurs with contact of contaminated animals, fish, or their products in soils. There are 28 known serotypes of *E rhusiopathiae*.[40] The infection is commonly known as "fish-handler's disease," or even "shrimp-picker's disease."[41] This marine infection can result from bites, abrasions, or even spines of fish causing a portal for microbial entry.[5] A study involving isolation of *E rhusiopathiae* from feed fish (including herring and capelin) and the gingival surface of a harbor seal demonstrated that most of the serotypes of this organism were able to survive long enough (at least 48 hours) to create visible cutaneous lesions when introduced to pigs via intradermal inoculation.[40] This proves that the organism is transmissible from the marine environment and able to produce infections, suggesting the ability of the organism to develop soft tissue infections in humans when exposed via fish or marine environment.

There are three known forms of *Erysipelothrix* disease in humans: a localized cutaneous form (erysipeloid), a diffuse cutaneous form, and septicemia with possible endocarditis. The erysipeloid form is a localized cutaneous infection, creating local cellulitis. The diffuse cutaneous form is more generalized and progresses to other sites of the body. The lesions are similar in appearance, although bullous lesions also occur in locations on the skin than the entry site. The most serious form of the infection is septicemia, which can lead to endocarditis. Incubation time for this infection is typically less than 4 days, but may present up to 7 days after initial exposure. Symptoms include localized swelling, itching, pain, fever, possibly joint aches, and lymphadenopathy.[39] Although these three types of infections are the most common presentations of *E rhusiopathiae*, there are documented cases of other types of infections including arthritis and necrotizing fasciitis.[42] In one case report, a 12-year-old boy was found to have *E rhusiopathiae* after developing erythema and swelling at the site of a dog bite that he had rinsed in a fresh water lake.[43]

Bacteremia from *E rhusiopathiae* has been linked to fish exposure. Case reports of *E rhusiopathiae* infection after fish exposure include a 73-year-old man with fever, chills, and somnolence who was discovered to have blood cultures containing *E rhusiopathiae* after cutting his thumb on the dorsal fin of a pet fish, and a case of necrotizing fasciitis after touching a pet goldfish and scratching the skin.[44,45]

Diagnosis

In cases of erysipeloid, biopsy samples should be taken of the entire dermis, because the bacterium lies in the deeper layers of the skin.[39] Diagnosis is made by Gram stain morphology, motility, biochemical properties, and wound culture. When sepsis or endocarditis is suspected, a standard blood culture should be performed.[39]

The infection rate may be underestimated considering how the infection may mimic other infections and problems with isolation and identification.[39] Because *E rhusiopathiae* is so rarely seen, it is often mistaken for more common infections unless laboratory personnel have a higher suspicion for the organism. It is misidentified as a gram-positive coccus or nonpathogenic gram-positive bacillus.[39]

Treatment

Because management of most SSTIs and bacteremia includes vancomycin, *E rhusiopathiae* may often be initially mistreated because this organism is resistant to vancomycin. The best treatment of *E rhusiopathiae* infections is penicillin G (12–20 million units/d).[41] The optimum dosage and duration of oral penicillin V is not defined but a dose of 2 g per day for 5 to 7 days is probably adequate for most uncomplicated cases. It is also highly susceptible to cephalosporins and clindamycin, and may be treated with ciprofloxacin.[39] In addition to vancomycin, strains are often resistant to aminoglycosides, TMP-SMX, and polymyxins.[39] The length of treatment and dosing varies by severity of infection. Erysipeloid can typically be treated with oral penicillin for 2 to 3 days. Septic arthritis and bacteremia treatment should continue for 4 to 6 weeks, although improvement has been shown with 2 weeks of treatment.[5,39,44,46] Safe work practices and hand hygiene are important methods of reducing exposure or infection. Clinical suspicion for this organism should be raised based on history to guide adequate treatment.

MYCOBACTERIUM MARINUM

Mycobacterium marinum is a type of slow-growing nontuberculous mycobacterium found in bodies of fresh and saltwater around the world. *M marinum* and has a short generation time of 4 to 6 hours. *M marinum* is a gram-positive, acid-fast, aerobic bacterium and grows at an optimal temperature of 30°C.[47] *M marinum* is one of the most identified nontuberculosis mycobacterial species associated with fish mycobacteriosis and is widely considered one of the most important fish pathogens.[48] The primary route of infection between fish is via consumption of infected fish, whereas secondary routes include contact with infected fish skin.[49] *M marinum* can cause human infection including granulomatous infection in human skin and tissues and cutaneous infections, such as ulcers, skin nodules, and lymphangitis, and can infect 150 species of freshwater and saltwater organisms.[50–54] This organism acts by stimulating actin polymerization within phagosomes that allows the organism to propel itself into adjacent cells and escape into the cytoplasm of the infected macrophage for cell-to-cell spread.[55]

M Marinum is most commonly acquired because of minor trauma associated with contact with a body of water. It was originally classified as "swimming pool granulomas," but the chlorination of water in swimming pools has reduced the rate of infection in humans.[56] *M marinum* is not transmittable from person to person.[57] Most infections occur because of exposure to bodies of water, but skin injuries can occur during processing or preparing seafood.[57–59] *M marinum* is also commonly referred to as "fish tank granuloma" and "fish-handler's disease" because of the infections relation to home aquariums and water-based activities.[56]

M marinum infections have a long incubation period and SSTIs may present from 3 weeks to 9 months after exposure.[50] SSTIs are classified into four distinct categories based on severity.[60] Type 1 *M marinum* infection is common in immunocompetent patients and varies between single or limited (<3) superficial skin infections. These infections often appear in the form of a crusted nodule or plaque.[58] Type II *M marinum* infection is classified as more than three lesions with inflammatory or spreading pattern with subcutaneous nodules. This classification of infection may also present with abscesses or granulomas in immune-suppressed patients.[61] Type III *M Marinum* infection is classified as deep infections that are seen with associated symptoms, such as arthritis or osteomyelitis. Type IV *M Marinum* infection presents with disseminated disease including lung or other systemic manifestations. Bacteremia is rare but may be seen in immunocompromised patients.[60]

Table 2
Recommended antibiotic regimens for aquatic infections

	Empiric Therapy	Duration
Vibrio	Ceftazidime 1–2 g IV/intramuscularly q 8 h AND doxycycline 100 mg IV/po bid	7–14 d
Aeromonas hydrophila	Doxycycline 100 mg IV q 12 h plus ciprofloxacin 500 mg IV q 12 h OR ceftriaxone 1–2 g IV q 24 h	7–10 d
Edwardsiella tarda	3rd/4th generation cephalosporin PLUS doxycycline	Determine clinically
Erysipelothrix rhusiopathiae	Penicillin G 12–20 million units/d	2–3 d for erysipeloid, 4–6 wk for septic arthritis or bacteremia
Mycobacterium marinum	Clarithromycin 500 mg bid, Bactrim DS bid, OR ciprofloxacin 500 mg bid	4–6 wk

Data from Refs.[5–7,15,23,37,39,41,58]

Diagnosis

Diagnosis is made by Gram stain and wound culture.

Treatment

M Marinum is a multidrug-resistant organism and this can make treatment of the disease fairly difficult.[62] Monotherapy with clarithromycin, 500 mg twice a day, Bactrim DS twice a day, or ciprofloxacin, 500 mg twice a day for 4 to 6 weeks, is effective in limited superficial infections. Deeper limited skin infections may require a combination therapy of two of these drugs to be effective. If the patient has subcutaneous nodules around the infection site, therapy with ethambutol and rifampin is recommended. *M marinum* is classically noted to be more resistant to streptomycin, isoniazid, and pyrazinamide so these medications should be avoided.[58] Therapeutic alternatives in deeper infections include electrodessication, cryotherapy, hyperthermic therapy, and photodynamic therapy.[48]

SUMMARY

Although SSTIs are usually caused by organisms that inhabit the skin, such as *Staphylococcus* and *Streptococcus*, a history including exposure to an aquatic environment should widen the differential to include unusual organisms. Guiding empiric treatment accordingly (**Table 2**) can prevent progression to serious consequences, such as necrotizing fasciitis. Individuals with conditions predisposing them to severe aquatic infections, such as a compromised immune system or liver disease, should take caution to avoid immersing open wounds in bodies of salt or fresh water.

REFERENCES

1. Hiransuthikul N, Tantisiriwat W, Lertutsahakul K, et al. Skin and soft-tissue infections among tsunami survivors in southern Thailand. Clin Infect Dis 2005; 41(10):e93–6.
2. Schwartz BS, Nydick JA, Abzug JM. Aquatic hand injuries. J Hand Surg Am 2014;39(8):1623–6 [quiz: 1627].

3. Kueh CS, Kutarski P, Brunton M. Contaminated marine wounds: the risk of acquiring acute bacterial infection from marine recreational beaches. J Appl Bacteriol 1992;73(5):412–20.
4. Crosby SN, Snoddy MC, Atkinson CT, et al. Upper extremity myonecrosis caused by *Edwardsiella tarda* resulting in transhumeral amputation: case report. J Hand Surg Am 2013;38(1):129–32.
5. Noonburg GE. Management of extremity trauma and related infections occurring in the aquatic environment. J Am Acad Orthop Surg 2005;13(4):243–53.
6. Diaz JH. Skin and soft tissue infections following marine injuries and exposures in travelers. J Travel Med 2014;21(3):207–13.
7. Horseman MA, Surani S. A comprehensive review of *Vibrio vulnificus*: an important cause of severe sepsis and skin and soft-tissue infection. Int J Infect Dis 2011;15(3):e157–66.
8. Sganga G, Cozza V, Spanu T, et al. Global climate change and wound care: case study of an off-season *Vibrio alginolyticus* infection in a healthy man. Ostomy Wound Manage 2009;55(4):60–2.
9. Maraki S, Christidou A, Anastasaki M, et al. Non-O1, non-O139 *Vibrio cholerae* bacteremic skin and soft tissue infections. Infect Dis (Lond) 2016;48(3):171–6.
10. Hundenborn J, Thurig S, Kommerell M, et al. Severe wound infection with photobacterium *Damselae* ssp. damselae and *Vibrio harveyi*, following a laceration injury in marine environment: a case report and review of the literature. Case Rep Med 2013;2013:610632.
11. Kotton Y, Soboh S, Bisharat N. *Vibrio vulnificus* necrotizing fasciitis associated with acupuncture. Infect Dis Rep 2015;7(3):5901.
12. Lee YC, Hor LI, Chiu HY, et al. Prognostic factor of mortality and its clinical implications in patients with necrotizing fasciitis caused by V*ibrio vulnificus*. Eur J Clin Microbiol Infect Dis 2014;33(6):1011–8.
13. Menon MP, Yu PA, Iwamoto M, et al. Pre-existing medical conditions associated with *Vibrio vulnificus* septicaemia. Epidemiol Infect 2014;142(4):878–81.
14. Hou CC, Lai CC, Liu WL, et al. Clinical manifestation and prognostic factors of non-cholerae *Vibrio* infections. Eur J Clin Microbiol Infect Dis 2011;30(6):819–24.
15. Kuo Chou TN, Chao WN, Yang C, et al. Predictors of mortality in skin and soft-tissue infections caused by *Vibrio vulnificus*. World J Surg 2010;34(7):1669–75.
16. Matsumoto K, Ohshige K, Fujita N, et al. Clinical features of *Vibrio vulnificus* infections in the coastal areas of the Ariake Sea, Japan. J Infect Chemother 2010; 16(4):272–9.
17. Ahmad A, Brumble L, Maniaci M. *Vibrio parahaemolyticus* induced necrotizing fasciitis: an atypical organism causing an unusual presentation. Case Rep Infect Dis 2013;2013:216854.
18. Morris JG, Horneman A. Aeromonas infections. UpToDate; 2018. Available at: http://www.uptodate.com/contents/aeromonas-infections. Accessed April 10, 2018.
19. Xu XJ, Ferguson MR, Popov VL, et al. Role of a cytotoxic enterotoxin in aeromonas-mediated infections: development of transposon and isogenic mutants. Infect Immun 1998;66(8):3501–9.
20. Smith JA. *Aeromonas hydrophila*: analysis of 11 cases. Can Med Assoc J 1980; 122(11):1270–2.
21. Sartor C, Limouzine-Perotti F, Legre R, et al. Nosocomial infections with *Aeromonas hydrophila* from leeches. Clin Infect Dis 2002;35(1):E1–5.
22. Hanson PG, Standridge J, Jarrett F, et al. Freshwater wound infection due to *Aeromonas hydrophila*. JAMA 1977;238(10):1053–4.

23. Stevens DL, Bisno AL, Chambers HF, et al. Executive summary: practice guidelines for the diagnosis and management of skin and soft tissue infections: 2014 update by the Infectious Diseases Society of America. Clin Infect Dis 2014;59(2):147–59.
24. Ramos JM, Cuenca-Estrella M, Esteban J, et al. Soft-tissue infection caused by *Aeromonas hydrophila.* Enferm Infecc Microbiol Clin 1995;13(8):469–72.
25. Jones BL, Wilcox MH. Aeromonas infections and their treatment. J Antimicrob Chemother 1995;35(4):453–61.
26. Wilson JP, Waterer RR, Wofford JD Jr, et al. Serious infections with *Edwardsiella tarda.* A case report and review of the literature. Arch Intern Med 1989;149:208–10.
27. Janda JM, Abbott SI. Infections associated with the genus *Edwardsiella*: the role of *Edwardsiella tarda* in human disease. Clin Infect Dis 1993;17:742–8.
28. Hirai Y, Asahata-Tago S, Ainoda Y, et al. *Edwardsiella tarda* bacteremia. A rare but fatal water- and foodborne infection: review of the literature and clinical cases from a single centre. Can J Infect Dis Med Microbiol 2015;26:313–8.
29. Slaven E, Lopez FA, Hart SM, et al. Myonecrosis caused by *Edwardsiella tarda*: a case report and case series of extraintestinal *E. tarda* infections. Clin Infect Dis 2001;32:1430–3.
30. Wyatt LE, Ranzell NH, Vanderzant C. *Edwardsiella tarda* in freshwater catfish and their environment. Appl Environ Microbiol 1979;38:710–4.
31. Hayato T, Fujita Y, Ogawa H, et al. Multiple brain abscesses in neonate caused by *Edwardsiella tarda.* Neurol Med Chir 2009;49:85–9.
32. Yousuf RM, How SH, Amran M, et al. *Edwardsiella tarda* septicemia with underlying multiple liver abscesses. Malays J Pathol 2006;28:49–53.
33. Kazuhiro N, Takahuru K, Ikki Y, et al. *Edwardsiella tarda* bacteremia with metastatic gastric cancer. IDCases 2016;5:76–7.
34. Frumberg DB, Epstein SE, Jauregui JJ, et al. Prosthetic hip infection with *Edwardsiella tarda* in sickle cell beta thalassemia disease: a case report. J Clin Orthop Trauma 2016;7(Suppl 1):130–3.
35. Funada H, Kameoka J, Machi T, et al. *Edwardsiella tarda* septicemia complicating acute leukemia. Jpn J Med 1988;27:325–8.
36. Janda JM, Abbott SL, Kroske-Bystrom S, et al. Pathogenic properties of *Edwardsiella* species. J Clin Microbiol 1991;29:1997–2001.
37. Stock I, Wiedemann B. Natural antibiotic susceptibilities of *Edwardsiella tarda, E. ictaluri,* and *E. hoshinae.* Antimicrob Agents Chemother 2001;45:2245–55.
38. Wang Q, Chang BJ, Riley TV. Erysipelothrix rhusiopathiae. Vet Microbiol 2010;140(3–4):405–17.
39. Brooke CJ, Riley TV. *Erysipelothrix rhusiopathiae*: bacteriology, epidemiology and clinical manifestations of an occupational pathogen. J Med Microbiol 1999;48(9):789–99.
40. Opriessnig T, Shen HG, Bender JS, et al. *Erysipelothrix rhusiopathiae* isolates recovered from fish, a harbour seal (Phoca vitulina) and the marine environment are capable of inducing characteristic cutaneous lesions in pigs. J Comp Pathol 2013;148(4):365–72.
41. Finkelstein R, Oren I. Soft tissue infections caused by marine bacterial pathogens: epidemiology, diagnosis, and management. Curr Infect Dis Rep 2011;13(5):470–7.
42. Mukhopadhyay C, Shah H, Vandana KE, et al. A child with *Erysipelothrix* arthritis: beware of the little known. Asian Pac J Trop Biomed 2012;2(6):503–4.

43. Alawdah LS, Campbell JN, Pollock N, et al. *Erysipelothrix rhusiopathiae* suppurative arthritis in a 12-year-old boy after an unusual fresh water exposure. Pediatr Infect Dis J 2017;36(4):431–3.
44. Asimaki E, Nolte O, Overesch G, et al. A dangerous hobby? *Erysipelothrix rhusiopathiae* bacteremia most probably acquired from freshwater aquarium fish handling. Infection 2017;45(4):557–62.
45. Simionescu R, Grover S, Shekar R, et al. Necrotizing fasciitis caused by *Erysipelothrix rhusiopathiae*. South Med J 2003;96(9):937–9.
46. Sinclair M, Hawkins A, Testro A. Something fishy: an unusual *Erysipelothrix rhusiopathiae* infection in an immunocompromised individual. BMJ Case Rep 2013;2013 [pii:bcr2013008873].
47. Clark HF, Shepard CC. Effect of environmental temperatures on infection with *Mycobacterium marinum (balnei)* of mice and a number of poikilothermic species. J Bacteriol 1963;86(5):1057–69.
48. Rallis E, Koumantaki-Mathioudaki E. Treatment of *Mycobacterium marinum* cutaneous infections. Expert Opin Pharmacother 2007;8(17):2965–78.
49. El Amrani MH, Adoui M, Patey O, et al. Upper extremity *Mycobacterium marinum* infection. Orthop Traumatol Surg Res 2010;96(6):706–11.
50. Jernigan JA, Farr BM. Incubation period and sources of exposure for cutaneous *Mycobacterium marinum* infection: case report and review of the literature. Clin Infect Dis 2000;31(2):439–43.
51. Lewis FM, Marsh BJ, von Reyn CF. Fish tank exposure and cutaneous infections due to *Mycobacterium marinum*: tuberculin skin testing, treatment, and prevention. Clin Infect Dis 2003;37(3):390–7.
52. Petrini B. *Mycobacterium marinum*: ubiquitous agent of waterborne granulomatous skin infections. Eur J Clin Microbiol Infect Dis 2006;25(10):609–13.
53. Beecham HJ 3rd, Oldfield EC 3rd, Lewis DE, et al. *Mycobacterium marinum* infection from shucking oysters. Lancet 1991;337(8755):1487.
54. Zeeli T, Samra Z, Pitlik S. Ill from eel? Lancet Infect Dis 2003;3(3):168.
55. Stamm LM, Morisaki JH, Gao LY, et al. *Mycobacterium marinum* escapes from phagosomes and is propelled by actin-based motility. J Exp Med 2003;198(9):1361–8.
56. Ang P, Rattana-Apiromyakij N, Goh CL. Retrospective study of *Mycobacterium marinum* skin infections. Int J Dermatol 2000;39(5):343–7.
57. Clark R, Spector H, Friedman D, et al. Osteomyelitis and synovitis produced by *Mycobacterium marinum* in a fisherman. J Clin Microbiol 1990;28(11):2570–2.
58. Aubry A, Chosidow O, Caumes E, et al. Sixty-three cases of *Mycobacterium marinum* infection: clinical features, treatment, and antibiotic susceptibility of causative isolates. Arch Intern Med 2002;162(15):1746–52.
59. Lawler A. Human *Mycobacterium marinum* Aronson infections. J Aquariculture Aquatic Sci 1994;6(4):93–5.
60. Bhatty MA, Turner DP, Chamberlain ST. *Mycobacterium marinum* hand infection: case reports and review of literature. Br J Plast Surg 2000;53(2):161–5.
61. Bartralot R, García-Patos V, Sitjas D, et al. Clinical patterns of cutaneous nontuberculous mycobacterial infections. Br J Dermatol 2005;152(4):727–34.
62. Edelstein H. *Mycobacterium marinum* skin infections: report of 31 cases and review of the literature. Arch Intern Med 1994;154(12):1359–64.

Infections During Pregnancy

Connie Leeper, MD, MPH[a,*], Andrew Lutzkanin III, MD[b]

KEYWORDS

- Congenital infection • Pregnancy complications • Vertical transmission • Zika • TORCH

KEY POINTS

- Some common infections affect pregnant women differently and treatment options must be chosen keeping safety in pregnancy in mind.
- Certain infections can be transmitted vertically and pregnancies affected by these infections must be monitored and managed to decrease transmission.
- Some infections can be acquired in utero and can cause congenital infections in newborns that lead to developmental anomalies, affect growth, and lead to significant neonatal morbidity and mortality.

INTRODUCTION

In pregnancy, potential effects of infections on both mother and fetus must be considered. Pregnant women are at increased risk of some infections due to physiologic changes of pregnancy. Infections may cause complications with the pregnancy, and some maternal infections are transmissible to the fetus. When determining treatment, potential effects on the fetus and the pregnancy must be taken into consideration including different effects by trimester. In this article, the authors discuss common infections that require special considerations in pregnancy, infections that can be vertically transmitted, and infections that can cause in utero and perinatal infection leading to birth defects (including the classic TORCH infections).

PREGNANCY CONSIDERATIONS WITH COMMON INFECTIONS

Urinary Tract Infections

Recurrent bacteriuria and pyelonephritis are more common in pregnancy. Smooth muscle relaxation and dilation of ureters with pregnancy increases the propensity for ascending infection. Screening and treatment of urinary tract infections (UTIs)

Disclosure: The authors have nothing to disclose.
[a] Department of Family, Internal, and Rural Medicine, University of Alabama, 850 Peter Bryce Boulevard, Tuscaloosa, AL 35401, USA; [b] Department of Family and Community Medicine, Penn State College of Medicine, 500 University Drive, Hershey, PA 17033, USA
* Corresponding author.
E-mail address: ccleeper@ua.edu

Prim Care Clin Office Pract 45 (2018) 567–586
https://doi.org/10.1016/j.pop.2018.05.013
primarycare.theclinics.com

are more intensive in pregnancy than in the general population. Infectious Disease Society of America guidelines recommend universal screening of pregnant women for asymptomatic bacteriuria with urine culture in early pregnancy and periodic rescreening in women with positive culture during pregnancy.[1] Diagnosis is made if greater than or equal to 10^5 colony-forming units of uropathogen or greater than or equal to 10^4 of Group B Streptococcus (GBS) is present in urine culture.[2,3] Pyelonephritis in pregnancy typically requires inpatient empirical intravenous antibiotics, with the patient switched to an oral regimen once improving and afebrile for 24 to 48 hours.[4] Appropriate antibiotics are given for 10 to 14 days followed by suppressive therapy for the remainder of pregnancy to prevent recurrence.[4] GBS growing in any amount in urine culture during pregnancy indicates significant anogenital colonization and therefore qualifies the woman for intrapartum antibiotics to prevent neonatal GBS disease.[5]

The pregnancy and trimester need to be considered when prescribing antibiotics. Penicillins, cephalosporins, and aztreonam are considered safe in pregnancy. Antibiotics with high protein binding, such as ceftriaxone, may cause hyperbilirubinemia in newborns if used within a day of delivery. Nitrofurantoin is associated with birth defects[6,7] and hemolytic anemia[8] and, therefore, is avoided in the first trimester and at term. Trimethoprim-sulfamethoxazole should be avoided in the first trimester and at term because trimethoprim is a folic acid antagonist and sulfonamides can displace plasma binding of bilirubin in newborns. Tetracyclines are avoided in pregnancy due to fetal bone and teeth developmental defects[9,10] and fluoroquinolones are avoided due to developmental defects of cartilage in animal experiments.[11]

Chlamydia and Gonorrhea

Chlamydia and gonorrhea are common infections that can affect pregnancy outcomes. Prevalence of chlamydia in pregnancy is 2% to 20% depending on the population.[12–14] Newborns born vaginally to women with chlamydia are at increased risk of chlamydia conjunctivitis and pneumonia. Signs of chlamydia conjunctivitis include swelling, eye discharge, and chemosis appearing 5 to 14 days after delivery. Signs of chlamydia pneumonia include staccato cough, nasal discharge, tachypnea, and rales without fever presenting at 4 to 12 weeks of life.

Rates of gonorrhea are highest in adolescents and young adults, particular racial minorities, and in the southeastern United States.[15] Gonorrhea has been associated with premature rupture of membranes, preterm birth, chorioamnionitis, small-for-gestational-age infants, and spontaneous abortion.[16–19] Newborns born to women with gonorrhea are at increased risk of gonococcal conjunctivitis, scalp abscesses (with fetal scalp electrode placement), and disseminated gonococcal infections, which may include arthritis, sepsis, or meningitis. Gonococcal conjunctivitis causes profuse purulent exudate and swelling 2 to 5 days after birth and can cause visual impairment if left untreated.

The Center for Disease Control (CDC) and US Preventative Services Task Force (USPSTF) recommend universal screening of pregnant women younger than 25 years and older than or equal to 25 years at increased risk for sexually transmitted infections (STIs) (**Box 1**) at the first prenatal visit for chlamydia and gonorrhea.[20–22] Retesting during the third trimester should be performed for women who remain at high risk.[20]

Pregnant women diagnosed with chlamydia should have a test of cure collected at least 3 weeks after treatment as cure rates are decreased in pregnancy and because continued infection places infants at risk of infection.

Rising antibiotic resistance makes treatment of gonorrhea more complicated. The CDC currently recommends single doses of ceftriaxone, 250 mg, intramuscularly

Box 1
Women at increased risk of sexually transmitted infections

Personal history of sexually transmitted infections (STI)

New sexual partner

Multiple sexual partners or a sexual partner with multiple partners

Sexual partner diagnosed with STI

Inconsistent condom use if not in a mutually monogamous relationship

Contact with sex workers or trading sex for money or drugs

Admission into a correctional facility

Data from LeFevre ML, U.S. Preventive Services Task Force. Screening for Chlamydia and gonorrhea: U.S. Preventive Services Task Force recommendation statement. Ann Intern Med 2014;161:902–10.

and azithromycin, 1gm, orally.[20] Doxycycline (potential alternative to azithromycin) should be avoided in pregnancy. Desensitization should be pursued for pregnant women with gonorrhea who have severe allergy to cephalosporins. Dual therapy with gentamicin and azithromycin is an alternative if desensitization is not possible. If alternative regimens are used, a test of cure is recommended. Culture with susceptibility testing is ideally used for test of cure starting at 7 days after treatment. If nucleic acid amplification testing is used for test of cure, it should be performed 14 days after treatment to avoid false-positive results.[23,24] The American Academy of Pediatrics (AAP) and the CDC recommend erythromycin ophthalmic ointment be given within 2 hours of birth to all newborns to prophylactically prevent gonococcal ophthalmia.[20,25]

Influenza

Pregnant women tend to have more severe illness and mortality from influenza than the general population.[26] This is theorized to be due to physiologic changes of pregnancy including decreased lung capacity, increased oxygen consumption, and decreased cell-mediated immunity. Infection in the first trimester increases risk of birth defects,[27] and maternal influenza has been associated with increased risk of miscarriage, preterm labor, small-for-gestational-age infants, and fetal death.[28–31]

Influenza vaccination is recommended for all pregnant women during influenza season.[32] Vaccination during pregnancy confers protection to a newborn for several months after birth[33–35] and antiinfluenza immunoglobulins are transferred to newborns through breast milk.[36] Pregnant women should not receive the live-attenuated influenza vaccine.

Pregnant women with suspected influenza should receive empirical antiviral treatment because it decreases morbidity and mortality. Although treatment within 2 days of symptom onset has the best data, benefit has still been shown after 2 days.[37] Neuraminidase inhibitors can be used in pregnancy and dosing and durations are the same as nonpregnant adults. Oseltamivir is preferred in pregnancy due to systemic absorption and more experience in pregnancy.

Vaginitis

The 3 main causes of vaginitis include bacterial vaginosis (BV), yeast vulvovaginitis, and trichomoniasis.

BV increases the risk of preterm labor.[38] However, screening and treatment of asymptomatic BV does not seem to reduce preterm birth and the American College of Obstetricians and Gynecologists (ACOG), USPSTF, and CDC recommend against routine screening for asymptomatic BV to prevent preterm birth.[20,39,40] Studies are currently being conducted to determine high-risk subpopulations (ie, women with history of preterm birth or with genetic polymorphisms affecting cytokine release) that may benefit from screening, but data are still lacking to determine which patients would benefit. Testing is recommended for symptomatic pregnant women and recommended treatment is with oral metronidazole or clindamycin for 7 days.

Yeast vulvovaginitis causes no pregnancy complications.[41] Vaginal treatment for 7 days with clotrimazole 1% cream or miconazole 2% cream or 100 mg suppositories is recommended over oral therapy due to potential risks of oral azoles in pregnancy. Oral azole use, particularly in the first trimester, may be associated with increased risk of miscarriage[42] and high doses may be associated with birth defects.[43,44]

Trichomoniasis is associated with premature rupture of membranes, preterm delivery, and low birth weight infants.[45,46] Newborns can become infected with trichomonas during delivery causing fever, nasal discharge, respiratory difficulty, UTIs, and vaginal discharge in female infants.[47–50] Routine screening for trichomonas in pregnancy is not recommended. A single oral dose of 2gm metronidazole is a preferred treatment in pregnancy, but 500 mg orally twice daily for 5 to 7 days is also acceptable if nausea/vomiting prevents 2g regimen.[51]

Vertically Transmissible Infections

These infections can be transmitted mother-to-child and therefore monitoring and, in some cases, treatment is warranted to prevent transmission to the newborn.

Hepatitis B

Hepatitis B can cause acute and chronic infections. Universal screening of pregnant women for chronic hepatitis B is recommended at the first prenatal visit with HBsAg testing. HBsAg-positive women should have testing for HBeAg, anti-HBe antibody, HBV DNA level, and aminotransferases. For pregnant women with chronic hepatitis B, antivirals are offered if HBV DNA is high to prevent mother-to-child transmission.[52] Tenofovir disoproxil fumarate is the preferred antiviral due to rare resistance and safety during pregnancy.[53,54] Women with chronic hepatitis B who do not require antiviral treatment should have repeat viral load tested at 26 to 28 weeks to determine if antiviral therapy is indicated to prevent mother-to-child transmission.

Pregnant women diagnosed with acute hepatitis B should be monitored for seroconversion indicating recovery instead of chronic infection. Recovery is indicated by disappearance of HBV DNA and seroconversion of HBeAg and HBsAg to anti-HBe and anti-HBs antibodies, respectively.

Cesarean delivery does not decrease risk of vertical transmission of hepatitis B.[55–57] Newborns born to women with positive HBsAg should receive their first dose of hepatitis B vaccine and HBIG within 12 hours of delivery.

Hepatitis C

Rates of hepatitis C have been increasing in young adults.[58,59] Chronic infection may not cause adverse pregnancy or newborn complications. However, newborns born to women with chronic hepatitis C are more likely to be low birth weight, small for gestational age, and require assisted ventilation or neonatal intensive care unit admission.[60] Antiviral therapy should not be used as safety and efficacy in pregnancy has not been established. In hepatitis C-infected pregnant women, invasive prenatal testing, prolonged rupture of membranes, and obstetric procedures (ie, fetal scalp electrode) should be avoided to decrease vertical transmission.[61,62] Hepatitis C is not an indication for cesarean delivery because it does not decrease vertical transmission.[63,64] Newborns born to women with hepatitis C should have HCV antibody checked after 18 months to test for vertical transmission.

Human Immunodeficiency Virus

Women make up an increasing percentage of AIDS cases in the United States.[65] Minority women have disproportionately higher rates of human immunodeficiency virus (HIV)/AIDS.[65,66] In the United States, an estimated 8700 women with HIV give birth yearly.[67] Perinatal transmission of HIV has significantly decreased to 2% or less in the United States with current recommendations for screening, treatment, and obstetric management.[68,69]

Universal screening for HIV is recommended in pregnancy.[70] For women with HIV, a CD4 count is measured at the initial prenatal visit and at least every 3 months. Viral load is measured at the initial prenatal visit, when antiretrovirals (ARVs) are initiated, 2 to 4 weeks after initiation of or change in ARVs, monthly until complete suppression achieved, then at least every 3 months during pregnancy. Resistance testing is measured before initiating or changing ARV regimens. Pregnant HIV-infected women should be screened for latent tuberculosis, Hepatitis C, and toxoplasmosis and immunity against Hepatitis A.[71]

All pregnant women with HIV should be treated with ARVs regardless of CD4 count to decrease vertical transmission.[71] Opportunistic infection prophylaxis should be prescribed at the same CD4 count cutoffs as nonpregnant patients. Pneumococcal, hepatitis A and B vaccination is indicated for pregnant women with HIV if they have not already received them.

Viral load should be measured at 34 to 36 weeks to assist with decisions regarding delivery as women with viral loads greater than or equal to 1000 copies/mL should be scheduled for cesarean delivery at 38 weeks.[71] Management of ARVs at delivery are reviewed in **Table 1**. Interventions including fetal scalp electrode placement and operative vaginal delivery should be avoided to decrease perinatal transmission. Breastfeeding is not recommended in resource-rich countries.

All newborns born to women with HIV should receive ARVs to reduce perinatal transmission. Exposed newborns should be tested with virologic tests (HIV RNA or DNA) at 2 to 3 weeks of life, 1 to 2 months of life, and 4 to 6 months of life.[71]

TORCH Infections

The classic group of perinatal infections known as the TORCH infections includes toxoplasmosis, other (syphilis), rubella, cytomegalovirus (CMV), and herpes simplex

Table 1
Peripartum management of HIV positive patients by viral load

Viral Load	IV Zidovudine at Delivery	Delivery Management
Undetectable: 49 copies/mL	Not indicated	Vaginal delivery safe unless obstetrically contraindicated
50–999 copies/mL	Can be considered	Vaginal delivery safe unless obstetrically contraindicated
≥1000 copies/mL	Given 3 h before cesarean	Cesarean delivery before labor at 38 wk recommended[71]

virus (HSV). This group has common presenting features of rash and ocular abnormalities.[72] Varicella-zoster virus and parvovirus B19 and Zika virus can also be grouped in this category.[73]

TOXOPLASMOSIS

Organism and Epidemiology

Toxoplasma gondii is a protozoan parasite spread through cat feces, contaminated soil, or by consuming undercooked meats. *T gondii* preferentially invades neural tissues (brain and retina), skeletal muscle, and/or cardiac muscle forming cysts that destroy host cells.[74] Approximately 201,000 cases of congenital toxoplasmosis are reported worldwide yearly with highest prevalence in tropical regions. Toxoplasmosis affects between 10 and 33/100,000 of live births in the United States.[75] Risk of fetal infection after maternal infection increases from 15% if infected at 13 weeks gestation to greater than 70% if infected at 36 weeks.[76]

Clinical Presentation

Maternal infections are predominately asymptomatic but symptoms can include fever, night sweats, cervical lymphadenopathy, myalgias, malaise, and hepatosplenomegaly.[77] Similarly, 70% to 90% of infants are asymptomatic at birth. The classic triad of chorioretinitis, hydrocephalus, and intracranial calcifications is rare. Fetal manifestations can present early (**Box 2**) or late (**Box 3**).[74]

Testing

There is no recommendation for universal screening of pregnant women.[77] When toxoplasma is suspected, maternal antibody testing is recommended. Immunoglobulin G (IgG) is the most sensitive test, because IgM antibodies have a high false-positive rate. IgM can remain elevated for up to 2 years following infection.[79]

Fetal testing either based on positive maternal tests or ultrasound findings can be done via polymerase chain reaction (PCR) analysis of the amniotic fluid after 18 weeks. At birth, affected infants should have repeat PCR or serology; a computed tomographic (CT) scan of head; and comprehensive eye, ear, and neurologic examinations.

Management

Before 18 weeks, pregnant women are treated with spiramycin until the diagnosis can be confirmed with ultrasound and PCR. Once the diagnosis is confirmed, patients are treated with a regimen of spiramycin, pyrimethamine, sulfadiazine, and folinic acid. Infected infants are treated for a total of 12 months with a regimen of pyrimethamine, sulfadiazine and folinic acid. One month after treatment the infant should be retested including serology, head CT, and detailed eye/ear/neuro examinations.[76]

Box 2
Early manifestation of fetal toxoplasmosis infection

Maculopapular rash

Fevers

Jaundice

Hepatosplenomegaly

Thrombocytopenia

Microcephaly

Box 3
Late manifestation of fetal toxoplasmosis infection

Chorioretinitis (occurs in 90% of cases)[78]

Cerebellar or motor dysfunction

Intellectual delay

Sensorineural hearing loss

Seizures

SYPHILIS

Organism and Epidemiology

Syphilis is a sexually transmitted infection caused by the spirochete *Treponema pallidum*. In 2016 there were 628 cases of congenital infection in the United States, rates being highest in the southern states and in minority populations.[80] Lack of adequate prenatal care carries the highest risk of congenital infection.

Clinical Presentation

Syphilis infection manifests over time in several stages. Primary syphilis presents 3 to 6 weeks after exposure with painless chancres in the genital areas at the site of infection. These may go unnoticed and resolve spontaneously. Secondary syphilis presents 6 to 8 weeks later with an erythematous papular rash on the palms and soles, condyloma lata in the mouth or groin, and systemic symptoms such as fever, lymphadenopathy, sore throat, muscle aches, weight loss, and fatigue. Again, these symptoms will typically resolve spontaneously. Syphilis may then remain latent from months to years before progressing to tertiary syphilis, which can affect the central nervous system, cardiovascular system, musculoskeletal system, or liver. Neurosyphilis and ocular syphilis can occur at any stage of infection.[74,80]

Most of the infants with congenital infection are asymptomatic at birth. Severe infections can result in hydrops fetalis, premature birth, and stillbirth. The clinical manifestations are categorized as early (age <2 years) or late (age >2 years) findings and are outlined in **Table 2**. Abnormalities in the placenta and umbilical cord include the placenta appearing enlarged and pale and the umbilical cord appearing inflamed with focal necrosis within the Wharton jelly.

Testing

Universal screening of pregnant women is recommended in the first trimester with repeat testing in the third trimester in high-risk areas/populations.[81] There are several different tests available including the following:

- Nontreponemal tests—Venereal Disease Research Laboratory (VDRL) and rapid plasma reagin (RPR)
- Treponemal tests—fluorescent treponemal antibodies and direct treponemal antibodies
- Treponemal culture, which requires dark field microscopy

The VDRL and RPR are fast and inexpensive but have higher false positives than treponemal-specific tests and thus these are used for confirmation and following treatment.

Fetal testing for treponemal antibodies can be performed after 18 to 22 weeks. After delivery, infants with suspected congenital syphilis are tested using the same 2-step

Table 2
Clinical manifestation of congenital syphilis infection

Organ System	Early Manifestations	Late Manifestations
Mucocutaneous	• Persistent rhinitis ("snuffles") • Maculopapular rash on palms and soles • Pemphigus syphiliticus • Condylomata lata	• Hutchinson teeth • Perforation of hard palate • Gummas • Rhagades
Neurologic (including eyes and ears)	• Meningitis • Hydrocephalus	• Chorioretinitis • Glaucoma • Sensorineural hearing loss • Intellectual/developmental delay • Seizures
Skeletal	• Symmetric long bone lesions • Periostitis • Metaphyseal serration • Pseudoparalysis	• Abnormal facies: ○ Frontal bossing ○ Saddle nose ○ Short maxilla ○ Protuberant mandible • Saber shins • Clutton joints
Reticuloendothelial	• Fever • Anemia • Leukopenia or leukocytosis • Thrombocytopenia • Hepatosplenomegaly • Jaundice • Generalized lymphadenopathy	

Data from Follett T, Clarke DF. Resurgence of congenital syphilis: diagnosis and treatment. Neonatal Netw 2011;30:320–8.

approach. The placenta and umbilical cord can be sent for pathologic evaluation including dark field microscopy.

Management

Primary, secondary, and early latent syphilis is treated with 2.4 million units of benzathine penicillin G given as a single dose intramuscularly. If the duration of latent infection is unknown, then 3 doses are given at 1-week intervals. Neurosyphilis and ocular syphilis are treated with 3 to 4 million units of aqueous crystalline penicillin G intravenously every 4 hours for 10 to 14 days. There is limited data on nonpenicillin alternatives. Pregnant women with penicillin allergy should be desensitized. Women should be retested and antibody titers followed throughout pregnancy to ensure effective treatment.[80]

Congenital infection is treated with intravenous aqueous penicillin G, 50,000 units/kg, every 12 hours (<1 week old) or every 8 hours (>1 week old) for 10 days. Intramuscular procaine penicillin G, 50,000 units/kg, daily for 10 days can also be used. If treatment is interrupted for more than 24 hours the course should be repeated. For more details regarding the evaluation and management of congenital syphilis, please refer to the AAP 2012 Report of the Committee on Infectious Diseases.[82]

RUBELLA

Organism and Epidemiology

Rubella is a single-stranded RNA virus spread via inhalation of infected particles. Routine vaccination worldwide has led to a 95% decrease in cases from 2000 to

2014 and The Pan American Health Organization declaring rubella eliminated from the Americas in 2015. The US National Congenital Rubella Registry does report 5 to 6 cases of congenital infection yearly, primarily in infants of mothers who emigrated from countries without adequate vaccine programs. Risk of congenital rubella is highest when primary infection occurs in the first trimester (80%–100%), decreases in the second trimester (10%–20%), and increases again in the third trimester (60%).[83]

Clinical Presentation

Maternal symptoms are mild and often go unrecognized. The primary manifestation is a diffuse maculopapular rash lasting around 3 days. Patients may have fever, sore throat, arthralgia, and fatigue. Fetal infection can result in miscarriage, stillbirth, or congenital rubella syndrome (CRS) (**Box 4**).[74]

Other findings include low birth weight, hepatosplenomegaly, thrombocytopenia, bone lesions, and a purpuric "Blueberry Muffin" rash. Late manifestations of CRS include diabetes mellitus, thyroid dysfunction, hypertension, intellectual and behavioral disorders, and panencephalitis.

Testing

Proof of rubella immunity should be documented at the first prenatal visit either through serologic testing or through documentation of immunization. Guidelines for fetal testing in suspected cases were developed by the CDC in 2009 and include the following:

- Viral PCR or culture
- Reverse transcription PCR for viral RNA from blood, cerebrospinal fluid, urine, or nasal swab
- Rubella IgM (usually positive at birth to 3 months in congenital infection)
  - Confirm with stable or rising IgG levels over first 7 to 11 months of age due to false-positive test results

Management

Women found to be nonimmune should be vaccinated immediately following delivery. No specific treatments are available for infants born with CRS. All cases should be reported to the National Congenital Rubella Registry at the CDC. Infants born with CRS are considered contagious through the first year of life unless serial cultures are negative after 3 months of age.[82]

CYTOMEGALOVIRUS

Organism and Epidemiology

CMV is the most common congenital viral infection, affecting up to 2% of live births.[84,85] In the United States, congenital CMV is the leading cause of long-term disabilities in children and is the most common cause of nonhereditary hearing loss worldwide.[86] Risk of vertical transmission is between 30% and 40% for a primary

Box 4
Clinical manifestations of congenital rubella syndrome

Sensorineural hearing loss

Ocular defects, including cataracts, glaucoma, retinopathy, and microphthalmia

Heart defects, including patent ductus arteriosus, pulmonary artery stenosis, and coarctation

infection; this risk increases with each trimester; however, more serious sequelae are typically seen with earlier infection.[77]

Clinical Presentation

Maternal infection with CMV is almost always asymptomatic, only about 5% will experience symptoms, including fever, myalgias, and lymphadenopathy. Between 12% and 18% of newborns will exhibit signs and symptoms at birth[77] (**Box 5**), and[87] the rest remain asymptomatic.

Late sequelae develop in up to 25% by 2 years of life and include hearing loss and intellectual delay. Severe infections have up to a 30% mortality rate.[77]

Testing

Routine testing is not recommended due to lack of effective treatment.[88] Serologic testing is the most common method with viral culture and PCR testing also available. Less than 30% of primary CMV infections will show a positive IgM with a high false-positive rate; thus IgG testing is performed in serial samples 3 to 4 weeks apart. Test result is positive if there is seroconversion from negative to positive or if the IgG titer increases more than 4-fold. Fetal infection may be suspected with ultrasound findings, such as intrauterine growth restriction, microcephaly, ventriculomegaly, liver calcifications, echogenic bowel, ascites, and/or fetal hydrops. Confirmation of infection can be made using CMV PCR testing of amniotic fluid at greater than 20 weeks gestation.[89]

Management

There are currently no approved treatments for either maternal or fetal CMV infection. One study of valganciclovir did demonstrate improvement at 6 months of age in neurodevelopmental and hearing measures.[90] Use of CMV hyperimmune globulin has also shown some initial promise but further study is needed.[91]

HERPES SIMPLEX VIRUS

Organism and Epidemiology

HSV is a sexually transmitted, double-stranded DNA virus that exists as 2 distinct subtypes, HSV-1 and HSV-2. A common infection, the prevalence of HSV-1 is higher (54%) when compared with HSV-2 (16%) in the United States amongst all individuals aged 14 to 49 years.[92] Despite a high prevalence, neonatal infections in the United

Box 5
Clinical manifestations of congenital cytomegalovirus infection

- Microcephaly
- Intracranial calcifications
- Sensorineural hearing loss
- Chorioretinitis
- Seizures
- Growth restriction
- Jaundice
- Thrombocytopenia
- Hepatosplenomegaly
- Petechial rash

States are uncommon occurring in around 1 out of every 3200 births.[93] In utero transmission is even more rare at 1 in 300,000 births.[94]

Infection with HSV-1 or HSV-2 in a patient seronegative to both HSV-1 and HSV-2 is known as a primary infection. A secondary infection occurs when a patient is seropositive to one type and acquires the other. The risk of vertical transmission is highest with primary infection (**Table 3**).[93,95–97]

Clinical Presentation

Up to two-thirds of women with genital infection are asymptomatic. Symptomatic infection presents with painful, erythematous, grouped, papular lesions on the external genitalia, which quickly convert to vesicles, then rupture forming small ulcerated lesions that resolve spontaneously. Burning or shooting pain often precedes the rash.[98] Congenital herpes infection only accounts for 5% of cases and presents with a characteristic triad of findings.[94]

- Cutaneous—vesicular rash, ulcerations, scarring, aplasia cutis
- Ocular—chorioretinitis, microphthalmia
- Neurologic—intracranial calcifications, microcephaly, hydranencephaly

Most cases of neonatal herpes are acquired in the peripartum or postpartum period during symptomatic maternal outbreak. There are 3 categories of clinical manifestations: skin/eyes/mouth (SEM), central nervous system (CNS), and disseminated disease, which account for 45%, 30%, and 25% of cases, respectively.[99] As many as two-thirds of cases of disseminated disease will have CNS involvement. The clinical findings for each category are outlined in **Table 4**.

Testing

Universal screening is not recommended. Viral culture of vesicular fluid is the gold standard for diagnosis of acute infection. Newer immunofluorescent and PCR tests are also available. Serologic testing for HSV-1 and HSV-2 antibodies is also useful for determining primary and secondary infection.

Management

Oral acyclovir and valacyclovir are the mainstays of treatment for active infection and can be used for suppression of recurrence during pregnancy. Suppressive therapy has been shown to decrease viral detection and active lesions at the time of delivery and thus the need for cesarean section but has not been shown to fully prevent neonatal disease.[98] Despite this, ACOG recommends women with known recurrent infection be offered suppressive therapy starting at 36 weeks.[100] Any patient with signs or symptoms of infection, whether primary or recurrent, should be delivered by cesarean section ideally before rupture of membranes to decrease the risk of transmission to the newborn.[100] Women with a history of infection but no signs of recurrence at delivery can safely deliver vaginally.

Table 3
Risk of maternal infection and vertical transmission of herpes simplex virus

	Risk During Pregnancy	Risk of Vertical Transmission
First episode, primary infection	4%	57%
First episode, secondary infection	2%[a]	25%
Recurrence	75%	2%

[a] Women with prior HSV-1 infection acquiring HSV-2.

Table 4
Clinical findings of neonatal herpes simplex virus infection

	Clinical Picture	Laboratory Findings
SEM Disease	• Vesicular rash • Conjunctivitis • Ulcerated lesions in oral mucosa	• Typically normal
CNS Disease	• Poor feeding, lethargy, irritability • Temperature instability • Bulging fontanelles • Tremor • Seizure • Skin lesions seen in up to 70% of cases	• CSF analysis: ◦ Mononuclear cell pleocytosis ◦ Normal or low glucose ◦ Mildly elevated protein • Focal or multifocal periodic epileptiform discharges on EEG • Edema, hemorrhage, or lytic lesions on CT/MRI
Disseminated Disease	• Septic appearance • Hyper/hypothermia • Respiratory distress • Hepatitis and liver failure • DIC • CNS findings in two-thirds of cases • Skin lesions seen in up to 80% of cases	• Elevated transaminases • Thrombocytopenia • CSF, EEG, and CT/MRI findings as mentioned earlier

Abbreviations: CSF, cerebrospinal fluid; DIC, disseminated intravascular coagulation; EEG, electroencephalogram.

Data from American Academy of Pediatrics. Committee on infectious diseases. Red book: 2012 report of the committee on infectious diseases. Elk Grove Village, (IL): American Academy of Pediatrics; 2012.

Neonatal infections are treated with intravenous acyclovir for 14 days in SEM disease and 21 days in CNS/disseminated disease followed by 6 months of suppressive therapy.[101] Guidelines for the testing and treatment of asymptomatic infants born vaginally during active infections have been developed by the AAP, the details of which are discussed elsewhere.[102]

VARICELLA-ZOSTER VIRUS AND PARVOVIRUS B19

Varicella-zoster virus is sometimes included with TORCH infections. The annual incidence of infection during pregnancy is low (0.4–0.7/1000) due to high rates of natural and acquired immunity. Between 10% and 20% of women infected during pregnancy develop pneumonia with a mortality rate up to 40%.[77] Manifestations of congenital varicella syndrome are shown in **Box 6**.[103]

Box 6
Manifestations of congenital varicella syndrome

Intrauterine growth restriction

Skin lesions or scarring in a dermatomal distribution

Chorioretinitis, congenital cataracts, and/or microphthalmos

Horner syndrome and/or nystagmus

Hypoplastic limbs

Cortical atrophy

Seizures

Intellectual disability

ACOG recommends oral acyclovir for treatment because it may reduce morbidity and mortality in patients with pneumonia; however, it does not prevent transmission to the fetus or treat the congenital manifestations.[77]

Parvovirus B19 is a common childhood infection with an annual incidence of new infections during pregnancy of 1% to 2%. Most fetal infections are self-limited and cause no harm to the fetus, but infection can cause spontaneous abortion, stillbirth, and hydrops fetalis.[74,77]

ZIKA

Organism and Epidemiology

Zika virus is a single-stranded RNA flavivirus transmitted to humans by Aedes mosquitoes. Person-to-person transmission is possible through sexual and mother-to-child transmission. Zika virus was first detected in the Western Hemisphere in 2014 and an outbreak has been ongoing in the Americas, Pacific, and Caribbean.[104–107] Between 2015 and February 2018, 5653 cases of symptomatic Zika virus have been reported in the United States with 95% of these in travelers to affected areas.[108]

Clinical Presentation

Acute maternal infection is characterized by fever, maculopapular rash, conjunctivitis, and arthralgia, but some patients may be asymptomatic. The manifestations of congenital Zika syndrome are shown in **Box 7**.[109–112]

Testing

All pregnant women should be questioned about potential exposure before and during the pregnancy and about symptoms of Zika virus. No testing is recommended for pregnant women with possible prior exposure without symptoms and without ongoing exposure. Testing algorithms are available from the CDC (https://www.cdc.gov/pregnancy/zika/testing-follow-up/testing-and-diagnosis.html), which includes testing pregnant women with possible exposure with symptoms and asymptomatic pregnant women with possible ongoing exposure.[113] Placental testing can be considered if diagnosis is unclear or if the newborn has possible Zika-associated birth defects.[114]

Management

Symptomatic treatment is provided for acute Zika infection in pregnancy. If Zika infection is suggested by maternal testing, serial ultrasounds are performed to evaluate for congenital infection. Recommendations exist for the first ultrasound 4 weeks after possible exposure, then every 4 weeks.[115,116] If ultrasound is concerning, amniocentesis can be considered to diagnose fetal infection. The timing and route of delivery is unchanged for affected pregnancies. Breastfeeding seems to be safe.[117]

Box 7
Manifestations of congenital Zika syndrome

Microcephaly

Central nervous system abnormalities (hypertonia, seizures)

Facial disproportion

Ocular abnormalities

Arthrogryposis

Sensorineural hearing loss

DISCUSSION

Some infections are highlighted in pregnancy due to having unique effects on the mother-child dyad. Research often lags or is lacking on the effects of diseases and medications in pregnancy. Research is constantly evaluating ways to decrease risk of vertical transmission. Some novel treatments such as direct-acting antivirals for hepatitis C have not yet been studied in pregnancy and may provide new options. Infections, such as Zika virus, that can cause in utero infection are emerging and being recognized as causing congenital syndromes. As more infections are recognized and studied for their effects on pregnancy, we may find more answers to causes of syndromes that are currently poorly defined, such as cerebral palsy.

REFERENCES

1. Nicolle LE, Bradley S, Colgan R, et al. Infectious Diseases Society of America guidelines for the diagnosis and treatment of asymptomatic bacteriuria in adults. Clin Infect Dis 2005;40:643–54.
2. Verani JR, McGee L, Schrag SJ. Division of bacterial diseases, National Center for Immunization and Respiratory Diseases, Centers for Disease Control and Prevention (CDC). Prevention of perinatal group B streptococcal disease–revised guidelines from CDC, 2010. MMWR Recomm Rep 2010;59:1–32.
3. American College of Obstetricians and Gynecologists Committee on Obstetric Practice. ACOG committee opinion no. 485: prevention of early-onset group B streptococcal disease in newborns. Obstet Gynecol 2011;117:1019–27.
4. American College of Obstetricians and Gynecologists. Antimicrobial therapy for obstetric patients. ACOG educational bulletin 245. Int J Gynaecol Obstet 1998; 61:299–308.
5. Centers for Disease Control and Prevention. Questions & answers about implementing the 2010 guidelines for obstetric providers. 2016. Available at: https://www.cdc.gov/groupbstrep/clinicians/qas-obstetric.html. Accessed April 16, 2018.
6. Crider KS, Cleves MA, Reefhuis J, et al. Antibacterial medication use during pregnancy and risk of birth defects: National Birth Defects Prevention Study. Arch Pediatr Adolesc Med 2009;163:978–85.
7. Ailes EC, Gilboa SM, Gill SK, et al. Association between antibiotic use among pregnant women with urinary tract infections in the first trimester and birth defects, National Birth Defects Prevention Study 1997 to 2011. Birth Defects Res A Clin Mol Teratol 2016;106:940–9.
8. Le J, Briggs GG, McKeown A, et al. Urinary tract infections during pregnancy. Ann Pharmacother 2004;38:1692.
9. Vennila V, Madhu V, Rajesh R, et al. Tetracycline-induced discoloration of deciduous teeth: case series. J Int Oral Health 2014;6:115.
10. Cohlan SQ, Bevelander G, Tiamsic T. Growth inhibition of prematures receiving tetracycline. Am J Dis Child 1963;105:453.
11. Bar-Oz B, Moretti ME, Boskovic R, et al. The safety of quinolones—a meta-analysis of pregnancy outcomes. Eur J Obstet Gynecol Reprod Biol 2009; 143:75.
12. American Academy of Pediatrics. Chlamydia trachomatis. In: Kimberlin DW, Brady MT, Jackson MA, et al, editors. Red book: 2015 report of the committee on infectious diseases. 30th edition. Elk Grove Village (IL): American Academy of Pediatrics; 2015. p. 288–94.

13. FitzSimmons J, Callahan C, Shanahan B, et al. Chlamydial infections in pregnancy. J Reprod Med 1986;31:19–22.
14. Much DH, Yeh SY. Prevalence of Chlamydia trachomatis infection in pregnant patients. Public Health Rep 1991;106:490–3.
15. Centers for Disease Control and Prevention. Sexually transmitted disease surveillance, 2016. Atlanta (GA): US Department of Health and Human Services; 2017.
16. Liu B, Roberts CL, Clarke M, et al. Chlamydia and gonorrhoea infections and the risk of adverse obstetric outcomes: a retrospective cohort study. Sex Transm Infect 2013;89:672–8.
17. Donders GG, Desmyter J, De Wet DH, et al. The association of gonorrhoea and syphilis with premature birth and low birthweight. Genitourin Med 1993;69: 98–101.
18. Maxwell GL, Watson WJ. Preterm premature rupture of membranes: results of expectant management in patients with cervical cultures positive for group B streptococcus or Neisseria gonorrhoeae. Am J Obstet Gynecol 1992;166: 945–9.
19. Heumann CL, Quilter LA, Eastment MC, et al. Adverse birth outcomes and maternal neisseria gonorrhoeae infection: a population-based cohort study in Washington state. Sex Transm Dis 2017;44:266–71.
20. Workowski KA, Bolan GA, Centers for Disease Control and Prevention. Sexually transmitted diseases treatment guidelines, 2015. MMWR Recomm Rep 2015;64: 1–137.
21. LeFevre ML, U.S. Preventive Services Task Force. Screening for chlamydia and gonorrhea: U.S. Preventive Services Task Force recommendation statement. Ann Intern Med 2014;161:902–10.
22. Centers for Disease Control and Prevention (CDC). Update to CDC's Sexually transmitted diseases treatment guidelines, 2010: oral cephalosporins no longer a recommended treatment for gonococcal infections. MMWR Morb Mortal Wkly Rep 2012;61:590–4.
23. Wind CM, Schim van der Loeff MF, Unemo M, et al. Test of cure for anogenital gonorrhoea using modern RNA-based and DNA-based nucleic acid amplification tests: a prospective cohort study. Clin Infect Dis 2016;62:1348–55.
24. Okah E, Westheimer EF, Jamison K, et al. Frequency of nucleic acid amplification test positivity among men who have sex with men returning for a test-of-cure visit 7 to 30 days after treatment of laboratory-confirmed neisseria gonorrhoeae infection at 2 public sexual health clinics, New York City, 2013 to 2016. Sex Transm Dis 2018;45:177–82.
25. American Academy of Pediatrics. Prevention of neonatal ophthalmia. In: Kimberlin DW, Brady MT, Jackson MA, et al, editors. Red book: 2015 report of the committee on infectious diseases. 30th edition. Elk Grove Village (IL): American Academy of Pediatrics; 2015. p. 972–4.
26. Mosby LG, Rasmussen SA, Jamieson DJ. 2009 pandemic influenza A (H1N1) in pregnancy: a systematic review of the literature. Am J Obstet Gynecol 2011; 205:10–8.
27. Luteijn JM, Brown MJ, Dolk H. Influenza and congenital anomalies: a systematic review and meta-analysis. Hum Reprod 2014;29:809–23.
28. Centers for Disease Control and Prevention (CDC). Maternal and infant outcomes among severely ill pregnant and postpartum women with 2009 pandemic influenza A (H1N1)–United States, April 2009-August 2010. MMWR Morb Mortal Wkly Rep 2011;60:1193–6.

29. McNeil SA, Dodds LA, Fell DB, et al. Effect of respiratory hospitalization during pregnancy on infant outcomes. Am J Obstet Gynecol 2011;204:S54–7.
30. Mendez-Figueroa H, Raker C, Anderson BL. Neonatal characteristics and outcomes of pregnancies complicated by influenza infection during the 2009 pandemic. Am J Obstet Gynecol 2011;204:S58–63.
31. Håberg SE, Trogstad L, Gunnes N, et al. Risk of fetal death after pandemic influenza virus infection or vaccination. N Engl J Med 2013;368:333–40.
32. Grohskopf LA, Sokolow LZ, Broder KR, et al. Prevention and control of seasonal influenza with vaccines: recommendations of the advisory committee on immunization practices - United States, 2017-18 influenza season. MMWR Recomm Rep 2017;66:1–20.
33. Madhi SA, Cutland CL, Kuwanda L, et al. Influenza vaccination of pregnant women and protection of their infants. N Engl J Med 2014;371:918–31.
34. Shakib JH, Korgenski K, Presson AP, et al. Influenza in infants born to women vaccinated during pregnancy. Pediatrics 2016;137 [pii:e20152360].
35. Nunes MC, Cutland CL, Jones S, et al. Duration of infant protection against influenza illness conferred by maternal immunization: secondary analysis of a randomized clinical trial. JAMA Pediatr 2016;170:840–7.
36. Schlaudecker EP, Steinhoff MC, Omer SB, et al. IgA and neutralizing antibodies to influenza a virus in human milk: a randomized trial of antenatal influenza immunization. PLoS One 2013;8:e70867.
37. Creanga AA, Johnson TF, Graitcer SB, et al. Severity of 2009 pandemic influenza A (H1N1) virus infection in pregnant women. Obstet Gynecol 2010;115: 717–26.
38. Leitich H, Kiss H. Asymptomatic bacterial vaginosis and intermediate flora as risk factors for adverse pregnancy outcome. Best Pract Res Clin Obstet Gynaecol 2007;21:375–90.
39. Committee on Practice Bulletins—Obstetrics, The American College of Obstetricians and Gynecologists. Practice bulletin no. 130: prediction and prevention of preterm birth. Obstet Gynecol 2012;120:964–73.
40. Nygren P, Fu R, Freeman M, et al. Evidence on the benefits and harms of screening and treating pregnant women who are asymptomatic for bacterial vaginosis: an update review for the U.S. Preventive Services Task Force. Ann Intern Med 2008;148:220–33.
41. Cotch MF, Hillier SL, Gibbs RS, et al. Epidemiology and outcomes associated with moderate to heavy Candida colonization during pregnancy. Vaginal infections and prematurity study group. Am J Obstet Gynecol 1998;178:374–80.
42. Mølgaard-Nielsen D, Svanström H, Melbye M, et al. Association between use of oral fluconazole during pregnancy and risk of spontaneous abortion and stillbirth. JAMA 2016;315:58–67.
43. Lopez-Rangel E, Van Allen MI. Prenatal exposure to fluconazole: an identifiable dysmorphic phenotype. Birth Defects Res A Clin Mol Teratol 2005;73:919–23.
44. US Food and Drug Administration Safety Communication: Use of long-term, high-dose Diflucan (fluconazole) during pregnancy may be associated with birth defects in infants. 2011. Available at: http://www.fda.gov/Drugs/DrugSafety/ucm266030.htm. Accessed February 9, 2018.
45. Cotch MF, Pastorek JG 2nd, Nugent RP, et al. Trichomonas vaginalis associated with low birth weight and preterm delivery. The vaginal infections and prematurity study group. Sex Transm Dis 1997;24:353–60.
46. Mann JR, McDermott S, Gregg A, et al. Maternal genitourinary infection and small for gestational age. Am J Perinatol 2009;26:667–72.

47. Smith LM, Wang M, Zangwill K, et al. Trichomonas vaginalis infection in a premature newborn. J Perinatol 2002;22:502–3.
48. Temesvári P, Kerekes A, Tege A, et al. Demonstration of trichomonas vaginalis in tracheal aspirates in infants with early respiratory failure. J Matern Fetal Neonatal Med 2002;11:347–9.
49. Carter JE, Whithaus KC. Neonatal respiratory tract involvement by Trichomonas vaginalis: a case report and review of the literature. Am J Trop Med Hyg 2008; 78:17–9.
50. Hoffman DJ, Brown GD, Wirth FH, et al. Urinary tract infection with Trichomonas vaginalis in a premature newborn infant and the development of chronic lung disease. J Perinatol 2003;23:59–61.
51. National guideline for the management of Trichomonas vaginalis. Clinical effectiveness group (Association for Genitourinary Medicine and the Medical Society for the Study of Venereal Diseases). Sex Transm Infect 1999;75(Suppl 1):S21–3.
52. Terrault NA, Bzowej NH, Chang KM, et al. AASLD guidelines for treatment of chronic hepatitis B. Hepatology 2016;63:261–83.
53. Chen HL, Lee CN, Chang CH, et al. Efficacy of maternal tenofovir disoproxil fumarate in interrupting mother-to-infant transmission of hepatitis B virus. Hepatology 2015;62:375–86.
54. Brown RS Jr, McMahon BJ, Lok AS, et al. Antiviral therapy in chronic hepatitis B viral infection during pregnancy: a systematic review and meta-analysis. Hepatology 2016;63:319–33.
55. Chang MS, Gavini S, Andrade PC, et al. Caesarean section to prevent transmission of hepatitis B: a meta-analysis. Can J Gastroenterol Hepatol 2014;28: 439–44.
56. Wang J, Zhu Q, Zhang X. Effect of delivery mode on maternal-infant transmission of hepatitis B virus by immunoprophylaxis. Chin Med J (Engl) 2002;115: 1510–2.
57. Yang J, Zeng XM, Men YL, et al. Elective caesarean section versus vaginal delivery for preventing mother to child transmission of hepatitis B virus–a systematic review. Virol J 2008;5:100.
58. Suryaprasad AG, White JZ, Xu F, et al. Emerging epidemic of hepatitis C virus infections among young nonurban persons who inject drugs in the United States, 2006-2012. Clin Infect Dis 2014;59:1411–9.
59. Ly KN, Jiles RB, Teshale EH, et al. Hepatitis C virus infection among reproductive-aged women and children in the United States, 2006 to 2014. Ann Intern Med 2017;166:775–82.
60. Pergam SA, Wang CC, Gardella CM, et al. Pregnancy complications associated with hepatitis C: data from a 2003-2005 Washington state birth cohort. Am J Obstet Gynecol 2008;199:38.e1-9.
61. Mast EE, Hwang LY, Seto DS, et al. Risk factors for perinatal transmission of hepatitis C virus (HCV) and the natural history of HCV infection acquired in infancy. J Infect Dis 2005;192:1880–9.
62. Society for Maternal-Fetal Medicine (SMFM), Electronic address: pubs@smfm.org, Hughes BL, Page CM, Kuller JA. Hepatitis C in pregnancy: screening, treatment, and management. Am J Obstet Gynecol 2017;217:B2–12.
63. Cottrell EB, Chou R, Wasson N, et al. Reducing risk for mother-to-infant transmission of hepatitis C virus: a systematic review for the U.S. Preventive Services Task Force. Ann Intern Med 2013;158:109–13.

64. McIntyre PG, Tosh K, McGuire W. Caesarean section versus vaginal delivery for preventing mother to infant hepatitis C virus transmission. Cochrane Database Syst Rev 2006;(4):CD005546.
65. Centers for Disease Control and Prevention. HIV surveillance report, 2015; vol. 27. 2016. Available at: http://www.cdc.gov/hiv/library/reports/hiv-surveillance.html. Accessed February 17, 2018.
66. Centers for Disease Control and Prevention (CDC). Diagnoses of HIV/AIDS–32 States, 2000-2003. MMWR Morb Mortal Wkly Rep 2004;53:1106–10.
67. Whitmore SK, Zhang X, Taylor AW, et al. Estimated number of infants born to HIV-infected women in the United States and five dependent areas, 2006. J Acquir Immune Defic Syndr 2011;57:218–22.
68. Townsend CL, Byrne L, Cortina-Borja M, et al. Earlier initiation of ART and further decline in mother-to-child HIV transmission rates, 2000-2011. AIDS 2014;28: 1049–57.
69. Centers for Disease Control and Prevention. Enhanced perinatal surveillance–15 areas, 2005-2008. HIV Surveill Supplemental Rep 2011 2011;16(no. 2). Available at: http://www.cdc.gov/hiv/topics/surveillance/resources/reports. Accessed February 2, 2018.
70. American College of Obstetrics and Gynecology Committee on Obstetric Practice. ACOG committee opinion No. 418: prenatal and perinatal human immunodeficiency virus testing: expanded recommendations. Obstet Gynecol 2008; 112:739–42.
71. Panel on treatment of HIV-infected pregnant women and prevention of perinatal transmission. Recommendations for use of antiretroviral drugs in transmission in the United States. Available at: http://aidsinfo.nih.gov/guidelines/html/3/perinatal-guidelines/0/. Accessed February 5, 2018.
72. Epps RE, Pittelkow MR, Su WPD. TORCH syndrome. Semin Dermatol 1995;14: 179–86.
73. Kinney JS, Kumar ML. Should we expand the TORCH complex? A description of clinical and diagnostic aspects of selected old and new agents. Clin Perinatol 1988;15:727–44.
74. Neu N, Duchon J, Zachariah P. TORCH infections. Clin Perinatol 2015;42: 77–103, viii.
75. Pappas G, Roussos N, Falagas ME. Toxoplasmosis snapshots: global status of Toxoplasma gondii seroprevalence and implications for pregnancy and congenital toxoplasmosis. Int J Parasitol 2009;39:1385–94.
76. SYROCOT (Systematic Review on Congenital Toxoplasmosis) study group, Thiébaut R, Leproust S, Chêne G, et al. Effectiveness of prenatal treatment for congenital toxoplasmosis: a meta-analysis of individual patients' data. Lancet 2007;369:115–22.
77. American College of Obstetricians and Gynecologists. Practice bulletin no. 151: Cytomegalovirus, parvovirus B19, varicella zoster, and toxoplasmosis in pregnancy. Obstet Gynecol 2015;125:1510–25.
78. Cortina-Borja M, Tan HK, Wallon M, et al. Prenatal treatment for serious neurological sequelae of congenital toxoplasmosis: an observational prospective cohort study. PLoS Med 2010;7(10) [pii:e1000351].
79. Murat J-B, Hidalgo HF, Brenier-Pinchart M-P, et al. Human toxoplasmosis: which biological diagnostic tests are best suited to which clinical situations? Expert Rev Anti Infect Ther 2013;11:943–56.

80. Syphilis - CDC Fact Sheet (Detailed). Centers for disease control and prevention. 2017. Available at: https://www.cdc.gov/std/syphilis/stdfact-syphilis-detailed.htm. Accessed February 23, 2018.
81. 2015 STD treatment guidelines - syphilis. Centers for disease control and prevention. 2016. Available at: https://www.cdc.gov/std/tg2015/syphilis.htm. Accessed February 23, 2018.
82. American Academy of Pediatrics. Committee on infectious diseases. Red book: 2012 report of the committee on infectious diseases. Elk Grove Village (IL): American Academy of Pediatrics; 2012.
83. Banatvala JE, Brown DWG. Rubella. Lancet 2004;363:1127–37.
84. Staras SAS, Flanders WD, Dollard SC, et al. Cytomegalovirus seroprevalence and childhood sources of infection: a population-based study among preadolescents in the United States. J Clin Virol 2008;43:266–71.
85. Kenneson A, Cannon MJ. Review and meta-analysis of the epidemiology of congenital cytomegalovirus (CMV) infection. Rev Med Virol 2007;17:253–76.
86. Cannon MJ, Davis KF. Washing our hands of the congenital cytomegalovirus disease epidemic. BMC Public Health 2005;5:70.
87. Bialas KM, Swamy GK, Permar SR. Perinatal cytomegalovirus and varicella zoster virus infections: epidemiology, prevention, and treatment. Clin Perinatol 2015;42:61–75, viii.
88. Grangeot-Keros L, Simon B, Audibert F, et al. Should we routinely screen for cytomegalovirus antibody during pregnancy? Intervirology 1998;41:158–62.
89. Feldman DM, Keller R, Borgida AF. Toxoplasmosis, parvovirus, and cytomegalovirus in pregnancy. Clin Lab Med 2016;36:407–19.
90. Kimberlin DW, Jester PM, Sánchez PJ, et al. Valganciclovir for symptomatic congenital cytomegalovirus disease. N Engl J Med 2015;372:933–43.
91. Nigro G, Adler SP, La Torre R, et al. Passive immunization during pregnancy for congenital cytomegalovirus infection. N Engl J Med 2005;353:1350–62.
92. Bradley H, Markowitz LE, Gibson T, et al. Seroprevalence of herpes simplex virus types 1 and 2–United States, 1999-2010. J Infect Dis 2014;209:325–33.
93. Brown ZA, Wald A, Morrow RA, et al. Effect of serologic status and cesarean delivery on transmission rates of herpes simplex virus from mother to infant. JAMA 2003;289:203–9.
94. Baldwin S, Whitley RJ. Intrauterine herpes simplex virus infection. Teratology 1989;39:1–10.
95. Brown ZA, Selke S, Zeh J, et al. The acquisition of herpes simplex virus during pregnancy. N Engl J Med 1997;337:509–15.
96. Watts DH, Brown ZA, Money D, et al. A double-blind, randomized, placebo-controlled trial of acyclovir in late pregnancy for the reduction of herpes simplex virus shedding and cesarean delivery. Am J Obstet Gynecol 2003;188:836–43.
97. James SH, Kimberlin DW. Neonatal herpes simplex virus infection. Infect Dis Clin North Am 2015;29:391–400.
98. Sheffield JS, Hollier LM, Hill JB, et al. Acyclovir prophylaxis to prevent herpes simplex virus recurrence at delivery: a systematic review. Obstet Gynecol 2003;102:1396–403.
99. Kimberlin DW, Lin CY, Jacobs RF, et al. Natural history of neonatal herpes simplex virus infections in the acyclovir era. Pediatrics 2001;108:223–9.
100. American College of Obstetricians and Gynecologists. ACOG Practice Bulletin No. 82: Management of herpes in pregnancy. Obstet Gynecol 2007;109:1489–98.

101. Kimberlin DW, Lin CY, Jacobs RF, et al. Safety and efficacy of high-dose intravenous acyclovir in the management of neonatal herpes simplex virus infections. Pediatrics 2001;108:230–8.
102. Kimberlin DW, Baley J, Committee on Infectious Diseases, Committee on Fetus and Newborn. Guidance on management of asymptomatic neonates born to women with active genital herpes lesions. Pediatrics 2013;131:383–6.
103. Gershon AA. Chickenpox, measles, and mumps. In: Infectious diseases of the fetus and newborn infant. Philadelphia (PA): Elsevier Saunders; 1987.
104. Chen LH, Hamer DH. Zika virus: rapid spread in the western hemisphere. Ann Intern Med 2016;164:613–5.
105. Fauci AS, Morens DM. Zika virus in the Americas–yet another arbovirus threat. N Engl J Med 2016;374:601–4.
106. Hennessey M, Fischer M, Staples JE. Zika virus spreads to new areas - region of the Americas, May 2015-January 2016. MMWR Morb Mortal Wkly Rep 2016;65:55–8.
107. Gatherer D, Kohl A. Zika virus: a previously slow pandemic spreads rapidly through the Americas. J Gen Virol 2016;97:269–73.
108. Centers for Disease Control and Prevention (CDC). Zika cases in the United States. 2018. Available at: https://www.cdc.gov/zika/reporting/case-counts.html. Accessed February 9, 2018.
109. Costello A, Dua T, Duran P, et al. Defining the syndrome associated with congenital Zika virus infection. Bull World Health Organ 2016;94:406.
110. Meneses JDA, Ishigami AC, de Mello LM, et al. Lessons learned at the epicenter of Brazil's congenital Zika epidemic: evidence from 87 confirmed cases. Clin Infect Dis 2017;64:1302–8.
111. de Fatima Vasco Aragao M, van der Linden V, Brainer-Lima AM, et al. Clinical features and neuroimaging (CT and MRI) findings in presumed Zika virus related congenital infection and microcephaly: retrospective case series study. BMJ 2016;353:i1901.
112. Miranda-Filho Dde B, Martelli CM, Ximenes RA, et al. Initial description of the presumed congenital Zika syndrome. Am J Public Health 2016;106:598–600.
113. Centers for Disease Control and Prevention. Zika and pregnancy: testing and diagnosis. 2018. Available at: https://www.cdc.gov/pregnancy/zika/testing-follow-up/testing-and-diagnosis.html. Accessed April 16, 2018.
114. Oduyebo T, Polen KD, Walke HT, et al. Update: interim guidance for health care providers caring for pregnant women with possible Zika virus exposure - United States (including U.S. territories), July 2017. MMWR Morb Mortal Wkly Rep 2017;66:781–93.
115. Vouga M, Baud D. Imaging of congenital Zika virus infection: the route to identification of prognostic factors. Prenat Diagn 2016;36:799–811.
116. Baud D, Van Mieghem T, Musso D, et al. Clinical management of pregnant women exposed to Zika virus. Lancet Infect Dis 2016;16:523.
117. Karwowski MP, Nelson JM, Staples JE, et al. Zika virus disease: a CDC update for pediatric health care providers. Pediatrics 2016;137(5) [pii:e20160621].

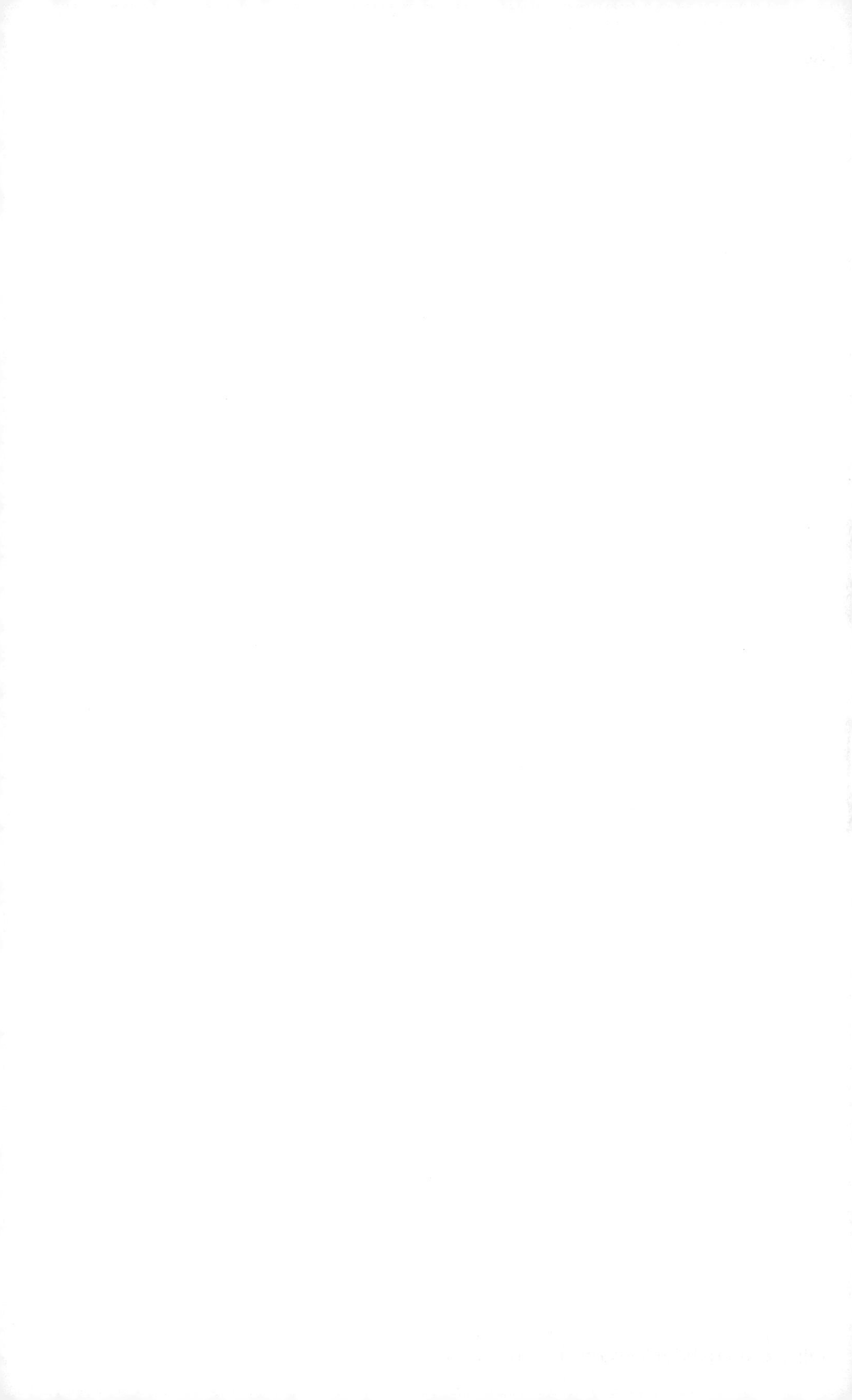

Printed and bound by CPI Group (UK) Ltd, Croydon, CR0 4YY

03/10/2024

01040849-0002